Handbook of Veterinary Science and Medicine

Handbook of Veterinary Science and Medicine

Edited by Ryan Jaxon

hayle
medical

New York

Hayle Medical,
750 Third Avenue, 9th Floor,
New York, NY 10017, USA

Visit us on the World Wide Web at:
www.haylemedical.com

ISBN: 978-1-63241-902-6

Cataloging-in-Publication Data

Handbook of veterinary science and medicine / edited by Ryan Jaxon.
   p. cm.
Includes bibliographical references and index.
ISBN 978-1-63241-902-6
1. Veterinary medicine. 2. Animals--Diseases. 3. Animal health. I. Jaxon, Ryan.
SF745 .H36 2020
636.089--dc23

Table of Contents

Preface

This book was inspired by the evolution of our times; to answer the curiosity of inquisitive minds. Many developments have occurred across the globe in the recent past which has transformed the progress in the field.

Veterinary science, also known as veterinary medicine, is the science concerned with the diagnosis, treatment and prevention of diseases which affect the health of animals. The control of such diseases is important because of the economic losses they cause and the potential transmission of pathogens to humans. Safe and effective vaccines are used for the prevention of companion animal diseases, such as feline distemper, canine distemper, etc. The study of anatomy, pathology, physiology, pharmacology, microbiology, toxicology and nutrition forms the foundation of veterinary science and medicine. Apart from these, diagnostic and clinical pathology, management of infectious and non-infectious diseases, radiology, obstetrics, anesthesiology and surgery are important dimensions of this field. Various instrumentation technologies may be applied for the diagnosis and treatment of diseases in animals. These include endoscopy, echocardiography, laser lithotripsy, nuclear scintigraphy, computed tomography, magnetic resonance imaging, etc. This book contains some path-breaking studies in the field of veterinary science and medicine. The topics included herein are of utmost significance and bound to provide incredible insights to readers. It aims to serve as a resource guide for students and experts alike and contribute to the growth of the discipline.

This book was developed from a mere concept to drafts to chapters and finally compiled together as a complete text to benefit the readers across all nations. To ensure the quality of the content we instilled two significant steps in our procedure. The first was to appoint an editorial team that would verify the data and statistics provided in the book and also select the most appropriate and valuable contributions from the plentiful contributions we received from authors worldwide. The next step was to appoint an expert of the topic as the Editor-in-Chief, who would head the project and finally make the necessary amendments and modifications to make the text reader-friendly. I was then commissioned to examine all the material to present the topics in the most comprehensible and productive format.

I would like to take this opportunity to thank all the contributing authors who were supportive enough to contribute their time and knowledge to this project. I also wish to convey my regards to my family who have been extremely supportive during the entire project.

Editor

Growth performance, feed conversion efficiency and blood characteristics of growing pigs fed on different levels of *Moringa oleifera* leaf meal

J. K. Serem[1]*, R. G. Wahome[1], D. W. Gakuya[2], S. G. Kiama[3], G. C. Gitao[4] and D. W. Onyango[3]

[1]Department of Animal Production, University of Nairobi, P. O. Box, 29053-00625, Kangemi, Nairobi, Kenya.
[2]Department of Clinical studies, University of Nairobi, P. O. Box, 29053-00625, Kangemi, Nairobi, Kenya.
[3]Department of Veterinary Anatomy and Physiology, University of Nairobi, P. O. Box, 29053-00625, Kangemi, Nairobi, Kenya.
[4]Department of Veterinary Pathology, Microbiology and Parasitology, University of Nairobi, P. O. Box, 29053-00625, Kangemi, Nairobi, Kenya.

To determine the effects of inclusion, at different levels of *Moringa oleifera* leaf meal (MOLM) in growing pig diets on pig's daily feed intakes (DFI), growth performance, feed conversion efficiency (FCE), haematology and plasma lipid indices, a total 24 pigs aged 2.5 months old were selected and assigned to 4 treatment diets (T) containing: 0% (T1), 3% (T2), 6% (T3) and 12% (T4) MOLM concentrations, each with 2 replications of 3 pigs. The DFI and weekly pig weights were monitored for 7 weeks, after which 2 sets of blood samples were drawn from 2 pigs per replication for haematology and serum lipid determination. The DFI for the T4 (3.16 kg) was significantly higher than T1 (2.90 kg), T2 (2.61 kg) and T3 (2.54 kg). Pigs in T2 had significantly higher daily weight gains (0.836 kg) compared to T1 (0.807 kg), T3 (0.810 kg) and T4 (0.810 kg) groups. Furthermore, pigs in T2 and T3 had significantly higher FCE (31.57 and 31.23% respectively) compared to T4 (28.05%) and T1 (30.31%). Inclusion of MOLM in the diet significantly increased haemoglobin concentration only to the level of T3 (14.70 g/dL) after which there was a reduction in T4 (12.70 g/dL). Higher mean corpuscular volume was also observed for T1 (60.0 fL) compared to T3 (52.30 fL). MOLM diet also improved the white blood cell counts; $16.70×10^9$/L in T2 compared to $14.50×10^9$/L from T1. Total cholesterol in T2 (2.80 mg/mL) were significantly reduced compared to T1 (3.90 mg/mL). This implies, MOLM at lower levels (<6%) in the diet improves haemoglobin concentration, white blood cell counts and exhibits hypocholesterolemic effects, thereby improving growth performance of the animals.

Key words: Growth, haematology, *Moringa oleifera,* total cell count, total cholesterol, pigs.

INTRODUCTION

Pig production is gaining importance in societies that currently are undergoing a shift from ruminant to non-ruminant livestock production in Kenya. However, increasing feed costs, especially the protein sources, have limited the expansion and profitability of the pig enterprise (FAO, 2012). As a result, farmers have adopted a variety of feed ingredients perceived to be cheaper without taking cognizance of their influences on the animals' body systems (Etim et al., 2014).

MO is a plant in the family Moringaceae introduced in East Africa in the 20th century from India and Pakistan (Foidl et al., 2001). Due to its rich nutritional value, the plant has been used for numerous purposes such as human food, animal feeds as an alternative growth promoter and medicinal purposes (Richter et al., 2003; Sanchez et al., 2006; Nkukwana et al., 2014; Babiker et al., 2017; Caturao et al., 2017). Nutritionally, MO leaves contain between 19.3 and 28.0% crude protein, 2.2% ether extracts, 19.2% crude fibre, 7.1% ash, 42.0% nitrogen free extractives, 0.3% phosphorus and 8.6% calcium (Foidl et al., 2001; Aregheore, 2002; Ferreira et al., 2008; Mustapha and Babura, 2009; Nuhu, 2010; Madukwe et al., 2013; Gakuya et al., 2014).

Haematological values can serve as baseline information for comparing conditions of nutrient efficiency, physiology and health status of farm animals (Ameen et al., 2007; Togun et al., 2007; Isaac et al., 2013; Etim et al., 2014). The phytochemicals from MO seeds, roots and leaves have been shown to have some effects on the haematological and plasma lipid profiles in humans and animals. For instance, El Tazi and Tibin (2014) recorded improved red blood cell indices in broiler chickens fed on MOLM diets. MOLM seed extracts also exerted blood hypocholesterolemic effects in chicken, mice and dogs (Fahey, 2005; Ghebreselassie et al., 2011; Garcia et al., 2015). However, Gakuya et al. (2014) reported that the plant leaves did not have any effects on total cholesterol and total triglycerides in chicken.

Despite the increased use of the plant as a nutritional supplement in humans and animals, there have been varied results on the effects of its inclusion at different concentrations in animal diets on growth performance, haematology and plasma lipids and thus, the need for the study. This study was therefore designed to determine the effects of inclusion of MOLM at varying levels in pig's diet on growth performance, feed conversion efficiency, haematological parameters and plasma lipid profiles in growing pigs.

MATERIALS AND METHODS

This study was conducted at the University of Nairobi, College of Agriculture and Veterinary Sciences, located in Nairobi County. The area receives an average of 869 mm annual rainfall with average daily temperature of 19°C. Growing pig diets were formulated using the NRC (2012) guidelines using maize meal, wheat pollard and vegetable oil as energy sources while MOLM, cotton seed cake, sunflower cake, fish meal and soybean meal served as protein sources. Vitamin mineral premix, Di calcium phosphate and limestone were also included as vitamin and mineral sources (Table 1). The nutritional compositions of the treatment diets are shown in Table 2.

This study was conducted in accordance with the University of Nairobi Faculty of Veterinary Medicine Research Animal Use and Ethics guidelines. Twenty four (24) large white growing pigs (2.5 months old) were selected and assigned to four treatment diets (T): 0% (T1) as the control, 3% (T2), 6% (T3) and 12% (T4) MOLM, each with 2 replicates of 3 pigs in a concrete floor housing system using the design of Reese et al. (2010).

Feeds were weighed each morning and fed in 3 portions to minimize wastage. At the end of the day, feed left in the troughs were weighed and subtracted from the total weight of feed provided for the day to get the daily feed intake. Average daily feed intake for each of the treatment groups was calculated for the entire experimental period. Water was provided ad libitum.

At the start of the experiment, each pig was weighed followed by weekly weighing for a total of 7 weeks. At the end of the experiment, pigs were starved for 12 h, with provision of drinking water only. Four pigs from each treatment were randomly selected and 2 sets of blood (5 ml each) drawn from jugular vein using 9 ml vacutainers; one treated with anticoagulant (EDTA) and the other with serum clot activator. Red blood cells, total white blood cell counts, granulocyte, lymphocyte and mid-range absolute count (MID) and differential counts were determined in the laboratory using an automated haematology analyser. Serum lipid profiling was undertaken after centrifuging blood for 15 min at 3,000 rpm (Li and Kim, 2014). Serum triglycerides, total cholesterol, HDL and LDL were analysed using the serum lipid profiling Kits.

Data on pigs' voluntary daily feed intake, weekly weights, haematological and lipid profiles were entered into Ms excel and exported to Statistical Analysis Software version 9 (SAS Inc, 2002) for descriptive statistics and analysis of variance (ANOVA). Tukey's test was used to determine whether there were significant differences between the means of the treatment groups.

RESULTS

MOLM used in formulating pig diets had 27.37% crude protein (CP), 8.90% crude fibre (CF), 46.01% nitrogen free extractives (NFE), 5.73% ether extract (EE) and 11.91% ash on dry matter basis.

In the feed trials, pigs from T4 registered a higher (P <0.05) daily voluntary feed intakes than those in T1, T2 and T3 groups. T1 group on the other hand had higher (P <0.05) daily feed intakes compared to T2 and T3 groups. The T2 group had a higher (P <0.05) average daily weight gains compared to T1, T3 and T4.

Furthermore, feed conversion efficiency (FCE) was higher in T2 and T3 compared to T1 and T4 (Table 3). All the blood parameters measured in this study (haematological and serum lipid profiles) were within the normal range for T1, T2, T3 and T4.

However, there were variations in haematological parameters and serum lipid profiles with variations of MOLM levels in the diet. From the study, the red blood cell (RBC) and haemoglobin concentration (Hb) was

*Corresponding author. E-mail: drjserem@gmail.com.

Table 1. Percentage (%) Compositions of the growing pig diets.

Ingredients	Dietary treatments (#MOLM inclusion levels, %)			
	T1 (0%)	T2 (3%)	T3 (6%)	T4 (12%)
Maize meal CP%	40.0	40.0	40.0	40.0
Moringa oleifera (27% CP)	0.0	3.0	6.0	12.0
Wheat pollard	30.0	26.0	23.0	16.8
Vegetable oil	1.0	2.5	3.3	3.5
Cotton seed cake (43% CP)	3.9	3.5	3.1	2.8
Sunflower meal (32% CP)	1.4	1.3	1.2	1.3
Fishmeal (50% CP)	10.0	10.0	10.0	10.0
Soybean meal (46% CP)	10.0	10.0	10.0	10.0
Di calcium phosphate	0.0	0.0	0.0	3.3
Limestone	3.4	3.4	3.1	0.0
Vitamin mineral premix	0.3	0.3	0.3	0.3
Total (%)	**100.0**	**100.0**	**100.0**	**100.0**

#MOLM = *Moringa oleifera.*

Table 2. Calculated nutritional compositions of the pig diets.

Nutrient	Dietary treatments (#MOLM inclusion levels, %)			
	T1 (0%)	T2 (3%)	T3 (6%)	T4 (12%)
Amino acid tabulations				
Lysine (%)	0.9	1	1.1	1.3
Threonine (%)	0.6	0.7	0.8	1
Methionine (%)	0.3	0.4	0.4	0.4
Methionine+Cysteine (%)	0.6	0.5	0.5	0.5
Tryptophan (%)	0.2	0.3	0.3	0.4
Isoleucine (%)	0.7	0.8	0.8	1.2
Leucine (%)	1.3	1.5	1.7	1.1
Valine (%)	0.8	0.9	1	1.3
Proximate tabulations				
Crude fibre (%)	5.2	5.2	4.2	5.6
Ash (%)	5.5	5.7	6.6	5.9
Ether extracts (%)	5.7	5.7	4.8	5.8
Digestible energy Mcal/kg	3.4	3.5	3.2	3.3

higher (P <0.05) in T3 group compared to T1, T2 and T4 (Table 4). Mean cell volume (MCV) was lower (P <0.05) in T3 compared to T1, T2 and T4; mean corpuscular haemoglobin (MCH) and mean corpuscular haemoglobin concentration (MCHC) on the other hand did not vary (P >0.05) with the diet (Table 4).

The T2 group had a higher (P = 0.05) concentration of white blood cells compared to T1, T4 and T3 treatment groups. There was also an increase in lymphocytic concentration with increase in MOLM in diet Table 5. Granulocyte cell concentration was, on the other hand, lower (P <0.05) in the MOLM treatment groups compared to the control (T1) groups. Differential cell counts showed that granulocyte proportions declined with increased MOLM in diet, but started to rise again with increased MOLM in T4 (12% MOLM). The mid-range absolute counts (MID) cell proportions further increased (P <0.05) with increase in MOLM in the diet and similarly for the lymphocytes (LMP).

Total cholesterol reduced (P <0.05) with the increase in MOLM in the diet but increased again at the higher levels of dietary MOLM (T3 and T4). T1 group also had the highest level of LDL (2.89 mg/ml) compared to T2 (2.27 mg/ml), T3 (2.26 mg/ml) and T4 (2.5 mg/ml), though not

Table 3. Mean voluntary daily feed intake, weight gains and feed conversion efficiency (FCE) of pigs fed on MOLM diets (± standard error of the mean).

Variable	Dietary treatments ([#]MOLM inclusion levels, %)			
	T1 (0%)	T2 (3%)	T3 (6%)	T4 (12%)
Starting weight (kg)	26.35 ± 0.10^a	25.95 ± 0.11^a	26.10 ± 0.11^a	26.31 ± 0.10^a
Final weight (kg)	66.46 ± 0.54^a	65.24 ± 0.55^a	66.55 ± 0.57^a	65.16 ± 0.53^a
Daily feed intake (kg/day)	2.90 ± 0.09^a	2.61 ± 0.09^b	2.54 ± 0.09^b	3.153 ± 0.09^c
Daily gains (kg/day)	0.807 ± 0.04^a	0.836 ± 0.05^b	0.810 ± 0.05^a	0.810 ± 0.05^a
Feed conversion efficiency (%)	28.05 ± 0.49^c	31.57 ± 0.48^a	31.23 ± 0.48^a	30.31 ± 0.48^b

T = treatment, [#]MOLM = *M. oleifera* leaf meal. The treatment means denoted by the same superscripts ([a, b and c]) in the same row did not have significant differences at $P <0.05$.

Table 4. Mean red blood cell parameters from pigs fed on diets with different levels of MOLM (± standard error of the mean).

Red blood cell parameters	Dietary treatments ([#]MOLM inclusion levels, %)				
	T1 (0%) (n=4)	T2 (3%) (n=4)	T3 (6%) (n=4)	T4 (12%) (n=4)	Normal references
RBC (x10^6/mm^3)	$7.50^a \pm 0.20$	$8.00^a \pm 0.42$	$8.70^b \pm 0.25$	$7.10^a \pm 0.09$	5.00-8.00
Hb (g/dL)	$13.50^a \pm 0.20$	$13.70^a \pm 0.25$	$14.70^b \pm 0.23$	$12.30^c \pm 0.26$	10.00-16.00
HCT (%)	$45.00^a \pm 0.40$	$44.30^a \pm 0.89$	$45.00^a \pm 0.42$	$43.40^a \pm 0.70$	32.00-50.00
MCV (fL)	$60.00^a \pm 0.01$	$56.70^a \pm 0.62$	$52.30^b \pm 0.25$	$58.00^a \pm 1.14$	50.00-68.00
MCH (pg)	$18.00^a \pm 0.01$	$17.30^a \pm 0.47$	$17.30^a \pm 0.25$	$17.00^a \pm 0.42$	17.00-21.00
MCHC (g/dL)	$30.50^a \pm 0.20$	$31.00^a \pm 0.42$	$32.30^a \pm 0.25$	$30.30^a \pm 1.73$	30.00-34.00

[#]MOLM = *M. oleifera* leaf meal, T = treatment, RBC = Red blood cell counts, Hb = Haemoglobin concentration, HCT = Haematocrit concentration; MCV = Mean cell volume, MCH = Mean corpuscular haemoglobin; MCHC = Mean corpuscular haemoglobin concentration. The treatment means denoted by the same superscripts ([a, b and c]) in the same row did not have significant differences at $P <0.05$.

Table 5. Mean white blood cell parameters of growing pigs fed on the different levels of MOLM in diet (± standard error of the mean).

White blood cell parameters	Dietary treatments ([#]MOLM inclusion levels, %)				
	T1 (0%) (n=4)	T2 (3%) (n=4)	T3 (6%) (n=4)	T4 (12%) (n=4)	Normal reference
WBC (10^9/L)	14.50 ± 0.20^a	16.62 ± 0.23^b	15.63 ± 0.23^a	14.87 ± 0.42^a	11.00-22.00
LYMPC (10^9/L)	7.50 ± 0.20^a	8.70 ± 0.23^b	9.30 ± 0.25^b	8.70 ± 0.23^b	3.80-16.50
MIDC (10^9/L)	1.00 ± 0.17^a	1.00 ± 0.17^a	1.00 ± 0.17^a	1.30 ± 0.25^a	0.10-5.00
GRANC (10^9/L)	6.50 ± 0.20^b	7.00 ± 0.23^b	5.00 ± 0.23^a	5.30 ± 0.25^a	5.00-13.90
LYMP (%)	50.00 ± 1.42^a	52.09 ± 1.7^a	60.70 ± 2.1^b	56.80 ± 1.30^c	39.00-62.00
GRA (%)	43.50 ± 1.40^a	41.90 ± 0.25^a	32.60 ± 0.42^b	34.64 ± 0.65^b	28.00-50.00
MID (%)	6.50 ± 0.54^a	6.00 ± 0.65^a	6.53 ± 0.23^a	8.40 ± 0.33^b	4.5.00-13.00

[#]MOLM = *M. oleifera* leaf meal, T = treatment, WBC = White blood cell counts, LYMPC = Lymphocyte cell counts, MIDC = Mid-range absolute counts, GRANC = Granulocyte cell counts, LYMP = Lymphocyte proportions, GRA = Granulocytic proportions, MID = Mid-range absolute count proportions. The treatment means denoted by the same superscripts ([a, b and c]) in the same row did not have significant differences at $P <0.05$

statistically significant. TGS and HDL however did not vary significantly with the diet(Figure 1).

DISCUSSION

The crude protein levels of MOLM in this study were close to 27.51% reported by Oduro et al. (2008), and 29.55% recorded by Nuhu (2010) in Ghana but higher than 23.30% reported by Gakuya et al. (2014), in Kenya. This could be attributed to differences in ecological zones and the physiological stage of harvesting where younger fresh materials could have had higher protein levels, NFE and lower crude fibre contents (Samkol et al., 2005; Gakuya et al., 2014).

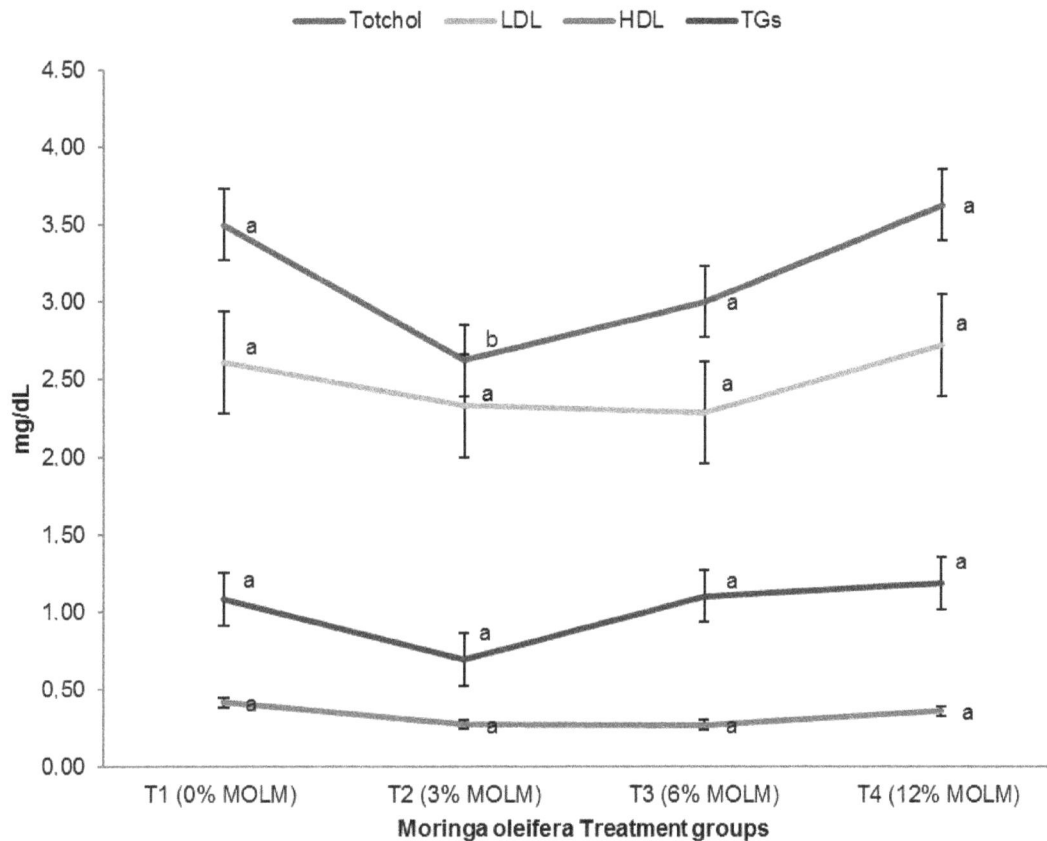

Figure 1. Effects of *M. oleifera* leaf meal diets on the mean serum lipid levels of growing pigs fed on MOLM leaf meal diets (n=16). Key: Totchol = Total cholesterol, LDL = Low density lipoproteins, TGs = Total triglycerides, HDL= High density lipoproteins, MOLM = *M. oleifera* leaf meal. The treatment means denoted by the same superscripts ([a, b and c]) in the same series did not have significant differences at $P < 0.05$

The MOLM diets in all treatment groups were well tolerated by the pigs and no mortalities were recorded. MO has shown a high safety margins both in human and animal research (Stohs and Hartman, 2015). Tolerance of MOLM has also been reported by Gakuya et al. (2014) in chicken, Nuhu (2010) in rabbits and Adedapo et al. (2009) in rats. The higher pig feed intake recorded in T1 and T4 groups may be attributed to limited nutrient availability in the diets as well as higher fibre contents which might have increased the rate of passage in the gut (Afuang et al., 2003). The highest average daily weight gain recorded in T2 was close to that of Mukumbo et al. (2014) who recorded the highest pig weight gain at 5% MOLM, attributed to high protein content from MOLM and higher digestibility. Nkukwana et al. (2014) reported the highest weight gains among broiler chicken fed on MO based diets attributing this to enhanced nutrient utilization. However the average daily gain weight in this study was different from that of Acda et al. (2010) who reported that MOLM up to 10% could substitute commercial pig pre-starter diets and Caturao et al. (2017)

Who reported enhanced growth of Oreochromis niloticus by inclusion of 10% dried MO in the diet.

Diet has been found to influence haematological parameters (Etim et al., 2014). MOLM improved the red blood cell counts and haemoglobin concentration in blood to a level of 6% after which the levels declined significantly. These results were similar to those of El Tazi and Tibin (2014) who recorded higher levels of Hb in broiler chickens fed on MOLM diets. This has been attributed to higher levels of protein and minerals, mostly iron, which are responsible for the formation of haemoglobin in the MO plant (Madukwe et al., 2013; El Tazi and Tibin, 2014). The higher the haemoglobin concentration the better the oxygen circulation in the body, hence, better performance of the animal (Olugbemi et al., 2010). At higher levels (greater than 6% MOLM) however, haemoglobin concentration declined and could possibly be due to the potential toxicities by high levels of flavanoids and tannins in the plant leaves (El Tazi and Tibin, 2014). Increased MOLM (12% MOLM) led to increased MCV implying that there might have been increased release of immature RBC or increased iron or folic acid levels that enhanced red blood cell formation (Fahey, 2005). This therefore implies that MOLM should be used in moderation since high levels may lead to toxicity and reduced efficiency in oxygen transportation in the body, hence, reduced performance. Higher levels of MCV could further imply existence of chronic liver diseases hence inefficiency of liver detoxification. This also could be as a result of increased levels of flavonoids which might have led to impairment of liver function at the highest MOLM in the diet (Fahey, 2005).

The T2 group had the highest white blood cell counts followed by T3 and T4 while T1 had the least counts. These results were similar to those of Gupta et al. (2012) which implied that higher vitamin and protein concentrations in MOLM may have led to improved immune system in animals; indicated by higher body defence cell levels. This is important since the treatment groups would be able to fight diseases compared to controls, hence, minimizing drug usage and thereby reducing the cost of production and subsequently, increasing the safety of pork (Pascoal et al., 2012). MID cells increased with increased MOLM in the diet, implying that the white blood cell precursors had increased therefore enabling the animal to readily counter any infections that may arise. These findings support those of Gaikwad et al. (2011) and Stohs and Hartman (2015) who documented that MO stimulate both cellular and humoral immune systems. This Immunomodulatory potential of *M. oleifera* leaves could be attributed to the presence of flavonoids, polyphenols and terpenoids which may modulate immune-mechanisms. Granulocytes in most instances are responsible for the immune defense against bacterial infections. In this case, MOLM antimicrobial properties may have led to suppression of the pathogenic microbes hence resulting decline in granulocyte levels.

Fahey (2005) and Ghebreselassie et al. (2011) reported that, MOLM exerts hopocholesterolemic effects when taken in the diet. This has also been supported by this study. Increased MOLM reduced cholesterol levels significantly, perhaps by lowering the serum concentrations of LDL by β-sitosterol; the bioactive phytoconstituents isolated from *M. oleifera* (Ghasi et al., 2000). However, pigs on the highest concentration of MOLM showed increased cholesterol levels therefore necessitating further studies to establish reasons for the increased cholesterol levels.

CONCLUSION AND RECOMMENDATIONS

This study therefore concludes that low levels of MOLM in the pig's diet could enhance haemoglobin and WBC formation which, could increase efficiency in oxygen circulation in the body and boost animal's immunity and

enhance better performance. However, higher levels beyond 6% could interfere with the normal haematological parameters and subsequently affect negatively the pig's performance. MOLM also at lower levels in diet has hypocholesterolemic effect which could reduce predisposition to cardiovascular diseases associated with higher levels of LDL and total cholesterol. Further studies however, ought to focus on the actual immune response in relation to specific infectious agents in pigs.

CONFLICT OF INTERESTS

The authors have not declared any conflict of interests.

ACKNOWLEDGEMENTS

The authors acknowledge Carnegie Foundation through the Rise AFNETT for funding the project, The University of Nairobi for provision of the research facilities.

REFERENCES

Acda SP, Masilungan HGD, Moog A (2010). Partial substitution of commercial swine feeds with malunggay (*Moringa oleifera*) leaf meal under backyard conditions. Philipp. J. Vet. Anim. Sci. 36(2):137-146.

Adedapo AA, Mogbojuri OM, Emikpe BO (2009). Safety evaluations of the aqueous extract of the leaves of *Moringa oleifera* in rats. J. Med. Plants Res. 3(8):586-591.

Afuang W, Siddhuraju P, Becker K (2003). Comparative nutritional evaluation of raw, methanol extracted residues and methanol extracts of moringa (*Moringa oleifera* Lam.) leaves on growth performance and feed utilization in Nile tilapia (*Oreochromis niloticus* L.). Aquac. Res. 34(13): 1147-1159.

Ameen SA, Adedeji OS, Akingbade AA, Olayemi TB, Oyedapo LO and Aderinola A (2007). The effect of different feeding regimes on haematological parameters and immune status of commercial broilers in derived savannah zone of Nigeria. Proceed. Annu. Confer. Niger. Soc. Anim. Prod. 32:146-148.

Aregheore EM (2002). Intake and digestibility of *Moringa oleifera*-batiki grass mixtures for growing goats. Small Rumin. Res. 46:23-28.

Babiker EE, Juhaimi FA, Ghafoor K, Abdoun KA (2017). Comparative study on feeding value of Moringa leaves as a partial replacement for alfalfa hay in ewes and goats. Livest. Sci. 195:21-26.

Caturao RD, Atilano MR, Urbina RB (2017). The Suitability of *Moringa oleifera* Leaf Meal Supplementation to Commercial Diets on the Growth and Survival of Oreochromis niloticus Fry. JPAIR Multidisciplinary Research. 27(1).

El Tazi SMA, Tibin IM (2014). Performance and blood chemistry as affected by inclusion of *Moringa Oleifera* leaf meal in broiler chicks diet. J. Vet. Med. Anim. Prod. 5(2):58-65.

Etim NN, Williams ME, Akpabio U, Offiong EE (2014). Haematological parameters and factors affecting their values. Agr Sci. 2(1):37-47.

Fahey WJ (2005). *Moringa oleifera*: A review of the medical evidence for Its nutritional, therapeutic, and prophylactic properties. Tree Life J. 15(1):1-15.

Ferreira PM, Farias DF, Oliveira JTA, Carvalho AFU (2008). *Moringa oleifera*: bioactive compounds and nutritional potential. Revista de Nutrição 21(4):431-437.

Foidl N, Makkar HPS, Becker K (2001). The potential of *Moringa oleifera* for agricultural and industrial uses. In: What development potential for moringa products? Dar Es Salaam October 20th - November 2nd 2001.

FAO (Food and Agricultural Organisation) (2012). Pig Sector Kenya. FAO Animal Production and Health Livestock Country Reviews, Rome. P 3.

Gaikwad SB, Mohan GK, Reddy KJ (2011). *Moringa oleifera* leaves: Immunomodulation in Winstar Albino Rats. Int. J. Pharm. Sci. 3(5):426-430.

Gakuya DW, Mbugua PN, Kavoi B, Kiama SG (2014). Effect of supplementation of *Moringa oleifera* leaf meal in broiler chicken feed. Int. J. Poult. Sci. 13(4):208-213.

Garcia CA, Malabanan NB, Flores MLS, Marte BRG, Rodriguez EB (2015). Hematologic profile and biochemical values in adult dogs given cholesterol with or without nanoliposome-encapsulated malunggay *(Moringa oleifera)* administration. Philippine J. Vet. Anim. Sci. 41(1):41-48.

Ghasi S, Nwobodo E, Ofilis JO (2000). Hypocholesterolemic effects of crude extract of the leaves of *Moringa oleifera Lam.* in high-fat diet fed Wistar rats. J. Ethnopharmacol. 69(1):21-25.

Ghebreselassie D, Mekonnen Y, Gebru G, Ergete W, Huruy K (2011). The effects of *Moringa stenopetala* on blood parameters and histopathology of liver and kidney in mice. Ethiop. J. Health Dev. 25(1):51-57.

Gupta A, Gautam MK, Singh RK, Kumar MV, Rao CV, Goel RK, Anupurba S (2012). Immunomodulatory effect of *Moringa oleifera* Lam. extract on cyclophosphamide induced toxicity in mice. Indian J. Exp. Biol. 48(11): 57-60.

Isaac LJ, Abah G, Akpan B, Ekaette IU (2013). Haematological properties of different breeds and sexes of rabbits. Proceed. Of 18th Annu. Confer. Anim. Sci. Assoc. Niger. pp. 24-27.

Li J, Kim IH (2014). Effects of levan-type fructan supplementation on growth performance, digestibility, blood profile, faecal microbiota, and immune responses after lipopolysaccharide challenge in growing pigs. J. Anim. Sci. 91(11):5336-5343.

Madukwe EU, Ugwuoke AL, Ezeugwu JO (2013). Effectiveness of dry *Moringa oleifera* leaf powder in treatment of anaemia. Int. J. Med. Med. Sci. 5(5):226-228.

Mukumbo FE, Maphosa V, Hugo A, Nkukwana TT, Mabusela TP, Muchenje V (2014). Effect of *Moringa oleifera* leaf meal on finisher pig growth performance, meat quality, shelf life and fatty acid composition of pork. South Afr. J. Anim. Sci. 44(4):388-400.

Mustapha Y, Babura SR (2009). Determination of carbohydrate and β-Carotene content of some vegetables consumed in Kano Metropolis,

Nigeria. Bayero J. Pure Appl. Sci. 2(1):119-121.

Nkukwana TT, Muchenje V, Masika PJ, Hoffman LC, Dzama K (2014). The effect of *Moringa oleifera* leaf meal supplementation on tibia strength, morphology and inorganic content of broiler chickens. South Afr. J. Anim. Sci. 44(3):228-239.

NRC (2012). Nutrient requirements of swine. Eleventh revised edition. National Academic Press, Washington, D.C. 20418 USA.

Nuhu F (2010). Effect of moringa leaf meal (MOLM) on nutrient digestibility, growth, carcass and blood indices of weaner rabbits. MSc thesis Kwame Nkrumah University of Science and Technology, Ghana.

Oduro I, Ellis WO, Owusu D (2008). Nutritional potential of two leafy vegetables : *Moringa oleifera* and *Ipomoea batatas* leaves. Sci. Res. Essays. 3(2):57-60.

Olugbemi TS, Mutayoba SK, Lekule FP (2010). Effect of *Moringa oleifera* inclusion in cassava based diets fed to broiler chickens. Int. J. Poult. Sci. 9(4):363-367.

Pascoal LAF, Maria CT, Pedro HW, Urbano SR, Pascoal JM, Ezequiel B, Amorim AB, Daniel E, Masson GI (2012). Fibre sources in diets for newly weaned piglets. Revista Brasileira de Zootecnia 41(3):636-642.

Reese ED, Eskridge KM, Stroupe WW (2010). How to conduct on farm pig experiments. University of Nebraska Linciloln Extension. Revised in October, 2010.

Richter N, Perumal S, Klaus B (2003). Evaluation of nutritional quality of moringa (*Moringa oleifera* Lam.) leaves as an alternative protein source for Nile tilapia (*Oreochromis niloticus* L.). Aquaculture 217:599-611.

Samkol P, Bun Y, Ly J (2005). Physico-chemical properties of tropical tree leaves may influence its nutritive value for monogastric animal species. Revista Computadorizada de Producción Porcina. 12(1):31-34.

Sanchez NR, Ledin S, Ledin I (2006). Biomass production and chemical composition of *Moringa oleifera* under different management regimes in Nicaragua. Agrofor. Syst. 66(3):231-242.

SAS Institute Inc (2002). SAS v 9.0. Cary, NC.

Stohs SJ, Hartman MJ (2015). Review of the safety and efficacy of *Moringa oleifera*. Phytother. Res. 29(6):796-804.

Togun VA, Oseni BSA, Ogundipe JA, Arewa TR, Hameed AA, Ajonijebu DC, Oyeniran A, Nwosisi I, Mustapha F (2007). Effects of chronic lead administration on the haematological parameters of rabbit - a preliminary study. Proceed. Confer. Agric. Soc. Niger. 41:341.

2

Antimicrobial resistance profile of *Staphylococcus aureus* isolated from raw cow milk and fresh fruit juice in Mekelle, Tigray, Ethiopia

Haftay Abraha[*], Geberemedhin Hadish, Belay Aligaz, Goytom Eyas and Kidane Workelule

College of Veterinary Medicine, Mekelle University, P. O. Box 2084, Mekelle, Ethiopia.

This study was conducted to evaluate drug resistance profile of *Staphylococcus aureus* in raw milk, fresh fruit juice and dairy farms settings of Mekelle, Tigray. A cross-sectional study was conducted on the total 258 samples of raw cow milk and fresh fruit juice. Antimicrobial resistance status was also checked for identified *S. aureus* using various commonly used antimicrobial discs. The overall viable staphylococcal count mean and standard deviation of samples from milk shop, fruit juice and dairy milk were found to be 8.86±107, 7.2 × 107, 8.65±107 cfu/ml, 33.87±106, 6.68±106 and 22.0±106, respectively. Among the total 258 samples, 75 (29.07%) samples were found positive for *S. aureus*. Proportion of the isolation from milk shop, fruit juice and dairy milk samples were 20 (23.26%), 32 (37.21%) and 23 (26.74%), respectively. Antimicrobial test of the high resistance revealed vancomycin (100%), ampicillin (90.9%). ciprofloxacin (90.9%), ceftaroline (63.6%), penicillin-G (81.8%) and clindamycin (72.7%) whereas they are highly susceptible to some antibiotics like gentamicin (100%), streptomycin (81.8%), norfloxacin (63.6%), chloramphenicol (81.8%), sulfamethoxazole (96%), kanamycin (72.7%), polymixin B (72.7%), erythromycin (72.7%) and tetracycline (81.8); also, some *S. aureus* also showed multi-drug resistance pattern. The present study, we isolated and determined the drug Resistance profile of S. aruesu in Mekelle city, Northern Ethiopia alarmingly, the S. aureus isolates circulating in the raw cow milk, fresh fruit juice and dairy milk. High level of S. aureus isolation from personnel and equipment besides food samples reveals that the hygiene practice is substandard. Prudent drug use and improved hygienic practice is recommended in the raw cow milk of dairy farms and fresh fruit juice to safeguard the public from the risk of acquiring infections and multiple drug resistance (MDR) pathogenic *S. aureus*.

Key words: Antibiogram, bacterial load, multiple drug resistance (MDR), Mekelle, Milk, *Staphylococcus aureus*.

INTRODUCTION

Foods borne illness are public health problem in developed and developing countries. *Staphylococcus aureus* is among the most significant pathogens causing a wide spectrum of diseases in both humans and animals. In humans, nosocomial and community acquired infections are common (Klotz et al., 2003). Pathogenic

*Corresponding author. E-mail: haftay.abraha@mu.edu.et or haftay24@gmail.com.

strains are usuallycoagulase-positive and cause disease in their hosts throughout the world. S. aureus is one of the most significant food-borne pathogens (Le Loir et al., 2003). Raw unpasteurized milk may become contaminated with enterotoxigenic coagulase-positive S. aureus either through contact with the cow's udder during milking or by cross contamination during processing (Normanno et al., 2005, Ekici et al., 2004).

Food-borne pathogens are recognized as a major health hazard associated with street foods, the risk being dependent primarily on the type of food and the method of preparation and conservation (CDC, 2011; FAO/WHO, 2005). S. aureus is a gram positive, catalase and coagulase positive microorganism responsible for various foodborne outbreaks. Contamination of food with entero-toxigenic S. aureus causes staphylococcal enterotoxins (SEs) intoxication hence the associated symptoms like vomiting and diarrhea (Veras et al., 2008). In countries where food borne illness were investigated and documented, the relative importance of pathogens like S. aureus, Campylobacter, Escherichia coli and Salmonella species were recorded as a major cause (WHO, 2004).

The ability of these microorganisms to survive under adverse conditions and to grow in the presence of low levels of nutrients and at suboptimal temperatures and pH values presents a formidable challenge to the agricultural and food processing industries. The continued prominence of raw meats, eggs, dairy products, vegetable sprouts, fresh fruits and fruit juices as the principal vehicles of human foodborne diseases poses a major challenge to coordinate sectorial control efforts within each industry (Knife and Abera, 2007). Studies conducted in different parts of Ethiopia also showed the poor sanitary conditions of catering establishments and presence of pathogenic organisms (Knife and Abera 2007; Mekonnen et al., 2012).

In addition to toxic effect of food borne microbial pathogens, antibiotic resistance remains a major challenge in human and animal health (Shekh et al., 2013). Food contamination with antibiotic-resistant bacteria can therefore be a major threat to public health, as the antibiotic resistance determinants can be transferred to other bacteria of human and animals, thereby has significant public health implications by increasing the number of food-borne illnesses and the potential for treatment failure (Adesiji et al., 2011). Studying antimicrobial resistance in humans and animals is important for detecting changing patterns of resistance, implementing control measures on the use of antimicrobial agents and preventing the spread of multidrug-resistant strains of bacteria. Up to now, many researchers have focused on the spread of resistant S. aureus in clinical settings (Ateba et al., 2010; Addo et al., 2011). However, limited number of investigations has been studied about the presence of antimicrobial resistance in food animals in Ethiopia (Mekonnen et al., 2005; Hundera et al., 2005). So far, there are no studies conducted on the burden and drug sensitivity profile of S. aureus in Mekelle city, Northern Ethiopia. In this study, S. aureus was isolated and the drug Resistance profile was determined.

MATERIALS AND METHODS

Study area

The study was conducted from October 2016 to June 2017 in Mekelle city. Mekelle is the capital city of Tigray Regional State located at about 783 km away north of Addis Ababa, Capital city of the Federal Democratic Republic of Ethiopia at geographical coordination of 39°28` East longitude and 13°32` North latitude. The average altitude of the city is 2300 m.a.s.l. with a mean annual rainfall and average annual temperature of 629 mm and 22°C, respectively (TBA, 2017). The population of the city is 406,338 (195, 605 male and 210,733 female) (TBA, 2017). The city has seven sub-cities and 33 Kebelles where over 139 juice houses, 48 dairy farms and 123 milk shops (street vender or retailer shops) are inhabited. Besides, the city possesses an extensive public transport network and active urban-rural exchange of goods with about 30,000 micro and small enterprises (Bryant, 2017).

Study design

A cross-sectional survey was conducted from October 2016 to June 2017 on raw cow milk and fresh fruit juice samples collected from different sources of raw milk shops and dairy milk supply centers, and juice houses in Mekelle. Purposive sampling technique was employed.

Sampling technique and collection

A total of 258 food samples were collected among which 172 are milk samples (86 from milk shops, 86 from dairy farms) and the remaining 86 are fresh juice samples (from 86 juice houses) in the seven sub-cities of Mekelle city. Samples were collected according to standards described by Oyeleke and Manga (2008). After aseptic collection, samples were labeled and packed with sterile bottles and transported with an ice box to Mekelle University, College of Veterinary Medicine, Microbiology and Public health laboratories for bacterial isolation and characterization. Samples were processed immediately for bacterial identification to species level using culture media and then isolates were kept in refrigerator at 4°C until microbial characterization with regular sub-culturing described (Oyeleke and Manga, 2008).

Enumeration of total viable

One milliliter and gram of raw milk and fruit juice samples respectively were homogenized into 9 ml of serial peptone water/NSS and 10 g/1 g of each food item was weighed out and homogenized into 90 ml/9 ml of sterile distilled deionized water. Then, serial dilutions were prepared. From the 10-fold dilutions of the homogenates; 1 ml of 10^{-4}, 10^{-5} and 10^{-6} dilutions were cultured in replicate on standard plate count agar (Hi Media, India), using the pour plate method. The plates were then incubated at 37°C for 24 – 48 h. At the end of the incubation period, colonies were counted using the illuminated colony counter. The counts for each plate were expressed as colony forming unit of the suspension (cfu/g) (Fawole and Oso, 2001). In order to determine the presence of S. aureus, 0.1 ml of samples from each dilution

Table 1. Antibiotics used, their concentration and drug sensitivity interpretive zone of inhibition diameters

Antibiotic	Disc code	Potency (µg)	Zone diameter		
			S	M	R
Erythromycin	ERY	15	≥23	14-22	≤13
Penicillin-G	P	10	≥29		≤28
Norflaxon	f	50	≥17	13-16	≤12
Sulphoxazole-trimethoprim	SXT-TMP	300	≥16	11-15	≤10
Streptomycin	S	10	≥15	12-14	≤11
Kanamycin	KAN	30	≥18	14-17	≤13
Chloramphenicol	CHL	30	≥18		≤18
Tetracycline	TE	30	≥22	19-21	≤19
Gentamicin	GM	10	≥18	-	≤18
Ampicillin	AMP	10	≥15	12-14	≤11
Ciprofloxacin	CIP	5	≥20		≤20
Ciftriaxone	CRO	30	≥23	20-22	≤19
Vancomycin	VA	30	≥12	10-11	≤19
Clindamycin	CC	10	≥21	15-20	≤14
Polymixin B	P	10	≥12	12-14	≤11

R= Resistant, I= intermediate, S = sensitive.
Source: CLSI (2008).

was introduced onto the Baird Parker agar (Oxorid). The plates were incubated at 37°C for 24 h. All the isolates were subjected to morphological and biochemical confirmation according to the prescribed method (Fawole and Oso, 2001).

Isolation and identification of *S. aureus*

About 10 ml of each raw cow milk and fresh fruit juice sample was suspended in 90 ml of Brain heart infusion broth supplemented with NaCl (6.5%) and incubated at 37°C for 24 h. A sterile loopful of the broth inoculum was streaked onto Baird Parker agar and incubated at 37°C for 24 h. Colonies that appeared black or greyish-black were Gram-stained and subjected to biochemical tests. Gram positive cocci that occurred singly and in pairs, tetrads, short chains and irregular grape-like clusters were suggestive of *S. aureus*. Conventional biochemical tests carried out for presumptive identification of *S. aureus* isolates included gram staining, catalase, coagulase, 5 % sheep blood agar, pigmentation (Mannitol salt agar) and DNase activity (McFaddin, 2000).

Antimicrobial susceptibility test

Antimicrobial susceptibility test, through Kirby diffusion test, was performed for all *S. aureus* isolates following the protocol of CLSI (2008). For susceptibility test, a pure culture of all *S. aureus* were taken and transferred to a tube containing 5 ml of sterile normal saline and mixed gently to make homogenous suspension which was adjusted to a turbidity equivalent to a 0.5 Mc Far land standard as measured by turbidity meter. The bacterial suspension was inoculated onto Muller–Hinton agar (Oxorid, UK) with the sterile swab to cover the whole surface of the agar. The inoculated plates were left at room temperature to dry. Before using the antimicrobial disks, they were kept at room temperature for 1 h and then

dispended on the surface of media. Following this, the plates were incubated aerobically at 37°C for 24 h (CLIS, 2012).

The diameters of the zone of inhibition around the disks were measured to the nearest millimeter using calibrated rulers, and the isolates were classified as susceptible, intermediate and resistant according to the interpretative accordance with the guidelines of (CLSI, 2008) as indicated in Table 1.

Data management and analysis

All data were checked against the standards and methods were used to perform the study. Data was entered in Microsoft Excel spreadsheet and analyzed using STATA Version 12. Descriptive statistics such as means, percentage and frequencies were computed to report desired outputs. The antimicrobial resistance test was analyzed using WHONET software version 5 statistical package (http://www.who.int/medicines/areas/rational_use/AMR_WHONET_SOFTWARE/en/). Analysis of Variance (ANOVA) was used to test the significant difference at $p < 0.05$.

RESULTS

Enumeration of total viable

The overall mean viable bacterial count recorded was 8.24 x 107. The individual sample type mean viable count and standard deviation of milk shop, fruit juice and dairy milk is indicated in Table 2.

Isolation and Identification of organism

Among the total 258 raw cow milk and fruit juice samples

Table 2. Total viable *S. aureus* count for different sample types.

Sample type	Mean bacterial count	±SD	Minimum bacterial count	Maximum bacterial count
Milk shop	8.86 ± 10^7	33.87 ± 10^6	1.5 ± 10^7	1.25 ± 10^8
Fruit juice	7.2 ± 10^7	6.68 ± 10^6	6.37 ± 10^7	8.5 ± 10^7
Dairy milk	8.65 ± 10^7	22.0 ± 10^6	6.4 ± 10^7	1.23 ± 10^8
Total	8.24 ± 10^7	23.8 ± 10^6	1.5 ± 10^7	1.25 ± 10^8

SD= standard deviation.

Table 3. Rate of isolation of *S. aureus* from raw cow milk and fruit juice samples.

Sample type	Number positive (%)	x^2	p-value
Milk shop (n=86)	20 (23.26)		
Fruit juice (n=86)	32 (37.21)	4.3987	0.111
Dairy milk (n=86)	23 (26.74)		
Overall (n=258)	75 (29.07)		

collected from different sources of Mekelle sub city, 75 (29.07%) samples were found positive for *S. aureus*. Proportion of the isolation from milk shop, fruit juice and dairy milk samples is described (Table 3). A statistically significant difference ($\chi2=4.3987$, P-value =0.111) was recorded among samples from the three sites (Table 3 and Figure 1).

Antimicrobial susceptibility profile of *S. aureus*

The antimicrobial resistance profile of the bacterial isolates from raw cow milk and fruit juice samples are summarized in Table 3. *S. aureus* showed high resistance to antibiotics like, vancomycin (100%), ampicillin (90.9%). ciprofloxacin (90.9%), ceftaroline (63.6%), pencillin-G (81.8%) and clindamycin (72.7%) whereas it was highly susceptible to some antibiotics like, gentamicin (100%), streptomycin (81.8%), norfloxacin (63.6%), chloramphenicol (81.8%), sulfamethoxazole (96%), kanamycin (72.7%), polymixin B (72.7%), erythromycin (72.7%) and tetracycline (81.8) (Table 4 and Figure 2).

The multi-drug resistance pattern of the bacterial *S. aureus* isolates is presented in Table 5. In general, antimicrobial susceptibility test revealed that gentamicin, streptomycin, norfloxacin, chloramphenicol, sulfamethoxazole, kanamycin, polymixin B, erythromycin, and tetracyclin were the antimicrobials indicated as active against *S. aureus* isolated from this study.

A total of 10 multiple drug resistance patterns were observed. The highest multiple drug resistance (MDR) noted was PEN, VAN, CIP and AMP (45.5%). The maximum multiple drug resistance registered was resistant to three and four antibiotics with the combination PEN, VAN, CIP and AMP.

DISCUSSION

The current finding indicates that samples from milk shop, fruit juice and dairy milk were found with a viable staphylococcal count load of 8.86 × 107, 7.2 × 107 and 8.65 × 107 cfu/ml respectively with an overall mean viable bacterial count of 8.24 × 107cfu/ml. The highest mean value of microbial load (8.86 × 107 cfu/ml) was found from milk shop samples.

The current study was found with higher viable staphylococcal count than previous reports such as viable bacterial count from raw cow milk and fresh fruit juice samples in 6.0 × 103 cfu/ml to 2.5 × 105 cfu/ml of (Lucky et al., 2016) in Bangladesh, 1.4 × 104 cfu/ ml (Tasnim, 2016) in Dhaka city; Staphylococcal count was from fresh vended fruit juices.

In the present study, out of 258 samples, 75 (29.07%) samples were found to be positive for *S. aureus* of which 20 (23.26%) were from milk shop, 32 (37.21%) from fruit juice and 23 (26.74%) from dairy milk. The result shows a high contamination rate, which might be attributed to poor hygeinic sanitation and handling improper. Statistically significant difference (P< 0.05) among the sample types in the prevalence of *S. aureus* was recorded. A similar report was also made by previous researchers (Abebe et al., 2013; Reta et al., 2016) that *S. aureus* was 15.5 and 24.2% in raw milk samples respectively in Ethiopia and in the other parts of the world which is contrary to this; different literatures revealed a very significant isolation rate of *S. aureus* from raw milk samples (Olatunji et al., 2009; Pourhassan and Taravat-Najafabadi, 2011; Mohanty et al., 2013; Sanaa et al., 2005).

The present overall isolation rate in raw cow milk products was 29.07% which seems to be higher than the findings of 6.25% by Thaker et al. (2013), 17% in Egypt (El-Gedawy et al., 2014), 18.2% in Turkey (Ekici et al.,

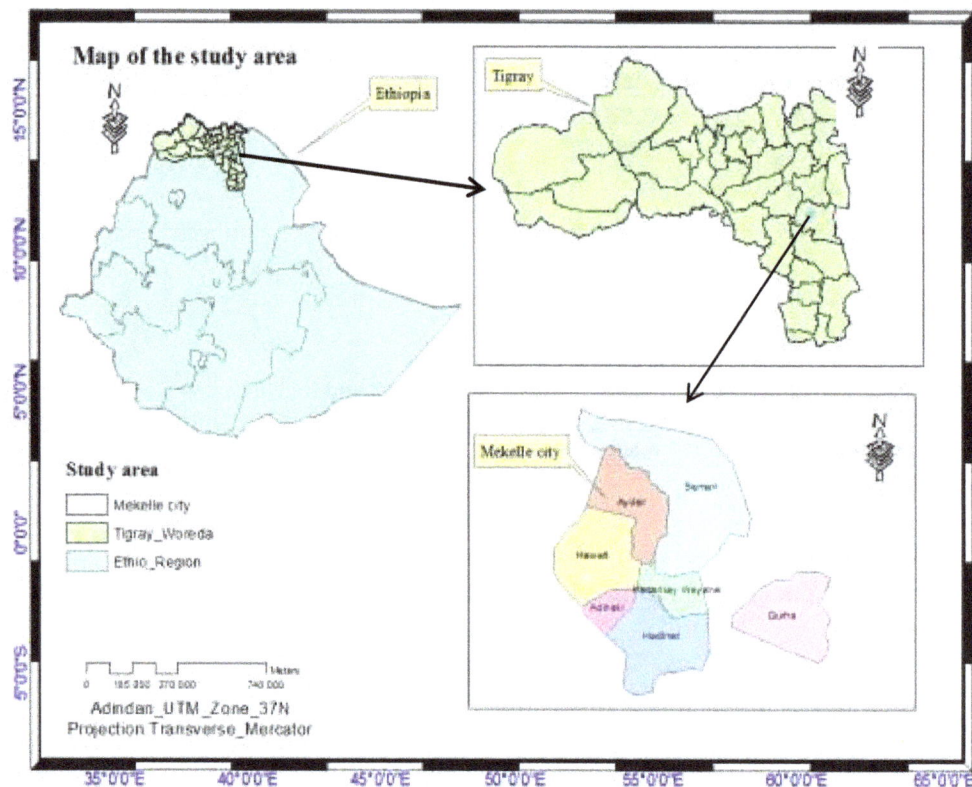

Figure 1. Map of the study area.

2004), 20.8% in Turkey (Aydin et al., 2011) and 21% in Iran (Ahmadi et al., 2009); were previously reported in milk samples collected from dairy farms. The present finding was much higher compared to the finding reported previously (Santana et al., 2010; Ekici et al., 2004) which found 17.39 and 18.18%, respectively; 4 (8%) of pasteurized milk samples, 9 (18%) of traditional butter samples and 12 (24%) of traditional cheese samples (Mirzaei et al., 2011) in Sarab whereas the new finding was much lower compared to the finding reported; 40% (Zakary et al., 2011), 22.5% (Hamid et al., 2017), 61.70% (Lingathurai and Vellathurai, 2011) and 44% (Mirzaei et al., 2011) from raw milk samples in Sarab.

The variation could be due to the reason that even when drawn under aseptic condition, milk always contains microorganisms which are derived from the milk ducts in the udder. In addition, contaminants coming from milking utensils, human handlers, unclean environmental conditions and poor udder preparation might expose raw milk to bacterial contamination.

Moreover, the present study showed the resistance of *S. aureus* to vancomycin (100%), ampicillin (90.9%), ciprofloxacin (90.9%), ceftaroline (63.6%), pencillin-G (81.8%) and clindamycin (72.7%) whereas was highly susceptible to some antibiotics like, gentamicin (100%), streptomycin (81.8%), norfloxacin (63.6%), chloramphenicol (81.8%), sulfamethoxazole (96%), kanamycin (72.7%), polymixin B (72.7%), erythromycin (72.7%) and tetracycline (81.8) (Table 4). Similarly, the present investigation indicated that the resistance pattern of penicillin was found to be 93.1% by Melese et al. (2016) which is similar to the finding (87.2 %) of Tariku et al. (2011) in Ethiopia, 80% in Sweden (Landin, 2006), 57% in Iran (Gooraninejad et al., 2007) and 50% in Finland (Myllys et al., 1998). This is in contrast to findings observed by (Adesiyun, 1994) who reported 23% of resistance to penicillin-G in West India.

The highest drug resistance recorded in the current study migh be due to high antimicrobial use in dairy farms and individual cows, to treat various diseases affecting the dairy sector. Similarly, several studies have indicated that *S. aureus* isolated from raw milk showed high resistance to vancomycin, ampicillin, ciprofloxacin, penicillin-G followed by ciprofloxacin and clindamycin thus indicating the safety of food products. However, few numbers of isolates exhibited resistance towards ampicillin (Thaker et al., 2013).

Antibiotic resistance development among the bacteria poses a problem of concern. Effectiveness of current treatments and ability to control infectious diseases in both animals and humans may become hazardous.

Different researchers reported antimicrobial resistant *S.*

Table 4. Antimicrobial resistant of S. aureus isolated from raw cow milk and fruit juice of sample.

Antibiotic	%R	%I	%S	%R 95%C.I.
Penicillin G	81.8	0	18.2	47.7-96.8
Ampicillin	90.9	0	9.1	57.1-99.5
Cefoxitin	63.6	0	36.4	31.6-87.6
Gentamicin	0	0	100	0.0-32.1
Kanamycin	18.2	9.1	72.7	3.2-52.3
Streptomycin	18.2	0	81.8	3.2-52.3
Ciprofloxacin	90.9	0	9.1	57.1-99.5
Norfloxacin	0	0	100	0.0-32.1
Sulfamethoxazole	27.3	9.1	63.6	7.3-60.7
Clindamycin	72.7	0	27.3	39.3-92.7
Polymixin B	27.3	0	72.7	7.3-60.7
Erythromycin	9.1	18.2	72.7	0.5-42.9
Vancomycin	100	0	0	67.9-100
Chloramphenicol	0	18.2	81.8	0.0-32.1
Tetracycline	18.2	0	81.8	3.2-52.3

R= resistance, I= intermediate, S= susceptibility.

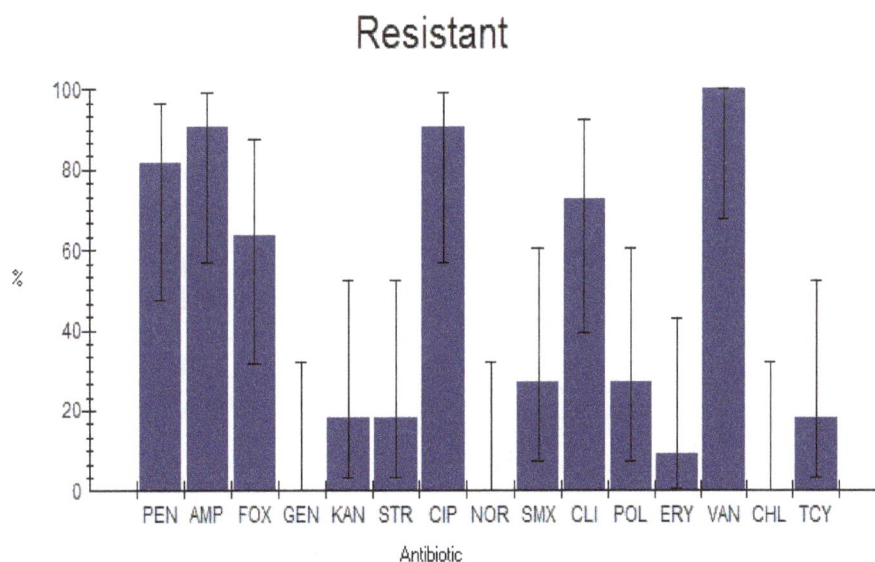

Figure 2. Antibiotic sensitivity pattern of S. aureus isolated from different samples.

aureus isolates of raw milk in their previous studies from Ethiopia. Reports from other researchers had also indicated S. aureus isolates resistance to vancomycin (100%), ampicillin (90.9%), ciprofloxacin (90.9%), ceftaroline (63.6%), penicillin-G (81.8%) and clindamycin (72.7%). Similar result was most frequently observed for penicillin (100%), ampicillin (100%), followed by erythromycin (95.7%) (Wang et al., 2014) in China, penicillin (100%), ampicillin (96%), amoxicillin (92%), and trimethoprim- sulphamethoxazole (88%) (Beyene, 2016) in Ethiopia, whereas the percent were found higher compared to what was reported by Hamid et al. (2017) of

94.4, 83.3 and 50% resistance for penicillin, ampicillin and ceftriaxone, respectively of S. aureus isolates with particular emphasis on penicillin G. The present observation agrees with preliminary finding conducted by Reta et al. (2016) of 93.1%. This is in accordance with the findings of Tariku et al. (2011) who reported resistance of S. aureus to chloramphenicol (16%), vancomycin (3%) it lower with compare the present finding while as (Khakpoor et al., 2011) in other study reported that all isolate of S. aureus from mastitis cattle were resistant to penicillin and 83.3% resistance to ampicillin in this study is much higher than that of 41.44%

Table 5. Multi-drug resistance of *S. aureus* isolated from raw cow milk and fruit Juices sample.

Number of AMR	MDR profile	% Isolates
1	VAN CIP	9.1
	VAN CIP AMP	9.1
2	PEN VAN AMP	9.1
1	PEN VAN CIP AMP	45.5
	PEN VAN CIP AMP STR	9.1
2	CHL PEN VAN CIP AMP	9.1
1	CHLPEN VAN CIP AMP STR	9.1

VAN= Vacomycin; PEN= penicillin G; AMP= ampicillin; STR= Streptomycin; CHL = chloramphenicol; CIP = ciprofloxacin.

as reported by (Mubarack et al ., 2012) and lower as compared to 100% resistance reported by (Khakpoor et al., 2011).The current study was highly susceptible to some antibiotics like, gentamicin (100%), streptomycin (81.8%), norfloxacin (63.6%), chloramphenicol (81.8%), sulfamethoxazole (96%), kanamycin (72.7%), polymixin B (72.7%), erythromycin (72.7%) and tetracycline (81.8); similar results were found for chloramphenicol, streptomycin and gentamycin (100, 94, and 90%), respectively by Beyene (2016) in Ethiopia but disagree with the observation made by Kassaify et al. (2013) in the case of streptomycin (95%), but it disagree with the observation made by Tariku et al. (2011) in the case of tetracycline (0%) and clindamycin (4%) in dairy farms in Jimma town, cefoxitin (100%) and clindamycin (each 100%) (Wang et al., 2014) in China. The probable explanation could be that *S. aureus* strains have the capacity to change their resistance behavior to the exposed antimicrobials.

The emergence degree of resistance to many drugs represents public health hazard due to the fact that food borne outbreaks would be difficult to treat and this pool of MDR S. aureus in food supply represents a reservoir for communicable resistant genes. The reason for the existence of antimicrobial resistant salmonella isolates could be due to the indiscriminate use of antimicrobials, self-medication, administration of sub therapeutic dose of antimicrobials to livestock for prophylactic purpose (Szyfers and Acha, 2001) and limited updating of the long used drug groups. Hence, due to the relatively limited access and high price to get the newly developed cephalosporin and quinolone drugs, the reports of prevalence of antimicrobial-resistant to relatively low-priced and regularly available antibiotics are alarming for a low-income society living in most developing countries, like Ethiopia.

Conclusion

The current study showed insights into the magnitude and incidence of *S. aureus* from raw cow milk and fresh fruit juice samples. The study revealed the development of antibiotic resistant against *S. aureus* which could pose serious threat for consumers as well as for health professionals in the study area. Hence, attention should be given to proper handling of the food items, and using recent antibiotics in the treatment of diseases both in humans and animals.

CONFLICT OF INTERESTS

The authors have not declared any conflict of interests.

Abbreviations: AMP, Ampicillin; **ANOVA,** analysis of variance; **CHL,** Chloramphenicol; **CIP,** Ciprofloxacin; **ERY,** Erythromycin; **I,** Intermediate; **MDR,** multiple drug resistance; **NSS,** normal saline solution; **R,** resistant; **S,** Sensitive; **SD,** standard deviation, **O,** Observation; **STR,** Streptomycin; **TCY,** Tetracycline.

REFERENCES

Abebe M, Daniel A, Yimtubezinash W, Genene T (2013). Identification and antimicrobial susceptibility of *S. aureus* isolated from milk samples of dairy cows and nasal swabs of farm workers in selected dairy farms around Addis Ababa, Ethiopia. Afr. J. Microbiol. Res. 7(27):3501-3510.

Addo KK, Mensah GI, Aning KG, Nartey N, Nipah GK, Bonsu C, Akyeh ML, Smits HL (2011). Microbiological quality and antibiotic residues in informally marketed raw cow milk within the coastal savannah zone of Ghana. Trop. Med. Int. Health 16(2):227-32.

Adesiji YO, Alli OT, Adekanle MA, Jolayemi JB (2011). Prevalence of Arcobacter, Escherichia coli, Staphylococcus aureus and Salmonella species in Retail Raw Chicken, Pork, Beef and Goat meat in Osogbo, Nigeria. J. Biomed. Res. 3(1):8-12

Adesiyun A (1994). Characteristics of *S. aureus* strains isolated from bovine mastitic milk: Bacteriophage and antimicrobial agent susceptibility and enterotoxigenecity. J. Vet. Med. 42:129-39.

Ahmadi M, Rohani SMR, Ayremlou N (2009). Detection of *Staphylococcus aureus* in milk by PCR. Comp. Clin. Pathol. 19(1):91-94.

Ateba CN, Mbewe M, Moneoang MS, Bezuidenhout CC (2010) Antibiotic-resistant Staphylococcus aureus isolated from milk in the Mafikeng Area, North West province. South Afr. J. Sci. 106:1-6.

Aydin A, Sudagidan M, Muratoglu K (2011). Prevalence of staphylococcal enterotoxins, toxin genes and genetic-relatedness of foodborne *Staphylococcus aureus* strains isolated in the Marmara

Region of Turkey. Int. J. Food Microbiol. 148(2):99-106.

Beyene GF (2016). Antimicrobial Susceptibility of Staphylococcus aureus in Cow Milk, Afar Ethiopia Int. J. Modern Chem. Appl. Sci. 3(1):280-283.

Bryant C. (2017). Investment opportunities in Mekelle, Tigray state, Ethiopia. Available at: https://www.ciaonet.org/attachments/15494

Centers for Disease Control and Prevention (CDC) (2011). Estimates of Foodborne Illness in the United States. Available at: http://www.cdc.gov/foodborneburden/index.html.

Clinical and Laboratory Standards Institute (CLSI) (2008). Performance standards for antimicrobial disk and dilution susceptibility tests for bacteria isolated from animals third edition. Approved standard M31-A3. CLSI, Wayne, PA.

Clinical and Laboratory Standards Institute (CLSI) (2012). Performance standards for antimicrobial susceptibility testing; twenty second informational supplements. CLIS document M100-S22 Wayne PA.

Ekici K, Bozkurt H, Isleyici O (2004). Isolation of some pathogens from raw milk of different milk animals. Pak. J. Nutr. 3(3):161-162.

El-Gedawy AA, Ahmed HA Awadallah MA (2014). Occurrence and molecular characterization of some zoonotic bacteria in bovine milk, milking equipments and humans in dairy farms, Sharkia, Egypt Int. Food Res. J. 21(5):1813-1823.

FAO/WHO (2005). Informal food distribution sector in Africa (street foods): importance and challenges CAF 05/4.

Fawole MO, Oso BA (2001) Laboratory manual of Microbiology: Revised edition, Spectrum Books Ltd, Ibadan. P 127.

Gooraninejad S, Ghorbanpoor M, Salati AP (2007). Antibiotic Susceptibility of Staphylococci isolated from bovine sub-clinical mastitis. Pak. J. Biol. Sci. 10:2781-2783.

Hamid S, Bhat MA, Mir IA, Taku A, Badroo GA, Nazki S, Malik A (2017). Phenotypic and genotypic characterization of methicillin-resistant Staphylococcus aureus from bovine mastitis. Vet. World 10(3):363-367.

Hundera S, Ademe Z, Sintayehu A (2005). Dairy cattle mastitis in and around Sebeta, Ethiopia. J. Appl. Res. Vet. Med. 3:1525-1530.

Khakpoor M, Safarmashaei S, Jafary R (2011). Study of milk extracted from cows related to Staphylococcus aureus by culturing and PCR. Global 7(6):572-575.

Klotz M, Opper S, Heeg K, Zimmermann S (2003). Detection of Staphylococcus aureus enterotoxins A to D by real-time fluorescence PCR assay. J. Clin. Microbiol. 41(10):4683-4687.

Knife Z, Abera K (2007). Sanitary conditions of food establishments in Mekelle town, Tigray, north Ethiopia. J. Health Dev. 21(1):3–11.

Landin H (2006). Treatment of mastitis in Swedish dairy production (in Swedish with English summary). Svensk Veterinärtidning 58:19-25.

Le Loir Y, Baron F, Gautier M (2003). Staphylococcus aureus and food poisoning. Genet. Mol. Res. 2(1):63-76.

Lingathurai S, Vellathurai P (2011). Bacteriological quality and safety of raw cow milk in Madurai, South India. Webmed Center Microbiol. 1:1-10.

Lucky NA, Nur IT, Ahmed T (2016). Microbiological quality assessment for drug resistant pathogenic microorganisms from the fresh vended fruit juices in Bangladesh, Stamford J. Microbiol. 6(1):7-10.

McFaddin JF (2000) Biochemical Tests for the Identification of Medical Bacteria, 3rd. Lippincott Williams & Wilkins, Philadelphia. pp. 94-95.

Mekonnen H, Habtamu T, Kelali A (2012). Contamination of "raw" and "ready-to-eat" foods and their public health risks in Mekelle City, Ethiopia. ISABB J. Food Agric. Sci. 2(2):20-29.

Mekonnen H, Workineh S, Bayleyegne M, Moges A, Tadele K (2005). Antimicrobial susceptibility profile of mastitis isolates from cows in three major Ethiopian dairies. Revue de médecine vétérinaire 176:391-394

Mirzaei H, Tofighi A, Karimi Sarabi, Mahdi Farajli (2011). Prevalence of Methicillin-Resistant Staphylococcus aureus in Raw Milk and Dairy Products in Sarab by Culture and PCR Techniques. J. Anim. Vet. Adv, 10(23):3107-11.

Mohanty NN, Das P, Pany SS, Sarangi LN, Ranabijuli S, Panda HK (2013). Isolation and antibiogram of Staphylococcus, Streptococcus and E. coli isolates from clinical and subclinical cases of bovine mastitis. Vet. World 6(10):739-743.

Mubarack HM, Doss A, Vijayasanthi M, Venkataswamy R (2012). Antimicrobial drug susceptibility of Staphylococcus aureus from

subclinical bovine mastitis in Coimbatore, Tamil Nadu, South India. Vet. World 5(6):352-355.

Myllys V, Asplund K, Brofeld E, Hirevela-Koski V, Honkanen-Buzalski T (1998). Bovine Mastitis in Filand in 1988 and 1995. Changes in Prevalence and Antimicrobial resistance. Acta Vet. Scand. 39:119–26.

Normanno G, Firinu A, Virgilio S, Mula G, Dambrosio A, Poggiu A, Decastelli L, Mioni R, Scuota S, Bolzoni G, Giannatale EDi, Salinetti AP, Salandra GLa, Bartoli M, Zuccon F, Pirino T, Sias S, Parisi A, Quaglia NC, Celano GV (2005). Coagulase-positive staphylococci and Staphylococcus aureus in food products marketed in Italy. J. Food Microbiol. 98:73-79.

Olatunji EA, Ahmed I, Ijah UJ (2009). Evaluation of microbial qualities of skimmed milk (nono) in Nasarawa State, Nigeria. Proceeding of the 14th Annual Conf. of Ani.Sc. Asso. Of Nig. (ASAN) LAUTECH Ogbomoso, Sept. 14th-17th.

Oyeleke SB, Manga SB (2008). Essentials of laboratory practical are in microbiology, to best publisher Minna, Nigeria. pp. 36-75.

Pourhassan M, Taravat-Najafabadi ART (2011). The spatial distribution of bacterial pathogens in raw milk consumption on Malayer City, Iran. Shiraz Med. J. 12:2-10.

Reta MA, Bereda TW, Alemu AN (2016). Bacterial contaminations of raw cow's milk consumed at Jigjiga City of Somali Regional State, Eastern Ethiopia. Int. J. Food Contamin. 3:4.

Sanaa OY, Nazik EA, Ibtisam EM, Zubeir EL (2005). Incidence of Some Potential Pathogens in Raw Milk in Khartoum North (Sudan) and Their Susceptibility to Antimicrobial Agents. J. Anim. Vet. Dev. 4(3):356-359.

Santana EHW, Cunha MLRS, Oliveira TCRM, Moraes LB, Alegro LCA (2010). Assessment of the risk of raw milk consumption related to staphylococcal food poisoing. Ciência Animal Brasileira pp. 643-652.

Shekh CS, Deshmukh VV, Waghamare RN, Markandeya NM, Vaidya MS (2013). Isolation of pathogenic Escherichia coli from buffalo meat sold in Parbhani city, Maharashtra, India. Vet. World 6(5):277-279

Szyfres B, Acha PN (2001). Zoonoses and communicable diseases common to man and animals: In Bacteriosis and Mycosis (3rd ed.), Washington DC: Pan Am. Health Organ. 1:233-246.

Tariku S, Jemal H, Molalegne B (2011). Prevalence and susceptibility assay of Staphylococcus aureus isolated from bovine mastitis in dairy farms in Jimma town South West Ethiopia. J. Anim. Vet. Adv. 10:745-749.

Tasnim M (2016). Isolation and identification of microbes from various fruit juices made and sold for immediate consumption at home and in the market of Dhaka city, MSc thesis.

Tigray bearou of administration (TBA) (2017). Tigray bearou of administration population census commission. Summary and statistical report of population and housing. Tigray bearou of Adimnstration.

Thaker HC, Brahmbhatt MN, Nayak JB (2013). Isolation and identification of Staphylococcus aureus from milk and milk products and their drug resistance patterns in Anand, Gujarat. Vet. World 6(1):10-13.

Veras JF, Carmo LS, Tong LC, Shop JW, Cummings C, Santos DA, Cerqueira MMOP, Cantini A, Nicoli JR, Jett M (2008). A study of the enterotoxigenicity of coagulase negative and coagulase positive staphylococcal isolates from food poisoning outbreaks in Minas Gerais Brazil. J. Infect. Dis. 12:410-415.

Wang X, Li G, Xia X, Yang B, Xi M, Meng J (2014). Antimicrobial susceptibility and molecular typing of methicillin-resistant staphylococcus aureus in retail foods in Shaanxi, China. Foodborne Pathog. Dis. 11(4):281-286.

World Health Organization (WHO) (2004). Regional office for Africa developing and maintaining food safety control systems for Africa current status and prospects for change, Second FAO/WHO Global Forum of Food Safety Regulators. Bangkok, Thailand. pp. 12-14.

Zakary EM, Nassif MZ, Mohammed GMO (2011). Detection of Staphylococcus aureus in Bovine Milk and its Product by Real Time PCR Assay. Glob. J. Biotechinol. Biochem. 6(4):171-177.

Zeina K, Pamela AK, Fawwak S (2013). Quantification of Antibiotic Residues and Determination of Antimicrobial Resistance Profiles of Microorganisms Isolated from Bovine Milk in Lebanon. Food Nutr. Sci. 4:1-9.

3

Prevalence, gross pathological lesions and financial losses of bovine Fasciolosis in Arba Minch Municipal Abattoir, Gamo Gofa Zone, Southern Ethiopia

Mandefrot Meaza*, Abayneh Keda, Biresaw Serda and Mishamo Sulayman

School of Veterinary Medicine, Wolaita Sodo University, Ethiopia.

A cross sectional study on bovine fasciolosis was carried out from October 2009 to April 2010 at Arba Minch Municipal abattoir with the aim of determining the prevalence and estimating financial loss. Out of the total 600 cattle examined during the study period, 203 were positive for *Fasciola* spp. infection with the prevalence rate of 33.83%. *Fasciola gigantica* was found to be the predominant *Fasciola* species affecting cattle slaughtered in the study area, 179 (88.18%) of the total livers positive for bovine fasciolosis were infected by *F. gigantica*, while 15 (7.39%) livers had *F. hepatica* and 9 (4.43) were infected by both species (*Fasciola hepatica* and *F. gigantica*). From positive livers for the parasite, 44.33, 33.50 and 22.17% of the livers had slight, moderate and severe gross lesions, respectively. There was a significant difference in the prevalence of fasciolosis (P<0.01) among different body conditions and also among different origins. Higher prevalence of the parasite was observed in animals with poor body condition and lowland origin. The total estimated annual financial losses due to fasciolosis in the abattoir during the study period was726,561.5 ETB ($52,649.38 US) of which 49,493.29 ETB ($3,586.47 USD) was due to liver condemnation (direct) and 677,068.21 ETB ($49,062.91 USD) was because of carcass weight loss (indirect). The estimated annual financial loss showed that fasciolosis is an economically important disease in the abattoir. Therefore, there is a need for further detailed studies on the epidemiology of the disease and snail intermediate hosts found in the area and strategic measure should be taken to control the disease.

Key words: Abattoir, Arba Minch, cattle, Ethiopia, Fasciolosis, financial loss, prevalence.

INTRODUCTION

Ethiopia owns huge number of ruminants with high contribution to the economy and livelihood to the people. Despite the significantly large livestock population, its contribution to the national economy is below the potential due to poor management practices, poor nutrition or low response to improved nutritional inputs, high disease incidence, and low genetic potential. Moreover, improper evaluation of public health importance is due to various individual parasitic disease and inadequate knowledge of epidemiology of disease

*Corresponding author. E-mail: meazamande@yahoo.com.

which otherwise is of great relevance where the distribution of disease determine the type and scope of control measures to be applied (Zegeye, 2003; Taylor et al., 2007; ILRI, 2009).

Fasciolosis is an important parasitic disease of domestic animals, especially cattle and the significance of fasciolosis as emerging helminthic zoonoses is highlighted (Chhabra and Singla, 2009). The two species most commonly implicated as the aetiological agents of fasciolosis are *Fasciola hepatica* and *Fasciola gigantic* (Pal, 2007). It is serious hazards to efficient production of cattle particularly in its sub clinical form (Radostitis et al, 2007). Occasionally, fasciolosis can infect human beings (CDC, 2013) and has recently been shown to be a re-emerging and widespread zoonosis affecting many people (Esteban et al., 2003).

Fasciola hepatica has a worldwide distribution but predominates in temperate zones, while *F. gigantica* is found on most continents, primarily in tropical regions (Andrews, 1999). Mixed infection by both species of *Fasciola* may occur in area where the ecology is conducive for replication of intermediate host. The economic impact of fasciolosis may greatly vary from year to year depending on the weather condition, management, level of infection, host immunity status and age of animals in endemic areas. In this, cumulative substantial loss could be very high in fluke remaining untreated and suffering from sub clinical fasciolosis (Taylor et al., 2007).

The development of infection in definitive host is divided into migratory phase and the biliary phase (Dubinsky, 1993). The parenchyma phase begins when encysted juvenile flukes penetrate the intestinal wall. After the penetration of the intestine, flukes migrate within the abdominal cavity and penetrate the liver or other organs and cause lesion. The young flukes tunnel through the parenchyma then enter the small bile ducts where they migrate to the larger bile ducts and cause lesion (Behm and Sangsten, 1999; Taylor et al., 2007).

Important economic losses associated with fasciolosis include great expenses on anthelmintics for treatment; liver condemnation; production loss due to mortality; lower production of meat, milk and wool; reduced weight gain; metabolic diseases and impaired fertility (Mason, 2004; Hillyer and Apt, 1997).

Economic losses in Africa and other parts of the world is due to the condemnation of liver as unsuitable for human consumption and associated with poor carcass conformation and predispose the animal to other infectious principally clostridium disease, weight loss, loss in productivity and loss due to death (Andrew et al., 2003)

A review of available literature strongly suggests that fasciolosis exists in almost all parts of Ethiopia. The prevalence and economic significance has been reported form different parts of the country by different researchers (Moje et al., 2015; Petros et al., 2013; Regassa et al.,

2012; Miheretab et al., 2010; Manyzewal et al., 2014; Terefe et al., 2012). Even though, different researchers in the country studied the parasite prevalence and economic significance, there is limited work in the southern part of Ethiopia, specifically, there was no work done at Arba Minch Municipal abattoir so far. Therefore, the main objectives of this study were to determine the prevalence of fasciolosis, identify the species of liver flukes involved in fasciolosis, compare the intensity of the infection with the liver lesion involved in fasciolosis and assess the financial loss due to fasciolosis in cattle slaughtered at Arba Minch Municipal Abattoir

MATERIALS AND METHODS

Study area

The study was conducted in Arba Minch, Southern Nation Nationality and People's Regional State (SNNPRS), from October, 2009 to April, 2010. The town is located geographically at 37°5' East of longitude and 6° North of latitude with altitude ranging from 1200 to 3125 m above sea level. The average annual rain fall ranges from 750 to 930 mm with mean average temperature of 30°C. The town is situated in the well-known East African Rift valley and surrounded by Lake Chamo and Abaya as well as the Nech Sar National Park. Mixed livestock agriculture farming system was practiced (GZARDO, 2007).

Study population

A total of 600 indigenous cattle are slaughtered at Arba Minch municipal abattoir. The animals were brought from district markets and brought to the abattoir for slaughtering purpose which originated from different origins with in Gamo Gofa Zonea and nearby areas mainly from highlands (Bonke, Chencha and highlands around Arba Minch), midlands (Kamba and Daramalo) and lowlands (in and around Arba Minch, Jinka and Borena).

Study design, sampling and sample size determination

A cross sectional study was carried out from October, 2009 to April, 2010 by collecting data on events associated with fasciolosis on cattle slaughtered at Arba Minch Municipality abattoir. The study was made on the slaughtered cattle at abattoir by the regular visiting. During abattoir survey includes both ante mortem and postmortem examination

The sample size was calculated according to Thrustfield (1995) by considering estimated prevalence of 50% since there was no previous abattoir survey conducted in the study area. The sample size calculated was 384 with 95% confidence interval and 5% expected error. However, in order to increase the precision, a total of 600 cattle were examined at Arba Minch Municipal abattoir by using systemtic sampling method.

The study animals were selected from the slaughter line using systematic random sampling and examined following ante-mortem and post mortem inspection procedure. Body condition was scored following the guidelines set by Nicholson and Butterworth (1986). Each animal was identified based on the enumerate marks on its body tagged before slaughter. Information regarding age, origin and body condition of the study animals was recorded during ante-mortem examination. Assessment of body condition was carried out using a modified method described by Nicholson and Butterworth

(1986). All cattle presented to the abattoir for slaughter were local indigenous breed and male cattle. The liver of each study animal was carefully examined through palpation and incision on each liver and bile duct for presence of lesions indicative of Fasciola infection externally and sliced for confirmation. Liver flukes were recovered for differential count by cutting the infected liver into fine, approximately 1 cm slices with a sharp knife.

Then, positive livers with adult parasites were collected by squeezing into universal bottle containing 10% formalin preservative and then examined to identify the involved fluke species by their size and morphological character. The size of *F. gigantica* is larger (20-75 x 3-12 mm) than *F. hepatica* (20-30 x 10 mm) and the anterior cone *F. gigantica* is not prominent as that of *F. hepatica* and the body is more transparent (Soulsby, 1982).

Characterization of gross liver lesion

Hepatic lesions in *Fasciola* positive livers were further grouped in to three different pathological categories depending on the severity of damage inflected by the parasite. The task of categorization was based on the criteria forwarded by Ogurinade and Ogurnrinade (1980). The criteria were:

Lightly affected liver: A quarter of liver was affected or one bile duct was prominently enlarged on the ventral surface of the liver and cutting revealed enlarged or calcified bile ducts and/or thick.

Moderately affected liver: Half of the organ was affected or two or more bile ducts are enlarged and visible before cutting.

Severely affected liver: The entire organ was involved or the liver was cirrhotic or the left lobe atrophy and hyperplasia of the right lobe is seen giving the liver triangular.

Financial loss assessment

The total financial loss due to fasciolosis in cattle slaughtered at Arba Minch municipal abattoir was estimated from the summation of annual liver condemnation (direct loss) and due to carcass weight reduction and poor quality (indirect loss).

Direct financial loss

All livers affected with fasciolosis were totally condemned. The annual direct financial loss was assessed by considering the overall prevalence rate of the disease, the total annual slaughtered animal in the abattoir and retail price during the time of sample collection of an average animal liver. The information obtained was subjected to mathematical compilation using the formula set by Ogurinade and Ogurnrinade (1980).

ALC= CSR*MLC*P

Where, ALC = Annual loss from liver condemnation; CSR = Mean annual cattle slaughtered per year at Arba Minch abattoir; MLC= Mean cost of one liver at Arba Minch town, P = Prevalence rate of the fasciolosis at Arba Minch abattoir.

Indirect financial loss

The indirect (carcass weight reduction) economic loss due to fasciolosis was calculated by considering an estimated 10% carcass weight loss due to fasciolosis in cattle as reported by Robertson (1976) and average carcass weight of an Ethiopian

zebu was taken as 126 kg (ILCA, 1992). According to Ogunrinade and Ogunrinade (1980), the annual economic loss because of carcass weight reduction due to bovine fasciolosis was assessed using the formula:

(ACW) = CSR* CL * BC * P*126 kg

Where, ACW is annual loss from carcass weight reduction; CSR, average number of cattle slaughtered at Arba Minch abattoir per year; CL, carcass weight loss in individual cattle due to fasciolosis; BC, an average price of 1 kg beef at the study abattoir; P, prevalence rate of fasciolosis at the study abattoir; 126 kg, average carcass weight of Ethiopia Zebu cattle.

Data management and analysis

The collected data were coded and stored in Microsoft Excel spread sheet. Statistical analysis was done using STATA Version 11.0 (Stata Corp. College Station, TX)) statistical software. Prevalence of fasciolola infection was calculated by descriptive statistics as percentage value, whereas association of Fasciola prevalence with origin, body condition score of the animals and others was analyzed using Chi-square analysis.

RESULTS

Prevalence of bovine fasciolosis

Out of 600 livers examined of cattle slaughtered at the abattoir during the study period, 203 were positive, indicating 33.83% over all prevalence rate. From the total positive livers for fluke 7.39% possess *F. hepatica*, 88.18% were found infected with *F. gigantica* and 4.43% have both *F. hepatica* and *F. gigantica* mixed infection (Table 2).

Prevalence of bovine fasciolosis from highland, midland and lowland origins were 15.93, 26.7 and 45.27%, respectively. Prevalence of bovine fasciolosis was significant (P< 0.01) based on three origins of animals from different ecological condition. There was significant statistical difference (p<0.001) among different body condition scores (good, medium and poor). More than half of the animals brought to the abattoir (58.02%) were with poor body condition which indicates that fasciolosis is chronic disease of cattle, and the main sign of is emaciation or loss of weight (Taylor et al., 2007). Statistical analysis of the effect of age on prevalence indicated no significance variation (P>0.05) among different age groups of animals.

Hepatic lesion characterization

Based on the severity of gross liver lesion, 44.33, 33.49 and 22.17% were lightly, moderately and severely affected, respectively (Table 1).

Direct financial loss assessment

The average annual cattle slaughtered were estimated to

Table 1. Classification of liver based on the extent of gross lesion.

Extent of lesions (judgment of condemnation)	Number of livers	Prevalence (%)
Lightly affected (1/4 condemned)	90	44.33
Moderately affected (1/2 condemned)	68	33.5
Severely affected (totally condemned)	45	22.17
Total	203	100

Table 2. The prevalence of bovine fasciolosis and associated risk factors.

	Number of examined animal	No of positive animals	Prevalence (%)
Species of *Fasciola*			
F. hepatica	600	15	7.39
F. gigantica	600	179	88.18
Mixed	600	9	4.43
Animal origin			
Low- land	296	134	45.27
Mid- land	191	51	26.70
High- land	113	18	15.93
Body condition			
Poor	81	46	58.02
Medium	242	100	41.32
Good	277	56	20.22
Age			
<6 years	228	72	31.58
6-10 years	258	92	35.66
>10 years	114	39	34.21
Total	600	203	33.83

Financial loss assessment.

be 4180, while mean retail price of bovine liver, 35 ETB and prevalence of fasciolosis was 33.83%, the estimated annual financial loss from liver condemnation was calculated as

ALC= CSR × LC × P

= 49,493.29 ETB or 3,586.47 $USD

Indirect financial loss assessment

It is the loss due to reduced carcass weight of Fasciola infected animals and was calculated by using average annual cattle slaughtered estimated to be 4180, while the price of carcass weight reduction (indirect) loss of 1 kg beef was 38 ETB. Then, the annual economic loss due to carcass weight reduction was assessed using the formula set by Ogunrinade and Ogunrinade (1980):

ACW = CSR* CL * BC * P*126 kg

= 677,068.21 ETB ($49,062.91 US)

Therefore, the total annual financial loss due to bovine fasciolosis in the Arba Minch Municipality abattoir was the summation of losses from organ condemnation (direct loss) and losses from carcass weight reduction (indirect loss) was about 726,561.5 ETB ($ 52,649.38).

DISCUSSION

Bovine fasciolosis is economically important and widely distributed disease in almost all region of Ethiopia. The result revealed that the disease is also problem in cattle slaughtered at Ariba Minch municipal abattoir causing high economic loss due to liver condemnation and carcass weight reduction. The overall prevalence of bovine fasciolosis (33%) from the current result was in agreement with the findings of Moje et al. (2015) (30%) in Areka, Mulat et al. (2012) (29.6%) and Miheretab et al. (2010) (32.3%) in Adwa, Ibrahim et al. (2009) (28%) in Kombolcha et al. (2004) (31.7%) from Zimbabwe and Badreldeen and Elfadil (2015) (31.6%) in Sudan.

The present prevalence was much lower than some studies in different parts of the country. In northern Ethiopia, Yilma and Mesfin (2000) reported 90.7% prevalence at Gondar abattoir and also Aregay et al. (2013) found 39.95% in Bahir Dar. In addition, Tolosa and Tigre (2007) recorded a prevalence of 46.2% at Jimma abattoir. Manyazewal et al. (2014) and Abebe et al. (2011) presented 47.1 and 53.7% in Southwest Ethiopia, respectively. The current prevalence findings are also lower than previous studies from other countries in sub-Saharan Africa with prevalence of 53.9% from Zambia, 63.8% from Tanzania and 38.5% from Uganda reported by Phiri et al. (2005), Keyyu et al. (2006) and Ssimbwa et al. (2014), respectively.

On the other hand, the finding is higher than some reports from different parts of Ethiopian and nearby east African country with prevalence of 14.0, 14.4, 24.3, 20.3, 21.9, 25.2, 21.5, 21.6, 24.4 and 26% in Wolaita Soddo (Abunna et al. 2009), Diredawa (Daniel, 1995), Mekele (Gebretsadik et al., 2009), Addis Ababa (Aragaw et al. 2012), Bishoftu (Regassa et al., 2012), Dessie, (Belay et al 2012), Adigrat (Afera, 2012), Nekemte (Petros et al., 2013), Haramaya (Yusuf et al., 2016) and Kenya (Mungube et al., 2006), respectively. Difference in prevalence among geographical locations is attributed mainly to the variation in the climatic and ecological conditions such as altitude, rainfall and temperature. Fasciola spp. prevalence has been reported to vary over the years mainly due to variation in amount and pattern of rainfall.

In relation to risk factors, there was a significant difference in the infection rate (P<0.05) among the animal origins and body condition scores condition groups but, revealed no statistical difference among age groups. The study revealed that there was a statistically significant association (P <0.001) in bovine fasciolosis prevalence among different body condition groups of the animals. Higher prevalence of fasciolosis in cattle with poor body condition as compared to cattle in medium and good body condition (Hagos, 2007; Terefe et al., 2012; Aragaw et al., 2012) as chronic fasciolosis is characterized by progressive loss of condition (Urquhart et al., 1996). However, it must be borne in mind that cattle coming from feedlots, which are expected to be in good body condition, are most likely to be de-wormed than cattle coming directly from grazing (Aragaw et al., 2012).

Out of the total positive livers for fasciolosis species identified, 88.18% of them were infected by F. gigantica where as 7.39% were infected by F. hepatica and 4.43% were mixed infections (both F. hepatica and F. gigantica). The predominant species involved in bovine fasciolosis in

the study area was F. gigantica. The high prevalence of F. gigantica as compared to F. hepatica may be associated with the presence of intermediate host L. natalensis and may be explained by the fact that most cattle for slaughter came from low land and mid altitude zones and also as described by Troncy (1989), the favorable condition the snail was border of lakes, flood prone area and low lying marshy and drainage ditches for favorable habitat. Aribaminch and the surroundings were surrounded by lakes Abaya and Chamo and rivers with spring and forest which may be conducive for the development of the intermediate host, L. natalensis.

Analysis of gross liver pathology showing 44.33, 33.5 and 22.17% were affected lightly, moderately and severely, respectively. According to Dwinger et al. (1982) and Yilma and Mesfin (2000), the number of fluke has no direct relationship with the liver gross lesion as it was observed that relatively less flukes in severely affected livers of beef cattle.

However, severe fibrosis impedes the passage of immature flukes and acquired resistance and calcification of bile ducts that impaired the further passage of young flukes and play a role by creating unfavorable microenvironment which results in the expulsion of flukes (Dwinger et al., 1982; Ramato, 1992).

The total annual financial loss estimated at 726,561.5 ETB ($ 52,649.38) which is summation of liver condemnation (direct) and carcass weight reduction (indirect) in this study account for 49,493.29 ETB ($3,586.47) and 677,068.21 ETB ($49,062.91). The direct financial loss due to liver condemnation is comparable to 47,124 ETB by Moje et al. (2015) but, lower than that of Manyzewal et al. (2014) (47,570 ETB) and Petros et al. (2013) (63,072 ETB) at Mettu and Nekemte abattoirs, respectively.

The total financial loss at Arba Minch municipal abattoir in this study was lower than the findings of Belay et al. (2012) at Dessie and Terefe et al. (2012) at Jimma. Moreover, the total financial loss is comparable to the report of Mulugeta et al. (2011) in and around Asella. The existing variation might be correlated with slaughter capacity and number of condemned organs at those specific areas.

Conclusion

The study revealed that bovine fasciolosis is a prevalent disease in the study area causing great financial loss due to condemnation of affected liver and carcass weight reduction. Predominant species involved in bovine fasciolosis in the study area was F. gigantica. This may be due to the fact that most cattle originated from low land and suitable ecological condition for the existence and multiplication of the intermediate host snail. Therefore, proper attention should be paid to control this disease in the study area in particular and in the country in general.

CONFLICT OF INTERESTS

The authors declare that there is no conflict of interest.

REFERENCES

Abebe F, Meharenet B, Mekibib B (2011). Major Fasciolosis infections of cattle slaughtered at Jimma municipality abattoir and the occurrence of the intermediate hosts in selected water bodies of the zone. J. Anim. Vet. Adv. 10:1592-1597

Abunna F, Asfaw L, Megersa B, Regassa, A (2009). Bovine fasciolosis: coprological, abattoir survey and its economic impact due to liver condemnation at Soddo municipal abattoir, Southern Ethiopia. Trop. Anim. Health Prod. 42(2):289-292.

Afera B (2012). Prevalence of bovine fascilosis in municipal Abbatoir of Adigrat, Tigray, Ethiopia. Available at: http://www.veterinaria.org/revistas/redvet/n090912/091202.pdf

Andrews S (1999).The Life Cycle of Fasciola hepatica. In Fasciolosis, Ed. Dalton, J.P. CABI Publishing. pp:1-29.

Aragaw K, Negus Y, Denbarga Y, Sheferaw De (2012). Fasciolosis in Slaughtered Cattle in Addis Ababa Abattoir, Ethiopia. Global Vet. 8 (2):115-118.

Aregay F, Bekele J, Ferede Y, Hailemelekot M (2013). Study on the prevalence of bovine fasciolosis in and around Bahir Dar, Ethiopia. Ethiop. Vet. J. 17(1):1-11.

Badreldeen BM, Elfadil AA (2015). A Cross-Sectional Survey of Bovine Fasciolosis at Elkadaro Abattoir, Khartoum State, Sudan. Glob. J. Med. Res. 15(2):1-9.

Behm C, Sangster N (1999). Pathology, pathophysiology and clinical aspects. In: Dalton, JP ed, Fasciolosis. CABI Publishing. Wallingford. pp: 185-224.

Belay E, Molla W, Amare A (2012). Prevalence and Economic Losses of Bovine Fasciolosis in Dessie Municipal Abattoir, South Wollo Zone, Ethiopia. Europ. J. Biol. Sci. 4 (2):53-59.

Centre of Disease Control and Prevention (CDC): Va. USA. (2013). Available at: https://www.cdc.gov/dpdx/fascioliasis/index.html

Chhabra MB, Singla LD (2009) Food-borne parasitic zoonoses in India: Review of recent reports of human infections. J. Vet. Parasitol. 23(2):103-110.

Daniel F (1995). Economic Importance of organ condemnation due to Fasciolosis and Hydatidosis in Cattle and Sheep slaughtered at Dire Dawa abattoir, DVM, Thesis, FVM, AAU Debre zeit, Ethiopia. pp: 18-26.

Dubinsky P (1993). Trematody atrematodozy. In: Jurasek V, Dubinsky P, kolektiv A, Vet. Parasitol. Priroda AS, Bratislava. pp:158-187.

Dwinger RH, Leriche PD, Kuhne GI (1982). Fascioliasis in beef cattle in North Western Argentina. Trop. Anim. Health Prod. 14(3):167-171.

Esteban JG, Gonzalez C, Curtale F, Mun˜oz-Antoli C, Valero MA, Bargues MD, El-Sayed M, El Wakeel A, Andel-Wahab Y, Montresor A, Engels D, Savioli L, Mas-Coma S (2003). Hyperendemic fascioliasis associated with schistosomiasis in villages in the Nile Delta of Egypt. Am. J. Trop. Med. Hyg. 69:429-437.

Gamo Goffa Zone Agricultural and Rural Development Office (GZARDO) (2007). Livestock Resource Development and Animal Health Department Annual Report, Arbaminch, Ethiopia.

Gebretsadik B, Kassahun B, Gebrehiwot T (2009). Prevalence and economic significance of fasciolosis in cattle in Mekelle Area of Ethiopia. Trop. Anim. Health Prod. 41:1503-1504.

Hagos A (2007). Study on prevalence and economic impact of bovine Hydatidosis and Fasciolosis at Mekelle Municipal Abattoir, DVM Thesis, FVM, AAU, Debre zeit, Ethiopia. pp:15-23.

Hillyer GV, Apt W (1997). Food-borne trematode infections in the Americas. Parasitol. Today 13:87-88.

Ibrahim N, Wasihun P, Tolosa T (2009). Prevalence of Bovines Fasciolosis and Economic Importance due to Liver Condemnation at Kombolcah Industrial Abattoir, Ethioipia. Internet J. Vet. Med. 8(2).

ILRI (2009). Management of vertisols in Sub-Saharan Africa, Proceedings of a Conference Post-mortem differential parasite counts FAO corporate document Repository.

International Livestock Center for Africa (ILCA) (1992). Debre Berhan experimental station annual report. P 46.

Keyyu JD, Kassuku AA, Msalilwa PL, Monrad J, Kyvsgaard CN (2006). Crosssectional prevalence of helminth infections in cattle on traditional, small-scale and large scale dairy farms in Iringa District, Tanzania. Vet. Res. Commun. 30:45-55.

Manyazewal AZ, Gurnesa M, Tesfaye T (2014). Economic Significance of Fasciolosis at Mettu Municipal Abattoir, Southwest, and Ethiopia. J. Adv. Vet. Res. 4(2):53-59.

Mason C (2004). Fasciolosis associated with metabolic disease in a dairy herd and its effects on health and productivity. Cattle Pract. 12:7-13

Miheretab B, Tesfay H, Getachew Y (2010). Bovine Fasciolosis: Prevalence and its economic loss due to liver condemnation at Adwa Municipal Abattoir, North Ethiopia. EJAST 1(1):39-47.

Moje N, Mathewos S, Desissa F, Regassa A (2015). Cross-sectional study on bovine fasciolosis: prevalence, coprological, abattoir survey and financial loss due to liver condemnation at Areka Municipal Abattoir, Southern Ethiopia. J. Vet. Med. Anim. Health 7(1):33-38.

Mulat N, Basaznew B, Mersha C, Achenef M, Tewodros F (2012). Comparison of coprological and postmortem examination techniques for the determination of prevalence and economic significance of bovine fasciolosis. J. Adv. Vet. Res. 2:18-23.

Mulugeta S, Begna F, Tesgaye E (2011). Prevalence of Bovine Fasciolosis and itsnEconomic Significance in and Around Assela, Ethiopia. Glob. J. Med. Res. 11(3):1-7.

Mungube EO, Bauni MS, Tenghagen BA, Wamae WL, Nginyi MJ, Mugambi MJ (2006). The Prevalence and Economic Significance of Fasciola gigantica and Stilesia hepatica in Slaughtered Animals in the Semi Arid Coastal Kenya. Trop. Anim. Health Prod. 38:475-483.

Nicholson MJ, Butterworth HM (1986). A guide to condition scoring of zebu cattle. International Livestock Center for Africa (ILCA), Addis Ababa, Ethiopia.

Ogunrinade A, Ogunrinade B (1980). Economic importance bovine fasciolosis in Nigeria. Trop. Anim. Health Prod.12(3):155-1590.

Pal M (2007). Zoonoses. (2nd edn.), Satyam Publishers, Jaipur, India

Petros A, Kebede A, Wolde A (2013). Prevalence and economic significance of bovine fasciolosis in Nekemt Municipal Abattoir. J. Vet. Med. Anim. Health 5(8):202-205.

Phiri AM, Phiri IK, Sikasunge CS, Monrad J (2005). Prevalence of fasciolosis in Zambian cattle observed at selected abattoirs with emphasis on age, sex and origin. J. Vet. Med. 52:414-416.

Radostitis OM, Gray CC, Hinchcliff KW, Constable PD (2007). Hepatic disease associated with trematods. In text book of cattle, horse, pigs and goats. Veterinary Medicine 10th ed. pp:1576-1580.

Ramato A (1992). Fasciolosis: clinical occurrence, coprological, abattoir and snail survey in Around Wolliso. DVM Thesis, FVM, AAU, Debre Zeit. P 35.

Regassa A, Woldemariam T, Demisie S, Moje N, Ayana D, Abunna F (2012). Bovine Fasciolosis: Coprological, Abattoir Survey and Financial loss Due to Liver Condemnation in Bishooftu Municipal Abattoir, Central Ethiopia. Europ. J. Biol. Sci. 4:83-90.

Robertson A (1976). Hand book on animal disease in tropics. pp: 3:304.

Soulsby EJL (1982). Helminths, Arthropods and Protozoa of Domesticated Animals,7th edition. Balliere Tindall, London, UK. pp: 40-52.

Ssimbwa G, Baluka AS, Ocaido M (2014). Prevalence and financial losses associated with bovine fasciolosis at Lyantonde Town abattoir. Livest. Res. Rural Dev. 26(9) Available at: http://www.lrrd.org/lrrd26/9/ssim26165.html

Taylor AM, Coop LR, Wall LR (2007). Veterinary Parasitology, 3rd Edition, UK, Wiley-Blackwell prublisher. pp:343-345.

Terefe D, Wondimu A, Dechasa GF (2012). Prevalence, gross pathological lesions and economic losses of bovine fasciolosis at Jimma Municipal Abattoir, Ethiopia. J. Vet. Med. Anim. Health 4:6-11.

Thrustfield M (1995). Veterinary epidemiology, University of Edinburgh, Black well Science. 2:180-188.

Tolosa T, Tigre W (2007). The prevalence and economic significance of bovine fasciolosis at Jimma abattoir, Ethiopia. J. Vet. Med.3(2):1-5.

4

Incidence and economic impact of fasciolosis in Wolkite town, Community Abattoir

Tesfaye Wolde* and Tigist Tamiru

Department of Biology, College of Natural and Computational Science, Wolkite University, Ethiopia.

The study was conducted to explore the incidence and economic loss related with fasciolosis in cattle at Wolkite town, Community Abattoir, Wolkite, Ethiopia. A cross-sectional study was conducted from February, 2016 - May, 2016 on bovine fasciolosis in Wolkite town, Community Abattoir. From a total of 392 cattle inspected coprologically 41.8% (164) were found positive for fasciolosis. The occurrence of cattle fasciolosis in the study sites was considerable (p<0.05) which is mainly determined based on body conditions. Post mortem assessment was conducted on a total of 392 bovine and 41.8% were found infected by Fasciola. *Fasciola hepatica* was the major *Fasciola* species causing bovine fasciolosis at the study areas. Analysis of the abattoir data indicated a total yearly liver disapproval was identified to result in 182582.4 Ethiopian birr. Likewise, the mean carcass weight loss was calculated to be 4984499.52 Ethiopian birr due to fasciolosis in cattle. The total yearly monetary loss due to fasciolosis in Wolkite town, Community Abattoir was calculated to be 5167081.92 birr. The results of the present study thus illustrated that the incidence and economic loss of fasciolosis in bovine slaughtered at Wolkite town, Community Abattoir was exceptionally elevated and necessitates urgent need for control and prevention of the parasite in the study area in specially and in Ethiopia as a whole.

Key words: Cattle, *Fasciolosis*, incidence, Wolkite town.

INTRODUCTION

Fasciolosis also named as distomitosis, or liver rot is an important helminth disease caused by trematode Fasciola commonly called "liver fluke". This disease belongs to plant born trematode (Mas-Coma et al., 2005). The definitive host range is very broad and includes many herbivores, mammals, including humans (Chhabra and Singla, 2009). The life cycle include fresh water snail as intermediate host of parasite (Torgerson and Claxton, 1999). The disease is a type of helminthsis and has been classified as Neglected tropical disease.

In recent times, worldwide fatalities in animal production because of *Fasciola hepatica* where predictably expected above 3.2 billion per annum. The WHO estimated at 180 million are at possibility of infection and 2.4 billion peoples are infected with *F. hepatica* (Spithil et al., 1999). In Europe, the American and Asia only *F. hepatica* is concerns but the distribution of the two species overlie in many areas of Africa as well as Asia (Mas-Coma et al.,

*Corresponding author. E-mail: tesfalem2002@gmail.com .

2005). The prevalence of fasciolasis in cattle in various parts of the world has been reviewed. In Africa, Ethiopia 30-90% (Magaji et al., 2014), Addis Ababa 20.3% (Kassaye et al., 2012), Nekemte 20% (Alula et al., 2013), Hossona 34.9% (Bekele et al., 2014). Ethiopia has enormous number of cattle having high role for meat expenditure and produces cash revenue from export of live cattle, carcass, organs and skin.

The monetary losses due to fasciolosis throughout the humanity are massive and these losses are coupled with death, illness, stunted growth condemnations of fluky liver, and greater than before vulnerability to secondary infection and outflow because of have power over a measure (Malone et al., 1998).

Despite the aforesaid existing condition and the incidence of a number of troubles due to fasciolosis, there is scarcity of well-documented information on the incidence of fasciolosis among cattle in Ethiopia. For that reason, the present investigation was intended with the objectives of assessing the incidence of fasciolosis in cattle and the extent of direct economic loss due to liver disapproval and not direct carcass loss at Wolkite community abattoir, Ethiopia.

MATERIALS AND METHODS

Study period and area

The investigation was carried out from March, 2016 to May and it was carried out at Wolkite municipal Abattoir. Wolkite is located at south western part of Ethiopia 152 km away from Addis Ababa.

Study design and population

The study population comprised of 392 adult cattle from different parts intended for slaughter at Wolkite municipal abattoir.

Study design and sampling procedure

The study was cross-sectional study whereby the study animals were prevalence of fasciolosis in cattle brought from selected from the slaughter line using systematic random sampling in such a way that 14 animals were examined per a day from a group of varying number of cattle slaughtered in one day. Information regarding sex, age, breed and body condition of the study animals was recorded during ante-mortem assessment. Body condition was scored following the guidelines set by Nicholson and Butterworth (1986). Accordingly, animals were classified into lean (score 2 and 3), medium (score 4, 5 and 6) and fat (score 7, 8 and 9) categories. There was no animal with score 1.

Liver examination

The liver of each study animal was carefully examined for presence of lesions suggestive of Fasciola infection externally and sliced for confirmation. Liver flukes were recovered for differential count by cutting the infected liver into fine, approximately 1 cm, slices with a sharp knife according to Hansen and Perry (1994). Each mature fluke was identified to species level according to its shape and size

(Soulsby, 1982). All intact immature and mature flukes and only fluke heads -when a portion of fluke was found- were counted.

Sample size determination and sampling methods

Simple random sampling method was used for selection of sampling units at equal intervals. The sampled cattle were screened for the presence of trematodes of interest by coprological and post-mortem examinations. The body condition score was estimated using techniques suggested by Nicholson and Bufferworth (1986), and accordingly, animals were classified into lean (score 2 and 3), medium (score 4, 5 and 6) and fat (score 7, 8 and 9) categories. Sample size for this study was determined using the formula described by Thrusfield (1995). Since no study has been carried out so far on the prevalence of Fasciola in cattle at this abattoir, the expected prevalence was taken as 50%. Thus, using the following formula the sample size for the study was calculated as 384. However, to increase the precision of the study, we decided to include 392 cattle in our investigation.

Abattoir survey

Examination of livers for Fasciola was done immediately after removal of internal organs. The livers were examined by inspection, palpation and systematic incision to recover immature and adult Fasciola flukes. Those livers condemned as unhealthy for human consumption due to fasciolosis during post mortem examination were registered.

Data analysis

The data was record on particularly intended types. The occurrence of fasciolosis was calculated as the number of cattle found to be infected by Fasciola expressed as a proportion of the total number of cattle slaughtered. Difference between the results by body condition score examination and by post-mortem examination was estimated. A 95% CI and 5% significance level was used to agree on whether there was considerable difference in the parameters calculated between different groups.

RESULTS

Postmortem examination

Three hundred and ninety-two liver sections were scrutinized in the present study. More than one or only one Fasciola species were identified by regular postmortem inspection of the liver. The identification results proved a prevalence of 41.8% (182/392) (Figures 1 and 2) fasciolosis. All the parasites identified as Fasciola were tested for species assignment using customary guiding principles. The explicit incidence of Fasciola species were known to be 32.6% (128/392) F. hepatica, 0.51% (20/392) F. gigantic, 0.3% (12/392) mixed (both F. hepatica and F. gigantic species) and 10.01% (4/392) unidentified immature flukes (Table 1).

Body state score was taken as possible threat reason for the incidence of fasciolosis in the present study cattle. Maximum contagion rate of fasciolosis was existed in low

Table 1. Prevalence of fasciolosis by species.

Species	Positive	Prevalence (%)
F .hepatica	128	32.6
F. gigantica	20	0.51
Mixed infection	12	0.3
Unidentified (immature flukes)	4	0.01
Total	164	41.8

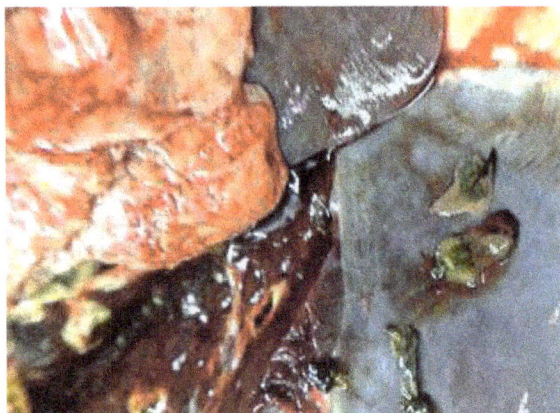

Figure 1. *Fasciola* in the liver of cattle.

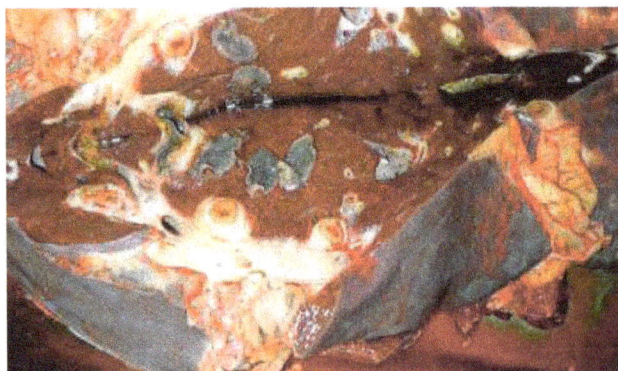

Figure 2. Bovine liver with heavy infection due to *Fasciola*.

body state cattle (68.2%) go after by average body state cattle (44.1%). The least incidence of fasciolosis was identified to happen in better body state cattle (21.5%). Arithmetical scrutiny of the figures indicated the existence of arithmetical considerable disparity (P<0.05) on the contagion rate of cattle with fasciolosis amongst the three dissimilar body stated examined cattle (Table 2).

Monetary loss

All the affected livers were condemned totally. Partial condemnation is not practiced. The data was collected from the abattoir to estimate the economic losses by considering annually condemned livers. Annual data of the last three years regarding animals slaughtered and livers condemned were collected from retrospective abattoir record. Current retail market price of single liver and 1 kg meat in Wolkite, at the study time was known to be around 60 and 130 Ethiopian birr, correspondingly was determined from interviews with local butchers in Wolkite town according to the formula set by Ogunrinade and Ogunrinade (1980).

Based on this information, the total yearly liver disapproval (ALD) was identified to cause in 36,516 Ethiopian birr (1826 United States Dollar) loss (ALD=7280×60×0.418) = 182582.4.

Likewise, the common carcass weight loss was known to be 99,690 Ethiopian birr (4984 United States Dollar) because of fasciolosis in livestock.

(IACW=7280 × (10%×126)×130× 0.418)= 4984499.52

The total yearly economic loss due to fasciolosis at Wolkite town, Community Abattoir was known to be 5167081.92 Ethiopian birr (240329 United States Dollar).

ALC=CSR x LC x P

DISCUSSION

The ecological and climatic condition of the countries such as temperature, altitude, rainfall though variations in livestock managing method and the capability to notice infection can play a part. On the other hand, when we compare prevalence of Fasciolasis with Africa country the highest prevalence (53.9%) was recorded from Zambia (Phiri et al., 2005).

The world losses of animals due to fasciolosis agricultural communities and commercial producers in urbanized countries as well as the occurrence of *F. hepatica* can be up to 77% in hot countries. Fasciolasis is taken as the solitary and largest part important helminthes interaction of cattle with shown prevalence of 30-90 (neglected tropic disease).

The aggregate incidence of cattle fasciolosis (41.8%) calculated in the present study is in contrary with the

Table 2. Proportion of Fasciolasis among dissimilar body stated animals.

Body state	Inspected	Positive	Proportion (%)	X^2 value	P-value
Better	140	32	21.5		
Moderate	184	72	44.1	8.48	0.001
Low	88	60	68.2		
Total	392	164	41.8		

work of Berhe et al. (2009) from northern part of the country who notified 24.3% proportion. Still, it is greatly less than that of many other reports of analogous studies from diverse abattoirs in the country and somewhere else in Africa. Yilma and Mesfin (2000) indicated a 90.7% prevalence of fasciolosis in cattle slaughtered at Gondar, whereas Tolosa and Tigre (2007) reported a prevalence of 46.2% at Jimma which was in concord with this study. The resemblance may be owing to the fact that two study places are so nearby and have more or less the same climatic conditions. Phiri et al. (2005) from Zambia and Pfukenyi and Mukaratirwa (2004) from Zimbabwe indicated 53.9 and 31.7% proportion respectively. On the other hand, a less occurrence of fasciolosis (14.0%) has been pragmatic in slaughter cattle at Wolaita Abattoir (Abunna et al., 2009). Dissimilarity in incidence amongst geographical locations is accredited primarily to the difference in the climate and ecology of the area. Fasciolosis commonness has been taught to be varying over the years largely due to deviation in quantity and pattern of rainfall (Mungube et al., 2006).

Similar to the present study's outcomes, numerous abattoir investigations in diverse localities of Ethiopia reported the high prevalence of F. hepatica to Fasciola gigantica (Tolosa and Tigre, 2007; Ibrahim et al., 2010; Berhe et al., 2009). Abunna et al. (2009), still, recorded privileged incidence of F. gigantica than F. hepatica in livestock butchered at Wolaita Abattoir in Ethiopia. The result of mixed infection with thus two species of Fasciola shows that there are places in the country where the climato-ecological conditions favor the existence of the intermediate snail hosts for both species. Disparity amongst the virtual incidence of the two species of Fasciola in cattle slaughtered in abattoirs situated in diverse regions of the country may possibly be clarified by the deviation in the climate-ecological conditions of the areas feeding the abattoirs. Quite a lot of studies in other African countries, however, indicated that F. gigntica is the leading if not only species ubiquitous (Phiri et al., 2005; Pfukenyi and Mukaratirwa, 2004; Kithuka et al., 2002; Opara, 2005).

This study showed there was a numerically considerable relationship (P <0.001) among Fasciola incidence and body states of the cattle. In an analogous investigation, Bekele et al. (2010) identified elevated incidence of fasciolosis in livestock with low body state contrasted to cattle in moderate and better body state.

Chronic fasciolosis is distinguished by continuous loss of state (Urquhart et al., 1996). Though, it should be noteworthy that livestock originated from feedlots, which are anticipated to be in better body state, and are nearly all probably to be de-wormed than livestock originating straightforwardly from grazing.

As cattle butchered at Wolkite Abattoir came from roughly all place of the zone it could be said that Fasciolasis is still ubiquitous in cattle in the surrounding area. The climates as well as ecological situations are sympathetic for continued existence and expansion of the intermediate snail hosts for the two species of Fasciola are also common in the study area.

Conclusion

The present study confirmed that fasciolosis is a significant disease cause substantial loss of income at Wolkite town Abattoir. The country was known to suffer loss of 5167081.92 Ethiopian Birr (240329 United States Dollar) annually due to liver disapproval and corpse weight loss that occurred from fasciolosis. For this reason, from the present study one can wind up that fasciolosis is among the key livestock parasitic disease of cattle which has a blow on the country's wealth further than its crash on the farmers. Consequently, stress should be given to management of its distribution while fasciolosis is one of the prominent parasitic diseases that have gigantic indirect and direct losses in domestic animals population.

CONFLICT OF INTERESTS

The authors have not declared any conflict of interests.

ACKNOWLEDGEMENT

The authors are thankful to Wolkite University for funding this research.

REFERENCES

Abunna F, Asfaw L, Megersa B, Regassa A (2009). Bovine Fasciolosis: Carpological, Abattoir Survey and its Economic Impact due to Liver Condemnation at Soddo Municipal Abattoir, Southern Ethiopia. Trop. Anim. Health Prod. 42:289-292.

Alula P, Addisu K, Amanuel W (2013). Prevalence and economic significance of bovine fasciolosis in Nekemte Municipal abattoir. J.Vet. Med. Anim. Health 5:202-205.

Bekele C, Menkir S, Desta M (2014). On farm study of bovine fasciolosis in lemo districts and its economic loss due to liver condemnation at Hossana Municipal Abattoir, Southern Ethiopia. Int. J. Curr. Microbiol. Appl. Sci. 3:1122-1132.

Bekele M, Tesfaye H, Getachew Y (2010). Bovine Fasciolosis: Prevalence and its Economic Loss due to Liver Condemnation at Adwa Municipal Abattoir, North Ethiopia. Ethiopia J. Appl. Sci. Technol. 1:39-47.

Berhe G, Berhane K, Tadesse G (2009). Prevalence and economic significance of fasciolosis in cattle in Mekelle area of Ethiopia. Trop. Anim. Health Prod. 41:1503-1405.

Chhabra MB, Singla LD (2009) Food-borne parasitic zoonoses in India: Review of recent reports of human infections. J. Vet. Parasitol. 23:103-110.

Hansen J, Perry B (1994). The Epidemiology, Diagnosis and Control of Helminth Parasites of Ruminants. Published by the International Livestock Center for Africa, Addis Ababa, Ethiopia.

Ibrahim N, Wasihun P, Tolosa T (2010). Prevalence of bovines fasciolosis and economic importance due to liver condemnation at Kombolcha Industrial Abattoir, Ethioipia. Internet J. Vet. Med. 8(2).

Kassaye A, Yehualashet N, Yifat D, Desie S (2012). Fasciolosis in slaughtered aattle in Addis Ababa Abattoir, Ethiopia. Glob. Vet. 8:115-118.

Kithuka JM, Maingi N, Njeruh FM, Ombui JN (2002). The Prevalence and Economic Importance of Bovine Fasciolosis in Kenya- an analysis of abattoir data. Onderstepoort J. Vet. Res. 69:255-262.

Magaji AA, Ibrahim K, Salihu MD, Saulawa MA, Mohammed AA, Musawa AI (2014). Prevalence of fascioliasis in cattle slaughtered in Sokoto Metropolitan Abattoir, Sokoto, Nigeria. Advan. Epidemiol. 2014:247258

Malone J, Gommes F, Nachet O, Agamen E (1998). A geographic information system on the potential and abundant of gigantica in east Africa based on food and agriculture organization data basis. Vet. Parasitol. 78:87-101.

Mas-Coma S, Bargues MD, Valero MA (2005). Fascioliasis and other plant-borne trematode zoonoses. Int. J. Parasitol. 35:1255-1278

Mungube EO, Bauni SM, Tenhagen BA, Wamae LW, Nginyi JM, Mugambi JM(2006). The prevalence and economic significance of Fasciola gigantica and Stilesia hepatica in slaughtered animals in the Semi-arid Coastal Kenya. Trop. Anim. Health Prod. 38:475-483.

Nicholson M, Bufferworth T (1986). A Guide to Condition Score in Zebu Cattle. International Livestock Center for Africa, Addis Ababa, Ethiopia.

Ogunrinade A, Ogunrinade BI (1980). Economic importance of fasciolosis in Nigeria. Trop. Anim. Health. Prod. 12:155-160.

Opara KN (2005). Population Dynamics of Fasciola gigantica in Cattle Slaughtered in Uyo, Nigeria. Trop. Anim. Health Prod. 37:363-36.

Pfukenyi D, Mukaratirwa S (2004). A Retrospective Study of the Prevalence and Seasonal Variation of Fasciola gigantica in Cattle Slaughtered in the Major Abattoirs of Zimbabwe between 1990 and 1999. Onderstepoort J. Vet. Res. 71:81-187.

Phiri AM, Phiri IK, Sikasunge CS, Monrad J (2005). Prevalence of fasciolosis in Zambian cattle observed at selected abattoirs with emphasis on age, sex and origin. J. Vet. Med. B 52:414-416.

Soulsby EJ (1982). Helminths, Arthropods and Protozoa of Domesticated Animals. 7th edition. Balliere Tindall, London, UK, pp. 40-52.

Spithil TW, Smoker PM, Copeman DB (1999). Fasciola gigantica, epidemiology, control, immunology and molecular biology. In: Dalton J.P. (ED), Fasciolosis, CAB International Publication Cambridge. pp. 465-525.

Thrusfield M (1995). Veterinary Epidemiology. (2nd edn.), Blackwell Science, London.

Tolosa T, Tigre W (2007). The Prevalence and economic significance of bovine fasciolosis at Jimma Abattoir, Ethiopia. Internet J. Vet. Med. 3(2):1937-1943.

Torgerson P, Claxton J (1999). Epidemiology and control. In Fasciolosis. Edited by Dalton JP. Oxon: CABI Publishing. pp. 113-149.

Urquhart GM, Duncan J, Armour L, Dunn J, Jenning AM (1996). Veterinary Parasitology. 2nd Editions, Blackwell Science, UK. pp. 103-113.

Yilma JM, Mesfin A (2000). Dry season bovine fasciolosis in North western Part of Ethiopia. Revue de Médicine Vétérinaire 151:493-500.

5

Serological evidence of African horse sickness virus infection of donkeys in Karamoja sub-region, North-eastern Uganda

Jesca Nakayima[1*], Mary L. Nanfuka[2], Daniel Aleper[1] and Duke Okidi[1]

[1]National Livestock Resources Research Institute (NaLIRRI), P. O. Box 96 Tororo, Uganda.
[2]National Animal Disease Diagnostics and Epidemiology Centre (NADDEC), P. O. Box 513, Entebbe, Uganda.

African horse sickness virus (AHSV) causes a non-contagious, infectious insect-borne disease of equids and it is endemic in many areas of sub-Saharan Africa but extends beyond its endemic zones to the Arabian Peninsula, Asia and Europe. The usual mode of transmission is by biting midge, a biological vector and *Culicoides imicola* appears to be the principal vector. Serum samples were screened from camels and donkeys for AHSV antibodies using competitive enzyme-linked immunosorbent assay (cELISA). Results revealed that 16/22 (73%) donkeys had been exposed to AHSV. All 85 camels screened in the study tested negative to AHSV. This was the first study of AHSV in Uganda and it was geared at creating awareness for the veterinary service needs of these animal species which is non-existent so far.

Key words: African horse sickness virus (AHSV), *Culicoides* spp., camels, donkeys, Uganda.

INTRODUCTION

African horse sickness (AHS) is caused by a double stranded RNA virus of the family *Reoviridae* of the genus *Orbivirus*. There are nine antigenically distinct serotypes of AHS virus (AHSV) identified by virus neutralization (Howell, 1962; McIntosh, 1958). The hosts for AHSV are equids: horses, mules, donkeys and zebra. Zebra is believed to be the reservoir host (Barnard, 1998). Antibody is found in camels, African elephants, and black and white rhinoceroses, but their role in epidemiology is unlikely to be significant (OIE, 2009). Dogs acquire peracute fatal infection after eating infected horse meat

(Bevan, 1911; Piercy, 1951), but are not a preferred host by *Culicoides* spp., therefore, are unlikely to play a role in transmission (McIntosh, 1955). Clinical manifestation of AHS in horses involve damage to the circulatory and respiratory systems resulting in serous effusion and haemorrhage in various organs and tissues (Awad et al., 1981; Coetzer and Erasmus, 1994; Lubroth, 1988). African horse sickness (AHS) is peracute, acute, subacute or mild but the disease is more severe in horses. Clinical manifestations of AHSV involve four forms: horse sickness fever, in the majority of cases (which usually

*Corresponding author. E-mail: jescan2001@yahoo.co.uk .

affects only mules, donkeys and partially immune horses); the subclinical cardiac form is suddenly followed by marked dyspnea and other signs typical of the pulmonary form. This could manifest as the cardio-pulmonary or mixed form or the peracute or pulmonary form (Maurer and McCully, 1963; Newsholme et al., 1983; Theiler, 1921). A nervous form may occur, though it is rare. All forms of disease can occur in any one outbreak but in susceptible populations of horses the mixed and pulmonary forms tend to predominate so mortality rates in these animals will be very high. Mortality rate ranges from 50 to 95% in horses to rare in African donkeys and zebra. Following recovery to AHSV, animals develop good immunity to the infecting serotype and partial immunity to other serotypes. There is no treatment for AHSV; the disease is managed by supportive treatment. Disease prevention is by vaccination with a polyvalent vaccine since all AHSV serotypes are present in South Africa and in most parts of sub-Saharan Africa. Several methods are employed for the diagnosis of AHSV, including virus inoculation of cell cultures, mice inoculation (Howell, 1962), postmortem, serology and molecular assays (Costa et al., 2016; Fowler et al., 2016; de Waal et al., 2016; Sánchez-Matamoros et al., 2016; Weyer et al., 2015). AHS is not contagious, but is known to be spread by insect vectors. The biological vector of the virus is the *Culicoides* (midges) species (Theal, 1900; Wetzel et al., 1970). *Culicoides* midges, in general, breed in damp soil rich in organic matter, however *C. bolitinos* breeds in bovine dung, and it therefore not as dependent on annual rainfall and soil-type. Adult midges become infected by taking blood meals from viraemic animals. However, this disease can also be transmitted by species of mosquitoes including *Culex*, *Anopheles*, and *Aedes*, and species of ticks such as *Hyalomma* and *Rhipicephalus*. Biting flies may also be able to transfer the virus. In Uganda, camels and donkeys are distributed in North-eastern Uganda in Karamoja and Sebei sub-regions. Zebras are found in the various conservation areas throughout the country while horses are sparsely distributed in Uganda. The horse medicine aspect of veterinary service in Uganda is not developed possibly because horses are not common in Uganda and their economic importance is limited. For this reason few people keep horses for prestige and deaths in these horses are common because during an emergency, the Ugandan veterinarians lack the expertise in horse medicine. This is the first report of AHSV in Uganda and it is geared at creating awareness for the need for equine veterinary intervention in these animals.

MATERIALS AND METHODS

Serum samples were collected from Karamoja sub-region in two districts namely: Moroto: N 2° 31' 41.604", E 34° 39' 28.794" and Amudat: N 1° 47' 29.841", E 34° 54' 23.583" districts, Uganda. The camels and donkeys were classified as: infant, juvenile, sub-adult and adult. Both sexes were sampled. Serum was collected from donkeys and camels from Karamoja sub-region in March, 2016.

Serological analysis

The animals were bled by the jugular vein following restraint. 2.5 ml blood was collected into plain vacutainer tubes without anti-coagulant. Serum was separated from the blood cells by centrifugation at 2500 rpm for 15 min and stored at -20°C until use in a competitive enzyme-linked immunosorbent assay (cELISA) (Inmunologia Y Genetica Aplicad, S. A. Madrid, Spain). In total, 110 serum samples were collected. These included 25 donkeys and 85 camels. Purposive sampling was employed due to the availability of the animals.

RESULTS AND DISCUSSION

16/22 donkeys tested positive to AHSV antibodies. All the 85 camels screened alongside the donkeys tested negative to the viral antibodies. Corrected optical densities (ODs) were calculated from sample ODs and blank ODs. Sample Id represents animal species, age, sex and sample number.

Results revealed that 16/22 (73%) of serum samples from donkeys tested positive to AHSV antibodies (Table 1). All the 85 camels tested negative to AHSV. No previous research has been done on AHSV in Uganda. Literature on AHSV research in Africa and other parts of the world is scanty although reports in South Africa exist (Liebenberg et al., 2016). Not much research interest on biting midges (*Culicoides* spp.) in Uganda (Mayo et al., 2016; Liebenberg et al., 2016; Probst et al., 2015) and not much interest in equine and cameline species in Uganda and their economic importance hence population structure is limited. Nakayima et al. (2017a, b) reported endo-parasites and equine piroplasmosis in these animals in Karamoja sub-region in the absence of veterinary care and these diseases are also prevalent around the globe (Singh et al., 2012; Sumbria et al., 2016; Singla and Sumbria, 2017).

The distribution of AHSV is determined by several factors including the efficiency of control measures, availability of vertebrate hosts or reservoirs, vector abundance, seasonality and climate. AHSV apparent infection rate rapidly fall to zero at temperatures below 15°C since virus replication does not seem to occur below this temperature (Wellby et al., 1996). However, overwintered midges could harbor "latent" virus in some of these surviving midges that will commence replication and transmission should temperatures rise to permissive levels for example during spring. The major vector of AHSV, *Culicoides imicola* adults are active at temperatures as much as 3°C lower than the minimum required for AHSV replication (Sellers and Mellor, 1993). The seasonality of AHSV is explained by vector activity; after the rainy season in the tropics, in the summer and autumn in temperate regions. Bluetongue virus shares the same vector species (*Culicoides)* (Boorman et al., 1975; Mellor, 2000; Mellor et al., 1975; Venter et al., 2000;

Table 1. Sero-prevalence of AHSV in donkeys from Karamoja sub-region, North-eastern Uganda.

S/N	Animal species	Sample ID	OD reading	Corrected OD	AHSV result
1	Donkey	D/A/F/02	0.152	101.7	Positive
2	Donkey	D/SA/F/03	0.459	83.2	Positive
3	Donkey	D/A/F/04	0.137	102.6	Positive
4	Donkey	D/A/F/05	0.11	104.3	Positive
5	Donkey	D/A/F/06	0.103	104.7	Positive
6	Donkey	D/A/F/07	1.827	0.4	Negative
7	Donkey	D/A/F/08	1.974	-8.5	Negative
8	Donkey	D/A/F/09	1.841	-0.5	Negative
9	Donkey	D/A/M/10	0.126	103.3	Positive
10	Donkey	D/A/M/11	1.972	-8.4	Negative
11	Donkey	D/A/F/12	0.098	105.0	Positive
12	Donkey	D/A/F/13	0.098	105.0	Positive
13	Donkey	D/A/F/14	0.121	103.6	Positive
14	Donkey	D/A/M/15	0.114	104.0	Positive
15	Donkey	D/A/M/16	0.132	102.9	Positive
16	Donkey	D/A/F/17	0.689	69.2	Positive
17	Donkey	D/A/F/18	0.097	105.1	Positive
18	Donkey	D/A/M/19	0.096	105.1	Positive
19	Donkey	D/SA/F/20	1.755	4.7	Negative
20	Donkey	D/A/F/55	0.605	74.3	Positive
21	Donkey	D/SA/F/56	0.335	90.7	Positive
22	Donkey	D/C/M/57	0.135	102.8	Positive

Du Toit, 1944). With the advent of climate change the midge vector has now significantly extended its range northwards into Europe. Since 1998, bluetongue virus has caused disease outbreaks and has become endemic in Europe. AHSV is widely distributed across sub-Saharan Africa (Mellor and Boorman, 1995; Howell, 1963), from Senegal and Gambia in the west to Ethiopia and Somalia in the east, and extending as far south as northern South Africa, and may extend at times to Egypt in the north (Howell, 1963). The Sahara desert serves as an effective geographical barrier preventing the infection from the South spreading north-wards. Probably AHSV has its first historical reference traced to an epizootic in Yemen which occurred in 1327 (Moule, 1896; Sailleau et al., 2000). However, the virus is believed to have originated from Africa following the introduction of susceptible equine breeds during exploration of central and eastern Africa (M'Fadyean, 1900). The earliest account of the disease in Africa traces back to 1569 (Theal, 1900). The first detection of AHSV in South Africa was in 1719, a major outbreak that killed 1,700 animals in the Cape region. However, before this, the wildlife reservoirs could have been circulating the disease (Mornet and Gilbert, 1968). The disease is endemic in these areas with subsequent outbreaks and massive horse deaths (Mellor and Hamblin, 2004). During outbreaks of AHS in endemic areas, different virus serotypes may be active simultaneously within an area,

but one serotype usually dominates during a particular season, followed in the following year by the dominance of another serotype. AHSV is a major challenge to horses in endemic areas in sub-Saharan Africa, but it repeatedly caused large epizootics in the Mediterranean region (North Africa and southern Europe in particular) as a result of trade in infected equids.

Conclusion

AHSV could be endemic in the equine population in Uganda but goes undiagnosed. Zebras in wildlife conservation areas and donkeys could be acting as reservoirs to the infection. No information about the disease is available in Uganda hence no control measures in place. This is a threat to the horse population in Uganda and neighboring countries. There is need to improve knowledge of equine and cameline medicine and welfare in Uganda.

CONFLICT OF INTERESTS

The authors have not declared any conflict of interests.

ACKNOWLEDGEMENT

This study was financially supported by the Government

of Uganda under National Agricultural Research Organization (NARO).

REFERENCES

Awad FI, Amin MM, Salama SA, Aly MM (1981).The incidence of African horse sickness in animals of various species in Egypt. Bull. Anim. Health Prod. Afr. 29:285-287.

Barnard JH (1998). Epidemiology of African horse sickness and the role of the zebra in South Africa. Arch. Virol. Suppl. 14:13-19.

Bevan LEW (1911). The transmission of African horse sickness to the dog by feeding. Vet. J. 67:402-408.

Boorman J, Mellor PS, Penn M, Jennings M (1975).The growth of African horse sickness virus in embryonated hen eggs and the transmission of virus by Culicoides variipennis Coquillett (Diptera: Ceratopogonidae). Arch. Virol. 47:343-349.

Coetzer JAW, Erasmus BJ (1994). African horse sickness, in: Coetzer JAW, Thomson GR, Tustin RC. (Eds.), Infectious diseases of livestock with special reference to southern Africa, Oxford University Press, Cape Town. 1:460-475.

Costa S, Sastre P, Pérez T, Tapia I, Barrandeguy M, Sánchez-Vizcaíno JM, Sánchez-Matamoros A, Wigdorovitz A, Sanz A, Rueda P (2016). Development and evaluation of a new lateral flow assay for simultaneous detection of antibodies against african horse sickness and equine infectious anemia viruses. J. Virol. Methods 237:127-131.

de Waal T, Liebenberg D, Venter GJ, Mienie CM, van Hamburg H (2016). Detection of African horse sickness virus in Culicoides imicola pools using RT-qPCR. J. Vector Ecol. 41(1):179-185.

Du Toit RM (1944). The transmission of bluetongue and horse sickness by Culicoides. Onderstepoort J. Vet. Sci. Anim. Ind. 19:7-16.

Fowler VL, Howson EL, Flannery J, Romito M, Lubisi A, Agüero M, Mertens P, Batten CA, Warren HR, Castillo-Olivares J (2016). Development of a novel reverse transcription loop-mediated isothermal amplification assay for the rapid detection of african horse sickness virus. Transbound. Emerg. Dis. Available at: http://onlinelibrary.wiley.com/doi/10.1111/tbed.12549/full

Howell PG (1962). The isolation and identification of further antigenic types of African horse sickness virus. Onderstepoort J. Vet. Res. 29:139-149.

Howell PG (1963). African horse sickness, in: Emerging diseases of animals, FAO, Rome FAO Agricultural Studies. 61:71-108.

Liebenberg D, Piketh S, Labuschagne K, Venter G, Greyling T, Mienie C, de Waal T, van Hamburg H (2016). Culicoides species composition and environmental factors influencing African horse sickness distribution at three sites in Namibia. Acta. Trop. 163:70-79.

Lubroth J (1988). African horse sickness and the epizootic in Spain 1987. Equine Pract. 10:26-33.

Maurer FD, McCully RM (1963). African horse sickness with emphasis on pathology. Am. J. Vet. Res. 26:235-266.

Mayo C, Venter E, Steyn J, Coetzee P, van Vuuren M, Crafford J, Schütte C, Venter G (2016). The prevalence of Culicoides spp. in 3 geographic areas of South Africa. Vet. Ital. 52(3-4):281-289.

McIntosh BM (1955). Horse sickness antibodies in the sera of dogs in enzootic areas. J. South Afr. Vet. Med. Assoc.26:269-272.

McIntosh BM (1958). Immunological types of horse sickness virus and their significance in immunization. Onderstepoort J. Vet. Res. 27:465-539.

Mellor PS (2000). Replication of arboviruses in insect vectors. J. Comp. Pathol. 124:231-247.

Mellor PS, Boorman J (1995). The transmission and geographical spread of African horse sickness and bluetongue viruses. Ann. Trop. Med. Parasitol. 89:1-15.

Mellor PS, Boorman J, Jennings M (1975). The multiplication of African horse sickness virus in two species of Culicoides (Diptera: Ceratopogonidae). Arch. Virol. 47:351-356.

Mellor PS, Hamblin C (2004). African horse sickness. Vet Res. 35:445-466.

M'Fadyean J (1900). African horse-sickness. J. Comp Pathol. 13:1-20.

Mornet P, Gilbert Y (1968). La pesteéquine. In Les maladies animales à virus. L'Expansion. 476:195.

Moule L (1896). Histoire de la MédecineVétérinaire, Maulde, Paris. P 38.

Nakayima J, Kabasa W, Aleper D, Okidi D (2017a). Prevalence of endo-parasites in donkeys and camels in Karamoja sub-region, North-eastern Uganda. J. Vet. Med. Anim. Health 9(1):11-15.

Nakayima J, Nanfuka LM, Aleper D, Okidi D (2017b). Serological prevalence of Babesia caballi and Theileria equi in camels and donkeys from Karamoja sub-region, North-eastern Uganda. J. Vet. Med. Anim. Health 9(6):137-142.

Newsholme O, Bedford GAH, Du Toit RM (1983). A morphological study of the lesions of African horse sickness. Onderstepoort J. Vet. Res. 50:7-24.

OIE: World Organization for Animal Health (2009). Available at: http://www.oie.int/

Piercy SE (1951). Some observations on African horse-sickness including an account of an outbreak among dogs. East Afr. Agric. J. 17:62-64.

Probst C, Gethmann JM, Kampen H, Werner D, Conraths FJ (2015). A comparison of four light traps for collecting Culicoides biting midges. Parasitol. Res. 114(12):4717-4724.

Sailleau C, Hamblin C, Paweska JY, Zientara S (2000). Identification and differentiation of the nine African horse sickness virus serotypes by RT-PCR amplification of the sero type specific genome segment 2. J. Gen. Virol. 81:831-837.

Sánchez-Matamoros A, Nieto-Pelegrín E, Beck C, Rivera-Arroyo B, Lecollinet S, Sailleau C, Zientara S, Sánchez-Vizcaíno JM (2016). Development of a luminex-based DIVA assay for serological detection of african horse sickness virus in horses. Transbound. Emerg. Dis. 63(4):353-359.

Sellers RF, Mellor PS (1993). Temperature and the persistence of viruses in Culicoides spp. during adverse conditions. Rev. Sci. Tech. Off. Int. Epizoot. 12:733-755.

Singh G, Soodan JS, Singla LD, Khajuria JK (2012). Epidemiological studies on gastrointestinal helminths in horses and mules. Vet. Practitioner 13(01):23-27.

Singla LD, Sumbria D (2017). Equine piroplasmosis: Belles-lettres update with special reference to Indian scenario. In: An Update on Diagnosis and Control of Parasitic Diseases, Ananda KJ, Pradeep BS, Rakesh RL and Malatesh DS (Eds), Department of Veterinary Parasitology, Veterinary College, Shimoga, KVAFSU, Bidar, Karnataka, India. pp. 372-400.

Sumbria D, Singla LD, Kumar S, Sharma A, Dhayia R, Setia RK (2016). Spatial distribution, risk factors and haematobiochemical alterations associated with Theileria equi infected equines of Punjab diagnosed by indirect ELISA and nested PCR. Acta Trop. 155:104-112.

Theal GM (1900). Records of South-Eastern Africa collected in various libraries and archive departments in Europe. Government of the Cape Colony. P 6.

Theiler A (1921). African horse sickness (Pestisequorum), Union S. Africa Dept. Agric. Pretoria, Sci. Bull. P 19.

Venter GJ, Graham SD, Hamblin C (2000). African horse sickness epidemiology: vector competence of South African Culicoides species for virus serotypes 3, 5 and 8. Med. Vet. Entomol. 14:245-250.

Wellby MP, Baylis M, Rawlings P, Mellor PS (1996). Effects of temperature on the rate of virogenesis of African horse sickness virus in Culicoides (Diptera: Ceratopogonidae) and its significance in relation to the epidemiology of the disease. Med. Vet. Entomol. 86:715-720.

Wetzel H, Nevill EM, Erasmus BJ (1970). Studies on the transmission of African horse sickness. Onderstepoort J. Vet. Res. 37:165-168.

Weyer CT, Joone C, Lourens CW, Monyai MS, Koekemoer O, Grewar JD, van Schalkwyk A, Majiwa PO, MacLachlan NJ, Guthrie AJ (2015). Development of three triplex real-time reverse transcription PCR assays for the qualitative molecular typing of the nine serotypes of African horse sickness virus. J. Virol. Methods 223:69-74.

6

Semen characteristics and fertility assessment of *Sennar* jackass (*Equus asinus*) in Ethiopia

Alemayehu Lemma

Department of Clinical Studies, College of Veterinary Medicine and Agriculture, Addis Ababa University, P. O. Box 34, Debre Zeit, Ethiopia.

The aim of this study was to evaluate the semen characteristics and fertility of *Sennar* jacks. Semen was collected between January and March using Missouri AV model and was subjected to gross and microscopic evaluation. Fertility was evaluated from pregnancy rate after AI was carried out with fresh semen on 12 Abyssinian jennies, 5 *Sennar* jennies and 17 local mares. Mean (±SD) total and gel-free volume; and spermatozoa concentration were 61.1±12.6 ml, 50.3±12.3 ml, and 257± 8.1 x 10^6/ml, respectively. Total and progressive sperm motility, sperm viability and abnormal sperm percentage were 84.2±2.1; 67.4 ± 6.1%, 89%, and 10.9±2.9, respectively. There was no significant individual difference in most semen parameters. Pregnancy rate was 40% (2/5) in *Sennar* jennie, 58.3% (7/12) in Abyssinian jennies and 64.7% (11/17) in mares. The study thus revealed that semen can be successfully collected and evaluated as part of a breeding soundness examination of *Sennar* jacks during cross breeding using AI. Further study on cryopreservation of semen and improving pregnancy rate after extending semen in optimized donkey semen extender is necessary in the future.

Key words: AI, fertility, *Sennar* jacks, semen, Ethiopia.

INTRODUCTION

With an estimated 6.2 million heads (CSA, 2011), donkeys are known to play a great role particularly in rural areas of Ethiopia, where they are used on a daily basis to carry out numerous tasks in the house and agricultural fields (Alemu et al., 1997). Classifications of Ethiopian donkeys based on size and coat colour, includes four major types namely *Abyssinian, Jimma, Ogaden,* and *Sennar* Donkeys (Fesseha, 1991). The *Sennar* donkey is by far the largest and the only one reputed for producing good mules. The natural habitat of the *Sennar* donkeys is the Northwestern lowland of Ethiopia. Donkey crossing with selected descendants of the Kessella Nubian asses is a very common practice, while mule production from Sudan *Sennar* donkeys is more common in the highlands around Ethio-Sudan border. Mating, in almost all cases, except for the crossing, is uncontrolled and hence usually associated with year-round foaling.

Due to their distinct phenotypic features, *Sennar* donkeys are expensive and are not easily available in all

E-mail: alemma2008@gmail.com.

areas of the country. Moreover, anecdotal information suggests that the work performance of *Sennar* donkeys is nearly twice that of Abyssinian types. Regardless, there is little published information on their genetic potential, selection, and reproductive management. Particularly, no work has been initiated to consider the use of AI, a technology which is relatively well developed in horses (Squires, 2005). At natural mating, the average fertile jack ass ejaculates 3.3-18 billion spermatozoa directly into the body of the uterus. Fewer than 100 spermatozoa pass through the uterotubal junction to reach the site of fertilization to give a per cycle conception rates of 60 – 70% (Allen et al., 2001; Hagstrom, 2004). AI in donkeys can improve the reproductive performance; however, expanded use of frozen semen is dependent on proper laboratory assessment of sperm quality as an essential procedure of the AI technology. Mares bred with frozen semen are often examined 4-6 times/day and inseminated immediately before or within 6 h post-ovulation because of lower survivability of spermatozoa in the reproductive tract (Squires et al., 2003; Contri et al., 2012). Another study (Samper, 2005) has shown that deep insemination into the horn ipsilateral to the ovary with the pre-ovulatory follicle results in 80% of the sperm remaining in that oviduct with-higher conception. On the other hand, with the apparent differences from horses, the efficient application of AI in donkeys requires an understanding of peculiar semen characteristics (Rota et al, 2012; Qeusada et al., 2012). This study was aimed at assessing *Sennar* donkey semen characteristics and evaluation of fertility of fresh ejaculate through AI.

MATERIALS AND METHODS

Animals

A total of 5 *Sennar* jacks previously selected for breeding at *Sennar* Donkey Multiplication Centre (Wekin, North Ethiopia) were used. The jacks were aged between 6 and 8 years, and had an average BCS of 7 (on 1-9 scale, Pearson and Quasat, 2000) body weight ranging 243 to 280 kg. The jacks were mainly used to produce donkey crosses and mules. Study jacks were allowed to graze in the field freely and were supplemented with ample amount of hay and concentrate. Water was provided *ad libitum*. All jacks were dewormed against common parasites, and vaccinated against African Horse Sickness and Anthrax before introduction to the stable.

Collection and evaluation of semen

The jacks were allowed to individually interact with jennies well into oestrus for 30 min. Semen was collected after the jacks were sufficiently stimulated using a Missouri model equine AV (Agtech, Manhattan, USA) twice a week for a total of 25 collections between January and March. Immediately after collection, the color and the total volume of the each ejaculate was recorded. Semen was then filtered and the gel-fraction removed and placed in water bath at 37°C. Aliquot of 5 µl semen was removed from the gel-free fraction for each of the following microscopic evaluation: total motility, progressive motility and sperm viability, abnormal sperm percent,

pH was determined using strip. Sperm concentration (10^6/ml) was measured using Neubauer hemocytometer. Total and progressive motility were evaluated by phase contrast microscopy at ×100 and ×200 magnifications. The differential staining was made after taking a 10 µl aliquot of the semen sample mixed at 1:1 ratio of with 3% sodium citrate buffer and 1% eosin and made into thin smear. The slide was quickly dried on a pre-warmed plate before evaluation. Live percent and percent abnormal sperm were determined under light microscope (oil immersion, x1000) after counting 200 spermatozoa. White (unstained) sperm was classified as live and those that showed pink or red coloration were classified as dead. Morphological defects were classified into head, mid-piece or tail defects.

Fertility assessment

Fresh semen was extended in 1:1 volume by volume ratio of semen and a modified equine semen extender (prepared from 100 ml skimmed milk, 2.5 ml egg yolk, 4 g of glucose, 150,000 IU crystalline penicillin and 150,000 µg streptomycin) (Davies-Morel, 1999). Sperm longevity was evaluated at 15 min intervals for the first one hour, followed by final evaluation after one hour. The semen was then evaluated again after 24 h of chilling in Equitainer-I Tube Style (Agtech, Inc., Manhattan, U.S.A.) at +6°C. Spermatozoa fertilizing ability was afterwards determined by inseminating 17 jennies (5 *Sennar* jennets, 12 Abyssinian jennets) and 17 mares that were induced for estrus prior to AI. Both the jennies and mares used for AI were selected based on their previous history of breeding and each received 1ml prostaglandin (Clorprostenol, Pharmacia and Upjohn Company, USA) for induction of estrus. Jennies and mares were followed for manifestation of estrus signs. Semen used for insemination was collected the day of AI, prepared to make up 100x10^6/ml (4 ml of semen; 400x10^6 sperm per insemination) Insemination was carried out after ovulation (but as close to time of ovulation as possible) which was determined by ultrasound. A catheter was inserted per vaginum into the uterus and semen was deposited using a plunger free syringe. Small amount of air was pushed into the catheter to gently drive out the remaining semen. Pregnancy was diagnosed using ultrasonography (Mindray, Hong Kong) after 30 days post insemination. Fertility assessment was performed from pregnancy rate per insemination.

Statistical analysis

All collected data was stored in Microsoft Excel data sheet. The statistical analysis was performed using SPSS for Windows (Version-15) and STATISTICA for Windows (version 6, Statsoft, USA). The data was summarized using descriptive statistics. Comparison between jacks in fresh semen parameters was done using One Way ANOVA. Correlation between variables was computed using Pearson correlation (r). Differences were considered significant when $P < 0.05$.

RESULTS

A total of 25 semen collection procedures were carried out. Summary of fresh semen parameters are given in Table 1. The most prominent pre-coital sexual displays observed during teasing included nibbling and/or sniffing of the vulva, head, neck and back of the knee, flank, perineum and tail; Olfactory investigation of voided urine, flehman response, mounting with and without erection (Figure 1) and naso-nasal contact. Once a jack gets

Table 1. Fresh semen characteristics in *Sennar* jacks (n=25 collections).

Parameter	Mean (±SD)	Range
Total semen volume (ml)	61.1 ± 12.6	25 - 100
Gel-free volume (ml)	50.3 ± 12.3	15 - 85
pH	7.4 ± 0.1	6.5 – 7.7
Semen concentration (10^6/ml)	257 ± 8.1	65 – 387
Total sperm motility (%)	84.2± 2.1	78 - 92
Progressive sperm motility (%)	67.4 ±6.1	60 - 75
Sperm viability (%)	89.1 ± 2.3	82 – 94
Morphologically normal sperm (%)	89.0 ± 2.9	80 - 94

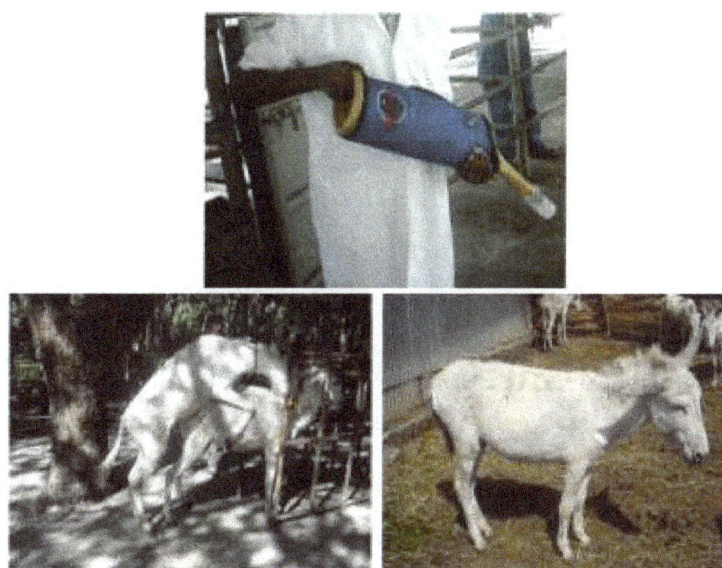

Figure 1. Semen collection in *Sennar* donkeys. Top: Missouri model equine AV used to collect *Sennar* jacks (Bottle cover removed), Left: False mount without erection during teasing, Right: Jack after semen collection displaying refractory isolation from estrous jennies.

erection, then it took on average less than two minutes to reach full erection and eventually being collected.Semen was collected successfully from all males on all occasions.Jacks entered into refractory period and often isolated themselves from the jenny in estrus after ejaculation.

Semen color was creamy white (91.5%), or milky (85%). There was no significant difference in semen parameters among individual jacks except for pH of semen. Live percent was successfully estimated in 1% eosin stain. Sperm abnormality was also fairly identifiable in the same slide prepared for determining sperm viability. The most common sperm defect was bent tail (40.9± 2.9%; p<0.05) as compared to head (17.6±01%) and other sperm defects. Sperm longevity declined with time and total motility was reduced to <60% at 2 h post ejaculation at 37°C water bath temperature. However,

after 24 h of chilling, total motility remained at 36.2±4.3% while progressive motility was 24 ±7.4%.

Pregnancy rate was 40% (2/5) in *Sennar* jennies, 58.3% (7/12) in Abyssinian jennies and 64.7% (11/17) in mares. Pregnancy confirmation at early stage using ultrasonography was fairly easier in all cases (Figure 2).

DISCUSSION

Although donkey population in Ethiopia is high population of *Sennar* donkeys is very low. Sparsely located within the country, they are mostly used in the production of best mule using hand mating. Their semen characteristics have never been assessed. Artificial insemination with cooled transported semen would allow the development of appropriate breeding plans and a

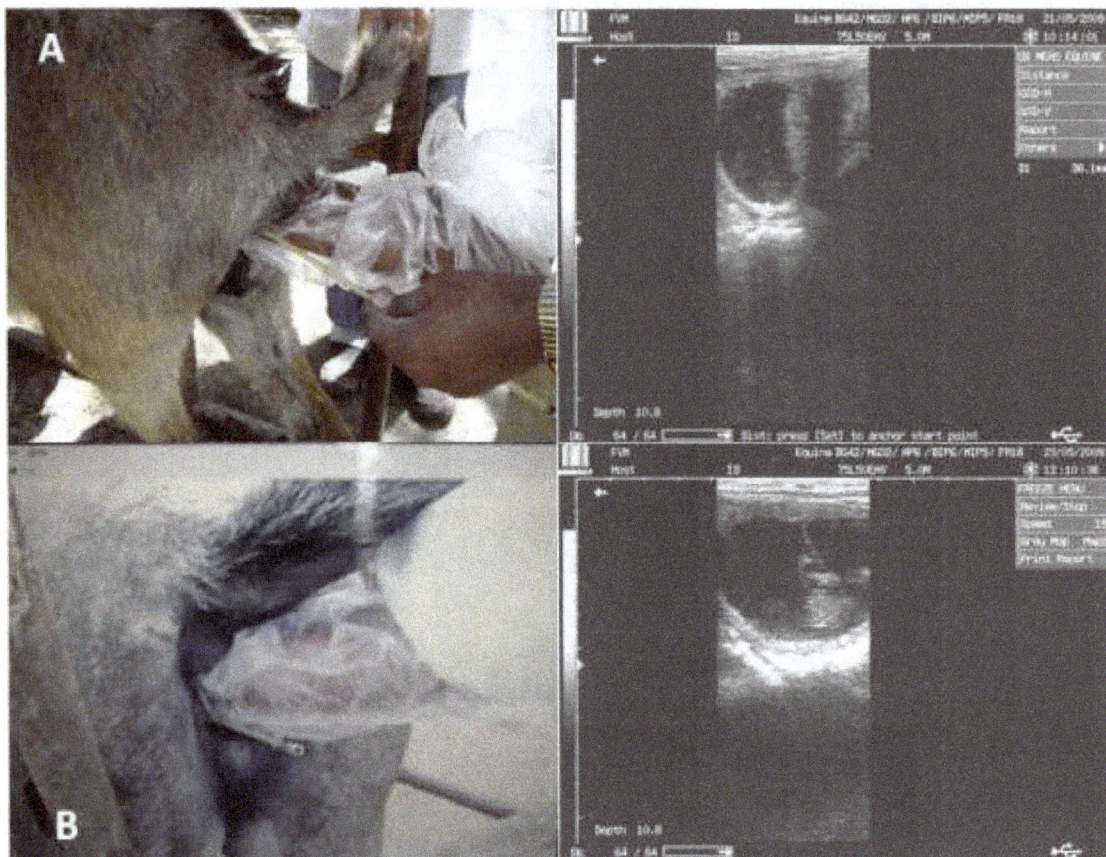

Figure 2. AI in Abyssinian donkey and 30-day embryo of the same jenny, AI in mare and 35-day embryo of the same mare.

better gene distribution, reducing the risks of excessive inbreeding in small populations (Canisso et al., 2011). Semen characteristics are very good showing comparatively better sperm motility; however this quickly deteriorates through time and particularly after chilling. Total volume and concentration are lower than Amiata breeds of donkeys (Rota et al., 2008), and are higher than Abyssinian donkeys (Lemma and Deressa, 2009) but comparable to report by Purdy (2005). Apart from semen characteristics, an important difference from stallion might be the continued reluctance of jacks to mount jennets during semen collection. Tail abnormality is much higher than previous reports for other donkeys (Henry et al., 1991). Pregnancy rate is affected by factors such as the freezing technique, extenders used, time of insemination, number of spermatozoa used for the AI (Rota et al., 2012; Saragusty, 2015). Previous study (Vidament et al., 2009) in donkey semen showed that pregnancy with fresh or chilled semen is similar for jennies and mares. Previous studies confirm freezing donkey semen with addition of glycerol can reduce pregnancy dramatically. An improved technique of freezing large volumes of semen as in directional freezing has been found to improve quality of frozen semen and

fertility (Arav and Saragusty, 2013). Some studies support the addition of homologous seminal plasma during re-suspension of frozen semen to improve fertility (Okazaki et al., 2012; Sabatiniet al., 2014). If seminal plasma has influenced the pregnancy rate in this study has to yet be verified. Pregnancy rate however is still much better than the 40% previously reported by Oliveira et al. (2006).

Conclusion

Evaluation of semen characteristic as part of the breeding soundness evaluation can give a more objective assessment of *Sennar* jacks breeding ability. Outcomes of semen analysis in the present study are generally good with acceptable level of fertility both in jennies and mares. The application of multiparametric evaluation could further improve quality of semen that can be used for AI. A notable setback observed in this study is the reluctance of the jacks to mount even on jennies well into estrous. AI both in mares and jennies also require meticulous ultrasonic evaluation of ovulatory follicle to match the time of ovulation with the time of insemination to get good pregnancy results.

CONFLICT OF INTERESTS

The author has not declared any conflict of interests.

REFERENCES

Alemu GW, Azage T, Alemu Y (1997). Research needs of donkey utilization in Ethiopia. Improving Donkey Utilization in Ethiopia. In: Proceeding of Animal Traction Network for Eastern and Southern Africa (ATNESA) Workshop held in Debre Zeit, Ethiopia, 5-9th May. pp. 77-81.

Allen WR, Tiplady C, Wilsher S, Lefranc AC, Morris LHA(2001). Videoendoscopic Low-Dose Uterotubal Insemination in the Mare; Proceedings of the Second Meeting of the, European Equine Gamete Group, Havemeyer Found. Monogr. Ser. 5:29.

Arav A, Saragusty J (2013). Directional freezing of spermatozoa and embryos. Reprod. Fertil. Dev. 26:83-90.

Canisso IF, Carvalho GR, Morel MD, Ker PG, Rodrigues AL, Silva EC, Coutinho Da Silva MA (2011). Seminal parameters and field fertility of cryopreserved donkey jack semen after insemination of horse mares. Equine Vet. J. 43:179-183.

Central Statistical Agency (CSA), (2011). Agricultural sample census, livestock sample census year 2010 by Central statistics agency, Addis Ababa, Ethiopia.

Contri A, Gloria A, Robbe D, Sfirro MP, Carluccio A (2012). Effect of sperm concentration on characteristics of frozen-thawed semen in donkeys. Anim. Reprod. Sci. 136:74-80.

Davies Morel MCG (1999). Equine Artificial Insemination. CABI Publishing, Wallingford, UK. P 416.

Fesseha G (1991). Use of equine in Ethiopia. Proceedings of Fourth Livestock Improvement Conference. Institute of Agricultural Research, 13-15 November, Addis Ababa, Ethiopia. 1:51-58.

Hagstrom DJMS (2004). Donkeys are Different; An Overview of Reproductive Variations from Horses, Equine Extension, University of Illinois. pp. 4-5.

Henry M, McDonnell SM, Lodi LD, Gastal EL (1991). Pasture mating behavior of donkeys (Equus asinus) at natural and induced estrus. J. Reprod. Fertil. 44:77-86.

Lemma A, Derresa B (2009).Study on Reproductive Activity and Evaluation of Breeding Soundness of Jacks (Equus asinus) in and Around Debre Zeit, Ethiopia. Age 8(1.21):1-21.

Okazaki T, Akiyoshi T, Kan M, Mori M, Teshima H, Shimada M (2012). Artificial insemination with seminal plasma improves the reproductive performance of frozen-thawed boar epididymal spermatozoa. J. Androl. 33: 990-998.

Oliveira JV, Alvarenga MA, Melo CM, Macedo LM, Dell'Aqua JA, Papa Jr. FO (2006). Effect of cryoprotectant on donkey semen freezability and fertility. Anim. Reprod. 94:82-84.

Pearson RA, Quassat M (2000). A guide to live weight estimation and body condition scoring of donkeys. UK, J. Thomson Colors Printers Ltd. P 21.

Purdy SR (2005). Artificial Insemination for Miniature Donkeys. In: Veterinary Care of Donkeys, Matthews N.S. and Taylor T.S. (Eds.). International Veterinary Information Service, Ithaca NY. Available at: http://www.ivis.org/home.asp

Qeusada F, Dorado J, Acha D, Ortiz I, Urbano M, Ramirez L, Galvez MJ, Alcaraz L, Portero JM, Gonzalez C, Demyda-Peyras S (2012). Freezing of donkey semen after 24 hours of cool storage: Preliminary results. Reprod. Fertil. Dev. 25:154.

Rota A, Magelli C, Panzani D, Camillo F (2008). Effect of extender, centrifugation and removal of seminal plasma on cooled-preserved Amiata donkey spermatozoa. Theriogenology 69:176-185.

Rota A, Panzani D, Sabatini C, Camillo F (2012). Donkey jack (Equus asinus) semen cryopreservation: studies of seminal parameters, post breeding inflammatory response, and fertility in donkey jennies. Theriogenology 78:1846-1854.

Sabatini C, Mari G, Mislei B, Love CC, Panzani D, Camill F, Rota A (2014). Effect of post-thaw addition of seminal plasma on motility, viability and chromatin integrity of cryopreserved donkey jack (Equus asinus) spermatozoa. Reprod. Domest. Anim. 49:989-994.

Samper JC (2005). Stallion semen cryopreservation: male factors affecting pregnancy rates. Proceedings of the Society for Theriogenology. San Antonio Texas. pp.160-165.

Saragusty J (2015). Directional freezing for large volume cryopreservation. In: Wolkers WF, Oldenhof H, editors. Methods in Cryopreservation and Freeze-Drying. New York: Springer Verlarg. pp. 381-397.

Squires EL, Barbacini S, Necchi D, Reger HP, Bruemmer JE (2003). Simplified Strategy for Insemination of Mares with Frozen Semen, 49th Annual Convention of the American Association of Equine Practitioners, 2003-New Orleans, LA, USA, (Ed.). Publisher: American Association of Equine Practitioners, Lexington KY. Internet Publisher: International Veterinary Information Service, Ithaca NY (www.ivis.org), 21-Nov; P0654.1103.

Vidament M, Vincent P, Martin FX, Magistrini M, Blesbois E (2009). Differences in ability of jennies and mares to conceive with cooled and frozen semen containing glycerol or not. J. Anim. Reprod. Sci. 112:22-35.

7

Genetic diversity of *Mycobacterium bovis* in Jalisco, Mexico: Tracing back sources of infection

Sara González-Ruiz[1], Susana L. Sosa-Gallegos[2], Elba Rodríguez-Hernández[3], Susana Flores-Villalva[3], Sergio I. Román-Ponce[3], Isabel Bárcenas-Reyes[2], Germinal J. Cantó-Alarcón[2] and Feliciano Milián-Suazo[2*]

[1]Doctorado en Ciencias Biológicas, Facultad de Ciencias Naturales, UAQ, Mexico.
[2]Facultad de Ciencias Naturales, UAQ, Mexico.
[3]Centro Nacional de Investigación Disciplinaria en Fisiología Animal-INIFAP. km 1 Carretera a Colón. Ajuchitlán, Querétaro, Mexico.

Bovine tuberculosis (bTB) is a disease of cattle that presents risk to public health, causing severe economic losses to the livestock industry and difficulty in eradication because of its complex epidemiology. The aim of this study was to identify relationships between *Mycobacterium bovis* strains from cattle in the State of Jalisco, and those of other States of México. Molecular fingerprints of 337 *M. bovis* isolates from Jalisco, and 1152 from other States of México were included in the study. Isolates were obtained from tubercles between 1997 and 2015. Evolutionary relationship was determined throughout spoligoforest (www.emi.unsw.edu.au/spoltools/). From 337 isolates from Jalisco, 59 spoligotypes were obtained, ten of them included 48% of all isolates in the state. Five spoligotypes were common to beef and dairy cattle. The molecular analysis showed eight clusters in a philogenetic three: one with three subclusters of nine isolates each, all from dairy cattle; four with two isolates, including dairy and beef cattle. All spoligotypes from Jalisco have been reported in other states, four of the most frequent ones: SB0673, SB0971, SB0669 and SB0140, were the same as in other states. The most frequent spoligotypes of *M. bovis* found in Jalisco were also the most frequent ones in other parts of Mexico. However, there is no evidence to conclude that Jalisco is the source of infection to other states since no information on movement and destination of cattle could be documented.

Key words: Tuberculosis, *Mycobacterium bovis*, spoligotyping, cattle, Jalisco, molecular epidemiology.

INTRODUCTION

Bovine tuberculosis (bTB) is an infectious disease caused by *Mycobacterium bovis,* a member of the *Mycobacterium tuberculosis* complex, which also includes *M. tuberculosis, M. cannettii, M. africanum, M. bovis, M. pinnipedii, M. caprae* and *M. microti.* Bacilli in this group are 99.9% genetically similar at the nucleotide level with identical 16S rRNA sequences (Boddinghaus et al., 1990; Sreevatsan et al., 1997) but with different host

*Corresponding author. E-mail: feliciano.milian@uaq.mx.

preferences; *M. bovis* has the broadest host range, causing disease in a wide range of mammals, including humans (O'Reilly and Daborn, 1995; Blischak et al., 2015). The proportion of cases due to *M. bovis* in humans in the last two decades has been variable, ranging from 0.5 to 13% depending on the study population, and it is estimated that nearly 10 million people are affected by tuberculosis worldwide every year (Müller et al., 2013; Olea-Popelka et al., 2017; Perea-Razo et al., 2017). Transmission to humans occurs by inhalation of infectious droplets from infected cattle, and consumption of contaminated unpasteurized dairy products (de la Rua-Domenech et al., 2006).

bTB causes direct and indirect economic losses to the livestock industry, infected animals have poor production performance, die or are culled prematurely. Free trade of animals and animal products in affected areas is prohibited, especially for exportation (Bawinek and Taylor, 2014; El-Sayed et al., 2016).

Like many countries, Mexico has a national program for the control and eradication of tuberculosis (NOM-031-ZOO-1995). This program is based on tuberculin testing and culling of reactors; however, after about two decades, the success has been partial, prevalence in beef cattle has been reduced to low levels (<0.5%) in 85% of the national territory, but in dairy cattle prevalence remains in about 16% (Plan Estratégico de la Campaña Nacional de la Tuberculosis Bovina en México, 2008-2012; Milián-Suazo et al., 2016). Poor participation of dairy farmers in the program, who are not willing to eliminate reactors is one of the main reasons. Nevertheless, the elimination of bTB in Mexico is a high priority task.

Another reason that has hampered the complete success of the bTB program in Mexico, and in other developing countries is the lack of a good system to trace back sources of infection and the indiscriminate movement of animals. Fortunately, in the last ten years, the arrival of molecular techniques to genotype strains of *M. bovis* has enormously supported epidemiological studies focused on detecting areas of risk. Because of simplicity and the low levels of DNA required in the analysis, spoligotyping is one of the methods most frequently used for studying genetic relationship between strains, and the spatial and temporal distribution of *M. bovis* (Kamerbeek et al., 1997; Rodríguez-Campos et al., 2011).

Spoligotyping detects presence or absence of spacers of the Direct Repeat (DR) locus in the *M. bovis* genome (Supply et al., 2006). The DR region contains a large number of DR´s of 36 bp interspersed by spacers from 35 to 41 bp in length. These repeats are present in isolates of the *M. tuberculosis* complex only, and it has been shown that this region is variable (Kemmerbeek et al., 1997). Presence or absence of DR´s allows phylogenetic analysis to determine genetic relationship between individual or groups of strains (Acosta-Salinas et al., 2009;

Jagielski et al., 2014).

Molecular genotyping suggests that isolates with similar fingerprints are epidemiologically related and differ from those epidemiologically unrelated (Maslow and Mulligan, 1993); however, the desirable characteristic for typing is related to its stability within the strain and its diversity within the species (Kemerbeek et al., 1997; Zhou et al., 2011; Kim et al., 2017). Strains with the same spoligotype are assumed to be individuals recently derived by clonal replication from a single ancestral cell; therefore, epidemiological related strains should have higher genetic similarity than those no related (Rodríguez-Campos et al., 2011; Milián et al., 2016). Furthermore, spoligotyping has been used successfully in epidemiological studies in many countries (Gibson et al., 2004; Parra et al., 2005; Duarte et al., 2010; Rodríguez et al., 2010; Skuce et al., 2010; Ruettger et al., 2012; Mwakapuja et al., 2013).

Bacilli of the *M. tuberculosis* complex are clonal, exchange of DNA between individual does not exist. Therefore, it is widely accepted that spoligotypes provide enough information to estimate recent evolution events to perform phylogenetic analysis for epidemiological purposes (Supply et al., 2006), and together with MIRU-VNTR has been recognized as the new gold standard for molecular epidemiological investigations of TB (Jagielski et al., 2014). Currently, there are many reports about the spatial and temporal distribution of *M. bovis* in different geographic areas around the world; however, no information on the role of specific geographic areas in the dissemination of bTB is available.

Therefore, the objective of this study was to use spoligotyping patterns to better understand the population structure of *M. bovis* in cattle in Jalisco, and to evaluate the role of this state as a source on infection for other regions in Mexico.

MATERIALS AND METHODS

Isolates data

Data from a total of 337 *M. bovis* isolates from cattle in the State of Jalisco, and 1,152 from other states in Mexico between 1997 and 2015 were included in the study. Isolates were obtained directly from bTB suspicious tissue collected from carcasses in slaughterhouses, and cultured in Stonebrink and Lowenstein-Jensen with pyruvate. Briefly, tissue samples were first decontaminated with 1:1000 solution of sodium hypochlorite and then macerated and decontaminated with a 10% solution of hydrochloric acid. DNA for spoligotyping was obtained by the CTAB-chloroform method, according to de Almeida et al. (2013). Briefly, a total of 500 μL of suspended colonies in TE 1X buffer was transferred into lysozyme (10 mg/ml) and incubated at 37°C for 1 h. Then, proteinase K and sodium dodecyl sulfate 10% were added, and the suspension was incubated at 65°C for 30 min. Subsequently, a solution consisting of a mixture of NaCl and CTAB (NaCl 5 M and CTAB 10%) was added, and the suspension was incubated for 30 min at 65°C. DNA was then extracted with chloroform/isoamyl alcohol (24:1). The supernatant was transferred to a new tube and isopropanol was added. The suspension was

Table 1. The most frequent *M. bovis* spoligotypes in Jalisco and other States of Mexico, by breed.

State	Breed	Spoligotype (SB)										Other	Total
		0673	0971	0669	0140	0145	0121	0663	0269	1116	0119		
Jalisco	Dairy	35	14	30	15	18	10	10	8	7	9	163	319
	Beef	0	0	0	1	0	0	2	0	0	0	2	5
	Unknown	2	0	0	0	0	0	0	1	2	1	7	13
	Total	37	14	30	16	18	10	12	9	9	10	172	337
Other States	Dairy	148	60	67	75	66	70	27	21	13	11	284	842
	Beef	8	19	13	4	0	0	7	5	10	1	24	91
	Unknown	22	33	13	14	10	4	4	7	10	3	99	219
	Total	178	112	93	93	76	74	38	33	33	15	407	1152
Grand total		215	126	123	109	94	84	50	42	42	25	579	1489

kept at -20°C for 2 h and centrifuged for 15 min at 14,000 g. The pellet was washed with 500 µL of 70% ethanol and centrifuged for 5 min at 14,000 g, and 50 µL of TE buffer was added.

Spoligotyping

Spoligotyping was performed according to Kamerbeek et al. (1997). The DR region was amplified using the primers DRa (GGTTTTGGGTCTGACGAC, 5_ biotinylated) and DRb (CCGAGAGGGGACGGAAAC). The amplified product was hybridized to a nylon membrane to which 37 spacer sequences from *M. tuberculosis* H37Rv and 6 spacer sequences from *M. bovis* BCG were covalently bound (Isogen Bioscience BV, Maarssen, The Netherlands). For the detection of hybridizing DNA, chemiluminescent ECL detection system (Amersham Biosciences; Piscataway, NJ) was used, followed by exposure to X-ray film (Kodak) for 45 min. Spoligotypes were named according to the website *M. bovis* spoligotype database (www.mbovis.org).

Phylogenetic analysis

Spoligotyping data were converted to binary character data (absent=0 and present=1) for the 43 probe hybridization positions. Genetic relationship between spoligotypes was determined by using the algorithm MIRU-VNTRplus available in www.miru-vntrplus.org. Evolutionary relationship was determined throughout spoligoforest in the spolTools webpage (www.emi.unsw.edu.au/spoltools/) for all spoligotypes clustering at least three isolates. Spoligoforest provides an evolutionary genetic tree showing the most probable relationship of all the spolgotypes in the data set (Reyes et al., 2008). This algorithm uses a model that considers mutations by irreversible deletions of spacers and assigns probabilities to the lengths of these deletions. The number of isolates in the cluster determines the size of each node in the tree. Edges between nodes reflect evolutionary relationships between spoligotypes with arrowheads pointing to descendants. Spoligotypes from Jalisco were matched to spoligotypes from other States of Mexico to determine the level of dissemination of *M. bovis* in the country.

RESULTS

Out of 337 isolates from Jalisco, a total of 59

spoligotypes were obtained, ten: SB0673, SB0971, SB0669, SB0140, SB0145, SB0121, SB0663, SB0269, SB1116, and SB0119 included 48% of all isolates from Jalisco; grouping between nine and 37 isolates. Ten spoligotypes grouped between two and three isolates, and 39 were orphans. When comparing spoligotypes from Jalisco with those from other states, it was found that the most frequent spoligotypes in Jalisco were also the most frequent ones in other States of Mexico. Five spoligotypes from Jalisco were common to beef and dairy cattle, suggesting related strains between these two breeds (Table 1).

Out of the 1,152 isolates from states other than Jalisco, a total of 159 spoligotypes were obtained, which included 56% of all isolates in the data set, 98 were orphans. The ten most frequent spoligotypes in Jalisco were also the ten most frequent ones in other parts of Mexico; two hundred and sixty-six were not found in the *www.mbovis.org* data set. From all the isolates in the data set, 1,161 came from dairy, and 96 from beef cattle; the rest had not information for this variable (Table 1).

Figure 1, shows the phylogenetic tree of spoligotypes from Jalisco, containing groups of at least three isolates each. Eight clusters were formed in this tree: one with three subclusters with nine isolates each, all from dairy cattle. Four with two isolates, including dairy and beef cattle, and three with one subcluster; one including an isolate from beef cattle. Isolates from other states matching spoligotypes from Jalisco are described in Table 2. All spoligotypes from Jalisco have been reported in other States, four of the most frequent spoligotypes in Jalisco: SB0673, SB0971, SB0669 and SB0140, were also the most frequent ones in other states. Some spoligotypes are common to dairy and beef cattle, suggesting related strains of bTB between these two breeds.

Figure 2 shows the spoligoforest hierarchical layout of isolates from Jalisco, where the continuity of lines indicates the weight of the hypothetical evolutionary

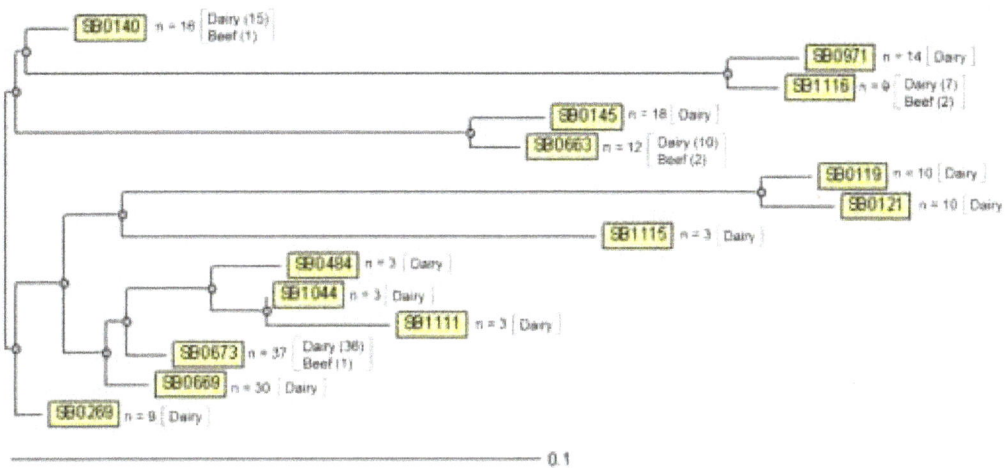

Figure 1. Phylogenetic tree of *M. bovis* isolates obtained from cattle in the State of Jalisco. Number in brackets indicates the number of isolates per breed.

relationship between spoligotypes; continuous line indicates stronger relationship. The spoligoforest shows two trees with connected components. The biggest tree, the one with the largest number of branches, is rooted by strain SB0140, suggesting this as the oldest strain in the tree.

A total of 141 isolates descended from SB0140, in four clearly defined clusters with 9 to 37 isolates each. The hypothetical evolutionary relationship between spoligotypes SB0140 and SB0673, the spoligotype with the largest cluster in the data set is strong, suggesting a small number of changes in the DR region sequence. Spoligotype SB0669, the second largest cluster, has a strong relationship with spoligotype SB0673 but is not directly connected to spoligotype SB0140, suggesting a new evolutionary route.

Spoligotypes SB0145, SB0269 and SB0971 all directly descended from SB0140. SB0145 and SB0971 have their own evolution route since other spoligotypes are derived from them (SB0663 and SB1116, respectively). From the second tree, rooted by spoligotype SB0121, only one lineage is formed, giving origin to strain SB0119.

Figure 3 shows the spoligoforest hierarchical layout of isolates from states apart from Jalisco in Mexico. Like the Jalisco's spoligotypes, the other States spoligoforest shows two separated trees, originating also from SB0121 and SB0140. The only big difference between the two spoligoforests is the presence of spoligotype SB0971 with a large number of isolates in a separated branch, suggesting a new genetic line. As before, spoligotype SB0140 seems to be the older spoligotype in the country.

DISCUSSION

Spoligotypes SB0673 and SB0669 were the most frequent spoligotypes in Jalisco. These spoligotypes SB0971 and SB0669 were also the most frequent ones in the rest of the country; however, this fact does not necessarily mean that Jalisco is the source of infection since no epidemiological evidence connecting strains from different sources in Mexico could be obtained. It is known that Jalisco is an important source of dairy replacements to other regions in Mexico under especial circumstances; however, this could not be confirmed due to the lack of information on movement of cattle. It is known from personal communication that Jalisco acted as a source of dairy heifers for other regions in the years 2003 to 2006, when Mexico closed the border to the importation of cattle from the United States (US) and Canada because of the bovine spongiform disease outbreak; the US and Canada are the main sources of replacements for dairy in Mexico. It was not known, however, what the distribution of *M. bovis* strains in the country was before that event, for comparison.

Beef and dairy cattle are maintained under different conditions in Mexico. Dairy cattle are raised in close intensive settings with a large number of cattle per square meter; in some regions it is possible to observe 10,000 cattle in a single unit operation. On the contrary, beef cattle are raised in open extensive areas with a low number of cattle per hectare. Because of this, the prevalence of bTB in dairy cattle is higher ≈16% (range 0 to 40%) than in beef cattle ≈0.5% (range 0 to 1%) (Plan Estratégico de la Campaña Nacional de la Tuberculosis Bovina en México, 2008-2012). Therefore, infected dairy populations are a risk to bTB-free or bTB-low prevalence areas of beef cattle. Fourteen of the isolates from beef cattle had spoligotypes SB0673 or SB0669, two of the most frequent spoligotypes in dairy cattle, suggesting transmission between breeds. From the epidemiological point of view, this is relevant because transmission from

Table 2. Frequency and relationship of *M. bovis* isolates from Jalisco and other States of Mexico by breed.

Spoligotypes from Jalisco	Number of isolates	State (number of isolates by State for States other than Jalisco)		
		Dairy	Beef	Unknown
SB0673	182	Ags (9), BC (3), Chih (6), Coah (16), EdoMex (17), Gto (9), Hgo (17), Qro (66), Sin (2), SLP (1), Ver (1), Zac (1).	Chih (1), Dgo (1), Gto (2,), Zac (4).	Ags (7), Coah (2), Col (1), Gro (1), Mich (1), Mor (7), Qro (7).
SB0971	109	Ags (6), BC (1), Chis (1), EdoMex (10), Gto (8), Hgo (8), Mich (1), Qro (22), SLP (1), Ver (1).	Gto (1), Mich (1), Qro (15), Son (1), Ver (1).	Ags (8), EdoMex (7), Gto (3), Gro (1), Mor (1), Nay (2), Qro (7), SLP (2).
SB0669	173	Ags (11), BC (1), Coah (10), Col (1), Dgo (3), EdoMex (18), Gro (2), Gto (5), Hgo (9), Qro (4), SLP (2), Tlax (1).	Gto (2), Mich (1), Nay (8) y Zac (2).	Gro (2), BL (1), Pueb (4), SLP (3), Son (1), Zac (1).
SB0140	90	Ags (10), Chih (8), Coah (2), Edo Mex (5), Gto (3), Hgo (9), Mich (3), Qro (33), Zac (2).	Gto (1), Mich (1), Zac (2).	Ags (6), EdoMex (2), Gto (2), Mor (1).
SB0145	74	Ags (4), BC (14), EdoMex (16), Gto (4), Hgo (5), Qro (20), Ver (2), Zac (1).	--	Ags (2), Nay (1), Qro (2), Sin (2), Ver (1),
SB0121	74	Ags (1), BC (1), Chih (29), Coah (2), EdoMex (3), Hgo (20), Qro (14).	--	Mich (3), Nay (1).
SB0663	37	Ags (5), BC (10), Chih (1), Dgo (1), Edo Mex (3), Gto (2), Qro (4), Zac (1).	Mor (1), Nay (4), Son (1) y Ver (1).	Sin (1), Son (1), Ver (1).
SB1116	33	Ags (5), Col (1), Dgo (1), Edo Mex (2), Mich (1), Qro (2), Zac (1).	Gro (1), Nay (1), Ver (8).	Pue (2), SLP (3), Sin (1), Tamps (2),Ver (2).
SB0269	33	Ags (5), Coah (1), Dgo (1), Edo Mex (2), Gro (1), Hgo (3), Qro (2), Ver (6).	Camp (3), Gto (1), Sin (1).	Col (1), Nay (1), Pue (2), SLP (3).
SB0119	14	Chih (4), Coah (2), Dgo (1), Hgo (3),y NL (1).	Gto (1).	Col (1), Sin (1).
SB0484	10	Edo Mex (3), Gto (1), Hgo (3) Qro (1), SLP (2).	--	--
SB1044	9	Edo Mex (3), Hgo (2), Qro (2).	--	Qro (1), Zac (1).
SB1115	1	Ags (1)	--	--
SB1111	1	Edo Mex (1)	--	--

dairy to beef cattle might jeopardize the goals of the national program to eradicate bTB, and the exportation of calves, an important source of currency for Mexican farmers. In this study, it is not known however if beef animals found infected are from cattle for beef operations or from dairy operations, where sometimes, beef bulls are used for breeding cows with reproductive problems, and beef calves are kept for fattening in the same farm.

Even though clustering of isolates occurred, the diversity of spoligotypes is wide. This agrees with previous reports (Cobos-Marín et al., 2005; Santillán-flores et al., 2006; Reyes et al., 2008; Pérez-Guerrero et al., 2008; Bobadilla-del Valle et al., 2015; Sandoval-Azuara et al., 2017), where in spite of studying samples from different and specific regions of Mexico, the diversity of strains has been evident, suggesting an intense and continuous exchange of animals, and new genetic

lines emerging as a consequence of the high prevalence of bTB in dairy cattle.

The spoligoforest demonstrates all possible relations of spoligotypes under the assumption of spoligotype mutation, with genetic instability ranging from 10 to 20 years (Brosch et al., 2002; Gutiérrez et al., 2005; Smith et al., 2006). In the data set, the largest root of the tree was spoligotype SB0140. Spoligotype SB0140 has infected cattle, deer, badgers and people in

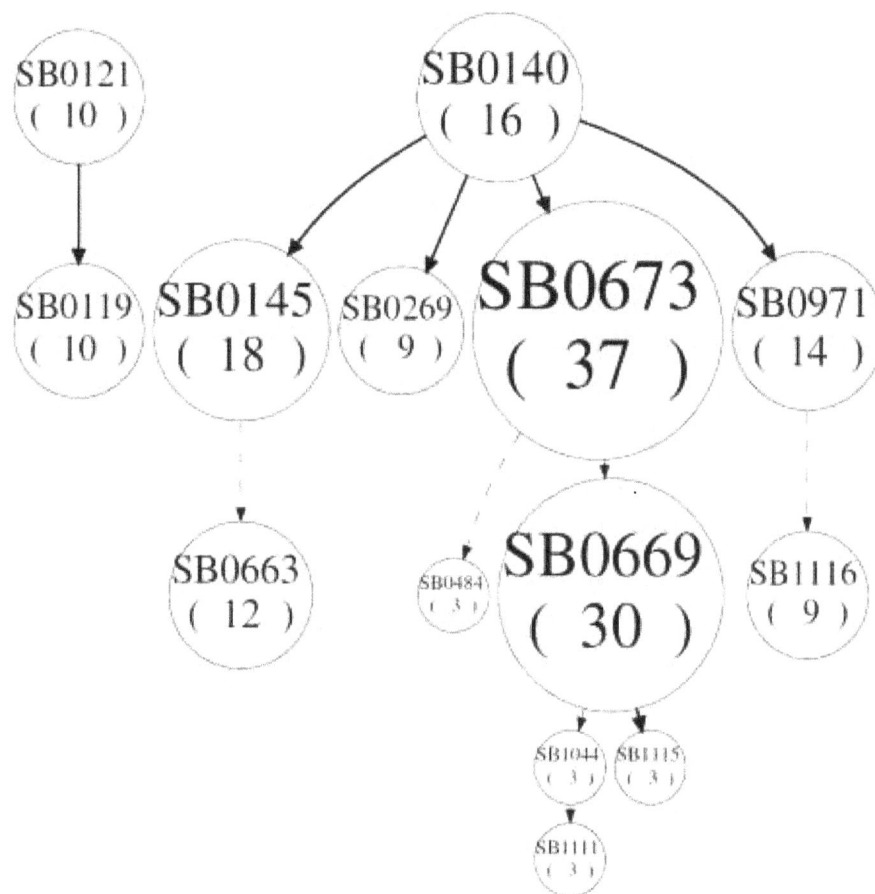

Figure 2. Spoligoforest of *M. bovis* spoligotypes obtained from cattle in Jalisco, Mexico. Nodes are labeled with the SB identifier as indicated in *mbovis.org*; numbers in parenthesis indicate cluster size. Lines between nodes reflect hypothetical evolutionary relationships among spoligotypes with arrows denoting descendence. Continuous lines indicate stronger relationship.
Source: http://spoltools.emi.unsw.edu.au/

Ireland (de la Rua-Domenech et al., 2006; McLernon et al., 2010), and cattle in the United Kingdom (de la Rua-Domenech et al., 2006; McLernon et al., 2010). It has also been reported as the most frequent spoligotype in pigs (Barandiaran et al., 2011), cattle and cats in Argentina (Zumárraga et al., 2009), and humans in the United States (Rodwell et al., 2008) and Mexico (Bobadilla-del Valle et al., 2015).

Spoligotype SB0140 has been studied profoundly in the United Kingdom (Smith et al., 2003). It was concluded that the frequency of strains with SB0140 in that country cannot be explained by random drift without selection. It has been concluded that some genotypes increase in number in a specific region in a "clonal expansion" by selection of favorable mutations when some cells find new host species or new geographical regions. In Mexico, it is believed that both situations are possible at least for the most frequent spoligotypes: selection of favorable mutations due to the high prevalence of *M. bovis* in the population and ecological opportunity by the indiscriminate movement of animals between regions.

Clusters with similar or highly similar *M. bovis* spoligotypes are considered the result or recent transmission, and that the orphans arise from migration or reactivation of acquired infections (Luciani et al., 2008). However, other factors may be involved in that clustering, that is, sampling and the mutation rate of the molecular marker used in fingerprinting (Tanaka and Francis, 2005). In the current study, both clustering and a high frequency of orphan spoligotypes occur. Clustering might well be a consequence of the conditions in which dairy cattle are maintained, in high density populations and orphans, the result of the indiscriminate movement of animals between regions or the high prevalence of the disease, which gives rise to new genetic lineages.

Something that is clear from the current study is that molecular information itself is not enough to explain the epidemiology of a disease. In the present study, no data on movement of animals from Jalisco could be obtained in spite of intensive search of data, and this is clearly a

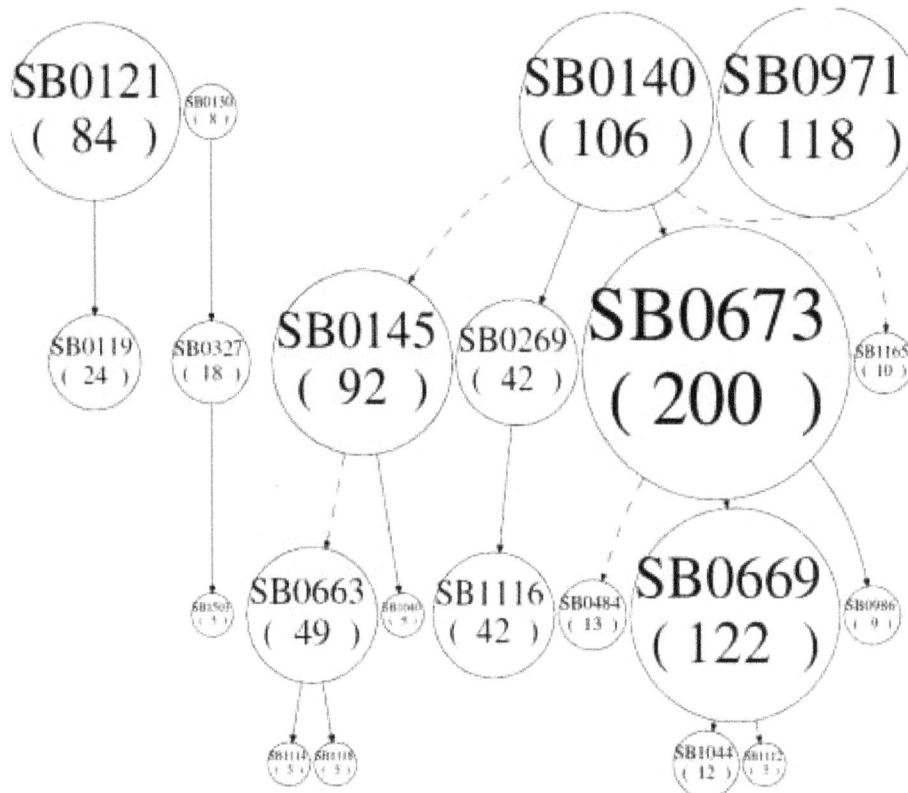

Figure 3. Spoligoforest of *M. bovis* spoligotypes obtained from States other than Jalisco in Mexico. Nodes are labeled with the SB identifier as indicated in *mbovis.org*; numbers in parenthesis indicate cluster size. Lines between nodes reflect hypothetical evolutionary relationships among spoligotypes with arrows denoting descendence. Continuous lines indicate stronger relationship.
Source: http://spoltools.emi.unsw.edu.au/

weakness of this study. This suggests that more knowledge on epidemiological methodologies, especially databases maintenance by bodies responsible for animal health care in Mexico, is required.

Conclusions

The most frequent spoligotypes of *M. bovis* found in Jalisco are also the most frequent ones in other parts of Mexico. However, there is no evidence to conclude that Jalisco is the source of infection since no information on movement and destination of animals could be documented. It is believed that similarity of spoligotypes around the country is in fact due to the indiscriminate movement of animals. The long history of bTB in Mexican herds, which favors the increase and dissemination of new and existing *M. bovis* strains in the population could be another reason.

CONFLICT OF INTERESTS

The authors have not declared any conflict of interests.

ACKNOWLEDGEMENTS

The authors thank the slaughter houses owners in the State of Jalisco, and MVZ Erick Fernando Rodríguez Durán for his support in samples collection.

REFERENCES

Acosta-Salinas R, Estrada-Chávez C, Milián-Suazo F (2009). Tipificación de cepas de *Mycobacterium bovis*. Revista Técnica Pecuaria en México 47(4):389-412.

Barandiaran S, Vivot MM, Moras EV, Meike V, Cataldi A, Zumárraga MJ (2011). *Mycobacterium bovis* in swine: Spoligotyping of isolates from Argentina. Vet. Med. Int. 2011:979647.

Bawinek F, Taylor NM (2014). Assessment of bovine tuberculosis and its risk factors in cattle and humans, at and around Dilla Town, Southern Ethiopia. Anim. Vet. Sci. 2(4):94-100.

Blischak JD, Tailleux L, Mitrano A, Barreiro LB, Gilad Y (2015). Mycobacterial infection induces a specific human innate immune response. Sci. Rep. 5:16882.

Bobadilla-del Valle M, Torres-González P, Cervera-Hernández ME, Martínez-Gamboa A, Crabtree-Ramírez B, Chávez-Mazari B (2015). Trends of *Mycobacterium bovis* isolation and first-line anti-tuberculosis drug susceptibility profile: A fifteen-year laboratory-based surveillance. PLOS Neglected Trop. Dis. 9(9):e0004124.

Boddinghaus B, Rogall T, Flohr T, Blocker H, Bottger EC (1990). Detection and identification of Mycobacteria by amplification of rRNA.

J. Clin. Microbiol. 28(8):1751-1759.

Brosch R, Gordon SV, Marmiesse M, Brodin P, Buchrieser C, Eiglmeier K, Garnier T, Gutierrez C, Hewinson G, Kremer K, Parsons LM, Pym AS, Samper s, van Soolingen D, Cole ST (2002). A new evolutionary scenario for Mycobacterium tuberculosis complex. Proceedings of the National Academy of Sciences of the United States of America 99(6):3684-3689.

Cobos-Marín L, Montes-Vargas J, Zumárraga M, Cataldi A, Romano MI, Estrada-García I, Gonzalez-Merchand JA (2005). Spoligotype analysis of Mycobacterium bovis isolates from Northern Mexico. Can. J. Microbiol. 51(11):996-1000.

de Almeida IN, Da Silva-Carvalho W, Rossetti ML, Costa ER, de Miranda SS (2013). Evaluation of six different DNA extraction methods for detection of Mycobacterium tuberculosis by means of PCR-IS6116: Preliminary Study BMC Research Notes 6:561.

de la Rua-Domenech R, Goodchild AT, Vordermeier M, Hewinson RG, Christiansen KH, Clifton-Hadley RS (2006). Ante mortem diagnosis of tuberculosis in cattle: A review of the tuberculin test, c-interferon assay and other ancillary diagnosis techniques. Res. Vet. Sci. J. Sci. 81(2):190-210.

Duarte EL, Domingos M, Amado A, Cunha MV, Botello A (2010). MIRU-VNTR typing discrimination value to groups of Mycobacterium bovis and Mycobacterium caprae strains defined by Spoligotyping. Vet. Microbiol. J. 143(2-3):299-306.

El-Sayed A, El-Shannat S, Kamel M, Castañeda-Vázquez MA, Castañeda-Vázquez H (2016). Molecular epidemiology of Mycobacterium bovis in humans and cattle. Zoonoses Public Health 63:251-264.

Gibson AL, Hewinson G, Goodchild T, Watt B, Story A, Inwald J (2004). Molecular epidemiology of disease due to Mycobacterium bovis in humans in the United Kingdom. J. Clin. Microbiol. 42(1):431-4.

Gutiérrez MC, Brisse S, Brosch R, Fabre M, Omais B, Marmiesse M, Supply P, Vincent V (2005). Ancient origin and gene mosaicism of the progenitor of Mycobacterium tuberculosis. PLoS Pathogens 1(1):0055-0061.

Jagielski T, van Ingen J, Rastogi N, Dziadek J, Mazur PK, Bielecki J (2014). Current methods in the molecular typing of Mycobacterium tuberculosis and other Mycobacteria. BioMed. Res. Int. 2014: 645802.

Kamerbeek J, Shouls L, Kolk A, van Agterveld M, van Soolingen D, Kujiper S, Bunschoten A, Molhuizen H, Shaw R, Goyal M, van Embden J (1997). Simultaneous detection and strain differentiation of Mycobacterium tuberculosis for diagnosis and epidemiology. J. Clin. Microbiol. 35(4):907-914.

Kim N, Jang y, Kyoung Kim J, Ryoo S, Hee Kwon K, Kim M, Seok Kang S, Seop H, Soo Lee H, Lim Y, Kim J (2017). Molecular and genomic features of Mycobacterium bovis strain 1595 isolated from Korean cattle. J. Vet. Sci. 18(S1):333-341.

Luciani F, Francis AR, Tanaka MM (2008). Interpreting genotype cluster sizes of Mycobacterium tuberculosis isolates typed with IS6110 and Spoligotyping. Infect. Genet. Evol. 8(2):182-190.

Maslow JN, Mullingan ME (1993). Molecular epidemiology: application of contemporary techniques to the typing of microorganisms. Clin. Infect. Dis. 17(2):153-164.

McLernon J, Costello E, Flyn O, Madigan G, Ryan F (2010). An evaluation of MIRU-VNTR analysis and spoligotyping for genotyping of Mycobacterium bovis isolates and a comparison with RFLP typing. J. Clin. Microbiol. 48:4551-4545.

Milián-Suazo F, García-Casanova L, Robbe-Austerman S, Canto-Alarcón GJ, Bárcenas-Reyes I, Stuber T, Rodríguez-Hernández E, Flores-Villalva S (2016). Molecular relationship between strains of Mycobacterium bovis from Mexico and those from countries with free trade of cattle with Mexico. PloS one 11(5):e0155207.

Müller B, Dürr S, Alonso S, Hattendorf J, Laisse CJ, Parsons SD (2013). Zoonotic Mycobacterium bovis –induces tuberculosis in humans. Emerg. Infect. Dis. 19(6):899-908.

Mwakapuja RS, Makondo ZE, Malakalinga J, Moser I, Kazwala RR, Tanner M (2013). Molecular characterization of Mycobacterium bovis isolates from pastoral livestock at Mikumi-Selous ecosystem in the eastern Tanzania. Tuberculosis 93(6):668-674.

Norma Oficial Mexicana (NOM-031-ZOO-1995) Campaña Nacional contra la Tuberculosis Bovina (Mycobacterium bovis) bovis).

O'Reilly LM, Daborn CJ (1995). The epidemiology of Mycobacterium bovis infections in animals and man: a review. Tuberc. Lung Dis. J. 76(1):1-46.

Olea-Popelka F, Muwonge A, Perera A, Dean AS, Mumford E, Erlacher-Vindel E (2017). Zoonotic tuberculosis in human beings caused by Mycobacterium bovis – a call for action. Lancet Infect. Dis. 17:e21-e25.

Parra A, Larrasa J, García A, Alonso JM, de Mendoza JH (2005). Molecular epidemiology of bovine tuberculosis in wild animals in Spain: a first approach to risk factor analysis. Vet. Microbiol. J. 110(3-4):293-300.

Perea-Razo CA, Milián-Suazo F, Bárcenas-Reyes I, Sosa-Gallegos S, Rodríguez-Hernández E, Flores-Villalba S, Canto-Alarcón GJ (2017). Whole genome sequencing for detection of zoonotic tuberculosis in Querétaro, Mexico. J. Infect. Dis. Prev. Med. 5:158.

Pérez-Guerrero L, Milián-Suazo F, Arriaga-Díaz C, Romero-Torres C, Escartín-Chávez M (2008). Epidemiología molecular de las tuberculosis bovina y humana en una zona endémica de Querétaro, México. Salud Pública de México 50(4):286-291.

Plan Estratégico de la Campaña Nacional de la Tuberculosis Bovina en México, 2008-2012. Dirección general de Salud Animal. Campaña Nacional Contra la Tuberculosis Bovina. Available at: http://www.senasica.gob.mx/?id=801.

Reyes JF, Francis AR, Tanaka MM (2008). Models of deletion for visualizing bacterial variation: an application to tuberculosis spoligotypes. BMC Bioinformatics 9(1):496.

Rodríguez S, Romero B, Bezos J, de Juan L, Álvarez J, Castellanos E, Moya N, Lozano F, González S (2010). High spoligotype diversity within a Mycobacterium bovis population: clues to understanding the demography of the pathogen in Europe. Vet. Microbiol. J. 141(1-2):89-95.

Rodríguez-Campos S, Aranaz A, de Juan L, Sáez-Llorente JL, Romero B, Bezos J, Jiménez A, Mateos A, Domínguez L (2011). Limitations of Spoligotyping and variable-number tandem-repeat typing for molecular tracing of Mycobacterium bovis in high diversity setting. J. Clin. Microbiol. 49(9):3361-3364.

Rodwell TC, Moore M, Moser KS, Brodine SK, Strathdee SA (2008).Tuberculosis from Mycobacterium bovis in binational communities, United States. Emerg. Infect. Dis. J. 14(6):909-916.

Ruettger A, Nieter j, Skrypnyk A, Engelmann I, Ziegler A, moser I, Monecke S, Ehricht R, Sachse K (2012). Rapid spoligoryping of Mycobacterium tuberculosis complex bacteria by use of a microarray system with automatic data processing and Assignment. J. Clin. Microbiol. 50(7):2492-2495.

Sandoval-Azuara S, Muñiz-Salazar R, Perea-Jacobo R, Robbe-Austerman S, Perera-Ortiz A, López-Valencia G, Bravo DM, Sánchez-Flores A (2017). Whole genome sequencing of Mycobacterium bovis to obtain molecular fingerprints in human and cattle isolates from Baja California, Mexico. Int. J. Infect. Dis. 63(2017):48-56.

Santillán-Flores MA, Flores J, Arriaga-Díaz C, Romero-Torres C, Suarez-Guemez F, Espitia C (2006). Polymorphism in the PE domain of PE/PE_PGRS sequences in clinical isolates of Mycobacterium bovis in Mexico. Vet. Microbiol. 115(4):364-369.

Skuce RA, Mallon TR, McCormick CM, McBride SH, Clarke G, Thompson A (2010). Mycobacterium bovis genotypes in Northern Ireland: herd-level surveillance (2003-2008). Vet. Rec. 1(1):112-112.

Smith NH, Dale J, Inwald J, Palmer S, Gordon SV, Hewinson RG, Smith JM (2003). The population structure of Mycobacterium bovis in Great Britain: clonal expansion. Proceed. Natl. Acad. Sci. 100(25):15271-15275.

Smith NH, Gordon SV, de la Rua-Domenech R, Clifton-Hadley RS, Hewinson RG (2006). Bottlenecks and broomsticks: the molecular evolution of Mycobacterium bovis. Nat. Rev. Microbiol. 4(9):670-681.

Sreevatsan S, Pan X, Stockbauer KE, Connel ND, Kreiswirth BN, Whittman TS, Musser JM (1997). Restricted structural gene polymorphism in the Mycobacterium tuberculosis complex indicates evolutionarily recent global dissemination. Proceed. Natl. Acad. Sci. 94:9869-9874.

Supply P, Warren RM, Banuls AL, Lesjean S, Van Der Spuy GD, Lewis LA, Tibayrenc M, Van Helden PD, Locht C (2006). Linkage disequilibrium between minisatelite loci support clonal evolution of

Mycobacterium tuberculosis in a high tuberculosis incidence area. Mol. Microbiol. 47(2):529-538.

Tanaka MM, Francis AR (2005). Methods for quantifying and visualizing outbreaks of tuberculosis using genotypic information. Infect. Genet. Evol. 5:35-43.

Zhou A, Nawaz M, Xue X, Karakousis PC, Yao Y, Xu j (2011).

Molecular genotyping of *Mycobacterium tuberculosis* in Xi´an, china, using MIRU-VNTR typing. Int. J. Tuberc. Lung Dis. 15(4):517-22.

Zumárraga MJ, Vivot MM, Marticorena D, Bernardelli A, Fasán R, Lachini R, Cataldi AA (2009). *Mycobacterium bovis* in Argentina: isolates from cats typified by spoligotyping. Revista Argentina de Microbiología 41(4):215-217.

8

Prevalence of gastrointestinal parasites in dry season on dairy cattle at Holeta Agricultural Research Center Dairy Farm, Ethiopia

Temesgen Kassa Getahun*, Tamirat Siyoum, Aster Yohannes and Melese Eshete

Ethiopian institute of Agricultural research, Holeta Agricultural Research Center, P. O. Box 31, Holeta, Ethiopia.

A cross sectional study was carried out in Holeta Agricultural Research Center Dairy Farm, Oromia Regional State, Ethiopia to determine the status of gastrointestinal (GI) parasites on dairy cattle, reveal the level of severity of GI parasites on the basis of mean egg per gram of faces (epg) count through McMaster technique and identify the different gastrointestinal parasites dominated by flotation and sedimentation techniques. A total of 206 faecal samples were collected from purposively selected cows, bulls and heifers. The overall prevalence of GI parasites was found to be 87.9%. The average epg was found to be 179.8, indicating light level of parasite infection. The sex-wise prevalence revealed 85.0 and 15.0% in female and male animals, respectively. The qualitative faecal examination techniques, showed a prevalence of coccidia (56.3%), *Fasciola* spp. (26.2%), *Paramphistomum* spp. (10.2%), *Bunostomum* spp. (8.7%), *Oesophagostomum* spp. (8.3%), and *Tricuris* spp. (1.5%). With statistically significant difference ($p < 0.05$), the prevalence was higher in milking cow (28.72%) than the rest of the animal categories and the lowest prevalence was observed on dry cow (12.15%). There was concurrent infection with two and more than two different GIT parasites with respective prevalence of 38.3 and 25.2%. The finding of the present study clearly suggests that GI parasites were higher in the farm with low severity, which contributes reduction in productivity. Hence, further and strengthened parasite control intervention is highly recommended taking into account the seasonality of parasite burden.

Key words: Animal category, breeds, epg, faeces, GI parasites, prevalence, Holeta

INTRODUCTION

Ethiopia, located in Eastern Africa, is predominantly an agricultural nation. Animal production is practiced in all ecological zones of the country (Tegegne and Crawford, 2000). The total animal population for the country is estimated to be about 53.99 million cattle out of which,

about 98.95% of the total cattle in the country are local breeds while the remaining are hybrid and exotic breeds that accounted for about 0.94 and 0.11%, respectively (Central Statistical Agency (CSA), 2008).

Ethiopia's great livestock potential is not properly

*Corresponding author. E-mail: temesgen.kassa@yahoo.com.

exploited due to many prevailing socio economic values and attitudes, traditional management methods, limited genetic potential and rampant disease (Etana, 2002). Parasitic infections are the major constraints for poor performance that causes great economic loss to dairy industry through retarded growth, low productivity and increased susceptibility of animals to other infections (Yadav et al., 2004).

The most important helminthes parasites in cattle include nematodes, trematodes and cestodes in which their impact is greater in small and large-scale farms of sub-Saharan Africa in general and Ethiopia in particular, due to the availability of wide range of agro-ecological factors suitable for diversified hosts and parasite species (Hailemariam, 2006).

In Holeta Agricultural Research dairy farm the exotic, cross and local dairy cows and calves are managed under semi-intensive rearing system. The prevalence, species composition and epidemiology of gastrointestinal (GI) parasites affecting dairy animals have not been investigated in detail in recent time. Hence, the objectives of this study were to determine the status of dry season GI parasites on dairy cattle of Holeta Agricultural Research Center dairy farm. Besides, the level of infection based on the mean epg count and the relationship between measurable parameters and GI parasites were assessed.

MATERIALS AND METHODS

Study area

The present study was conducted in Holeta Agricultural Research Center dairy farm; in west Shoa Zone Wolmera District Oromia Regional State, Ethiopia. Wolmera is a district dominated by highland temperature. Holetais is an administrative town of Wolmera district in central Ethiopia, located in West Shoa zone surrounding Finfinne of the Oromia Region. It has latitude and longitude of 9°3′N 38°30′E and an altitude of 2391 m above sea level. The host town of the study area is Holeta Agricultural Research Center dairy farm of the Ethiopian Institute of Agricultural Research.

Study animal

The study was conducted on 206 (31 male and 175 female) Holstein Friesian cows, bulls and heifers maintained under intensive and semi-intensive management production system. Different age and sex groups were represented as much as possible. Selection was conducted irrespective of age and sex based on body condition. Their body conditions which score less than 1.5 were selected purposively.

Study design

A cross sectional study design was conducted in dry season from December to February 2015 to identify, assess and estimate the prevalence of GI parasites.

Sample size determination and sampling methodology

Sample size was calculated with an expected prevalence of 50%. The desired sample size for the study was calculated using the formula given by Thrusfield (2005) with 95% confidence interval and 5% absolute precision.

$$n = \frac{1.96^2 \times Pexp\,(1- Pexp)}{d^2}$$

Where;
Pexp = expected prevalence,
d = absolute precision;
n = sample size.
206 animals were selected purposively from respective barns of the farm.

Sample collection and examination

Faecal sample collection

Faecal samples were collected per-rectum using plastic rectal gloves. Each sample was labeled with the animal number, date of collection, age, and sex in edible pen. The collected samples were kept in icebox with the lid tightly placed, and were transported to laboratory. Except on occasions where immediate processing was not possible, samples will be kept in four refrigerators and processed within 12 h.

Faecal sample examination

Faecal examination was done by different qualitative and quantitative examination technique for the presence of parasitic eggs and their level (Gupta and Singla, 2012).

Qualitative faecal examination was carried out by sedimentation and floatation technique. The floatation fluid used in this study was saturated solution of sodium chloride (Nacl) prepared in the laboratory. The procedure given by Urquhart et al. (1996) was monitored using the above parasitological methods.

Quantitative faecal examination was also conducted using McMaster egg counting technique. Severity of infection as obtained from the number of epg was determined as follows: ≤5000 epg is regarded as mild infection; 5000 to 10000 epg as moderate infection; and >10000 epg as severe infection (Jorden, 1994).

Data analysis

The entire data were entered into Microsoft Excel spread sheet and coded. Statistical analyses were performed using SPSS version 20 software packages. Percentage was used to calculate prevalence while Chi-square was used to calculate the degree of association between risk factors and prevalence of gastrointestinal parasites. In the analysis, a difference was taken as significant at p-value <0.05 and confidence level at 95%.

RESULTS

The result revealed an overall prevalence of 87.9%. The parasites encountered included *Fasciola* spp (26.2%), *Paramphistomum* spp (10.2%), coccidia (56.3%), *Bunostomum* spp (8.7%), *Oesophagostomum* spp (8.3%)

Table 1. Overall prevalence of gastrointestinal parasites.

Parasites	Number positive	%
Fasciola spp.	54	26.2
Paramphistomum spp.	21	10.2
Coccidia	116	56.3
Bunostomum spp.	18	8.7
Oesophagostomum spp.	17	8.3
Tricuris spp.	3	1.5
Mixed of more than two parasites	52	25.2
Mixed of two parasites	79	38.3
Total	**181**	**87.9**

Table 2. Prevalence of gastrointestinal parasites by sex.

Sex	Frequency	%	X^2-value	P-value
Female	153	85.0	0.150	0.698
Male	29	15.0		

Table 3. Prevalence of gastrointestinal parasites between animal categories.

Animal category	Number positive	%	X^2-value	P-value
Bull	27	14.9		
Dry Cow	22	12.15		
Heifer	33	18.23	46.702	0.000
Milking Cow	52	28.72		
Pregnant	47	25.96		

Table 4. Mean epg of GI parasites.

Parasite species	Average EPG and degree severity		
	Mild (<5000epg)	Moderate(5000-10,000)	Severe (>10,000)
Fasciola spp.	219	-	-
Coccidian	207	-	-
Paramphistomum spp.	205	-	-
Oesophagostomum spp.	240	-	-
Bunostomum spp.	176	-	-
Trichuris spp.	207	-	-
Mean epg.		179.8	

and *Tricuris* spp (1.5%) (Table 1). Mixed infections with two parasites were also more common (38.3%) than infections with more than two parasites (25.2%) (Table 1).

Out of examined female and male, 29 (15%) and 153 (85 %) were found to be positive, respectively. Accordingly, the prevalence of GI parasites in female was higher than male with no significant variation (p>0.05) (Table 2). Of all the positive animals, (14.9%) were bull, (12.15%) were dry cow, (18.23%) were heifer, (28.72%)

were milking cow and (25.96%) were dry cow. Accordingly, the highest prevalence was recorded in pregnant category. There were highly significant difference between animal categories on infection with GI parasites (p<0.05) (Table 3).

The McMaster technique revealed an average epg value of 179.8. Similarly, the study showed that the mean epg of *Oesophagostomum* spp. is greater than the other GI parasites (Table 4). Animal category has a potential risk factors, which are associated with gastrointestinal

Table 5. Prevalence of gastrointestinal parasites against different age categories.

Animal category	Fasciola spp. No. positive (%)	Paramphistomum spp. No. positive (%)	Coccidia No. positive (%)	Oesophagostomum spp. No. positive (%)	Bunostomum spp. No. positive (%)	Trichuris spp. No. positive (%)	X^2-value	P-value
Bull	0	0	15 (12.9)	0	4 (22.2)	2 (66.7)	46.702	0.000
Dry cow	11 (20.4)	0	7 (6)	1 (5.9)	0	0		
Heifer	7 (13)	0	26 (22.4)	3 (17.6)	1 (11.1)	0		
Milking cow	36 (66.7)	2 (9.5)	35 (30.3)	6 (3.5)	8 (44.4)	0		
Pregnant	0	19 (90.5)	33 (28.4)	7 (4.1)	4 (22.2)	1 (33.3)		

parasites at the dairy farms. The highly prevalent parasite among different categories with an individual prevalence rate was *Fasciola* spp. 66.7%, coccidia 30.3%, and *Bunostomum* spp. 44.4% in milking cow, *Paramphistomum* spp. 90.5% in pregnant cow, *Oesophagostomum* spp. 17.6% in heifers, and *Trichuris* spp. 66.7 in bull (Table 5).

DISCUSSION

The overall prevalence of gastrointestinal parasites in the present study was 87.9%. This finding is higher than 41.2% prevalence by Epherem (2007) and 26.3% by Darsema (2009) in Western Amhara region, Ethiopia. In addition, Keyyu et al. (2006) reported an overall prevalence of 44.4 and 37.0% for large and small scale dairy cattle, respectively in Tanzania.

This higher prevalence in the study area could be due to the fact that cattle from farmers surrounding farm have frequent exposure to the same communal grazing land that causes contamination of pasture, most favorable environmental condition for the development of larvae, variation in management and husbandry practices, climate, and management of pastures. In this study, lower prevalence of *Fasciola* spp.

(26.2%) was obtained when compared with 34% prevalence reported by Tesfa (1994) in Gojjam with 61.97% prevalence. This difference may be due to variation in management system, absence of swampy area, effect of deworming and variation in the study period.

The overall prevalence of coccidia in this study was 56.3%, which is higher than previous findings of 31.9% reported by Alemayehu et al., (2013) in Kombolcha. This variation is most likely attributed to the differences in agro-ecology and husbandry practices of the study animals and the resistance level of animal increase as age increase.

The prevalence of *Paramphistomum* spp found in the present study (10.2%) was lower than the finding by Fromsa et al (2011) in Jimma (45.2%), which reported 6.7% in dairy farm in Hawassa town. Many studies conducted in different parts of the world reported prevalence of 22% in Pakistan by Raza et al. (2009). This lower prevalence may be due to agro ecological factors and management system.

In the current study, the prevalence of *Oesophagostomum* spp. was found to be 8.3% which is lower than (11%) as reported by Hiko and Wondimu (2011) in Haramaya University Dairy Farm. This difference could be due to, difference in deworming habit and higher susceptibility of exotic cattle in cross and local breeds. The lower

prevalence of *Bunostomum* spp. (8.7%) and *Trichuris* (1.5%) in farm was due to the effect of deworming practice, which is given as three times per year and also, the study season in which most gastrointestinal parasites can't resist dry environment.

The study shows that gastrointestinal parasite in the study area is higher in female (85%) than male (15%). As reported by Ram (2009), the difference in parasite prevalence between sexes was due to the fact that,females are found to have higher infection rates due to their low immunity in gestation and lactation period. The co-infection pattern observed in this study showed that, dairy animals have a high chance of related exposure of different GI parasites.

In relation with animal category, the occurrence of GI parasites has a significant difference which is relatively lower in dry cow (12.15%) and higher in milking cow (28.75%), with a respective highly prevalent parasite species of *Ascaris* spp. (13.8%) and *Fasciola* spp. (66.7%). Such finding may be due to the fact that, in milking cow the immune response of the host to gastrointestinal nematodes is partially suppressed, leading to an increase in the population of the worms.

According to the McMaster quantitative result, the mean epg of the overall gastrointestinal parasite encounter during the study period was 179.8 while the minimum and maximum epg scored was 176 for *Bunostomum* spp. and 240 for *Oesophagostomum* spp. Jorgen (1994) reported that, the epg level of the present study has a mild infection. This finding might be due to the effect of the seasonal deworming in the farm.

CONCLUSION AND RECOMMENDATIONS

The overall prevalence of gastrointestinal parasite in the study area indicated that, gastrointestinal helminthosis was found to be an important health problem due to its high prevalence and occurrence of polyparasitism. The majority of cattle were infected by more than one parasite type with some animals showing pure infection. Therefore, the farm is prone to health problems related to gastrointestinal helminthosis which might subsequently reduce the economic output from cattle production.

Most of the animals examined during the present study relatively harbor low to moderate parasite eggs. In view of these conclusions, the following recommendations are forwarded;

1) Strategic parasitic control programs should be designed.
2) The role of veterinarians in giving professional advices regarding preventive and control measures against gastrointestinal helminthes should be prominent to prevent any abuses.
3) To improve the management and feeding condition of those cattle residing in the farm.

Further study on epidemiology and determinant factors for, the occurrence of helminthes parasites and implementation of appropriate control and prevention methods in GI parasites, identified the cause economic losses and diseases of animals in this study.

CONFLICT OF INTERESTS

The authors have not declared any conflict of interests.

9

Status of mange infestation in indigenous sheep and goats and their control practices in Wag-Himra zone, Ethiopia

Adane Agegnehu, Basaznew Bogale*, Shimelis Tesfaye and Shimelis Dagnachew

College of Veterinary Medicine and Animal Sciences, University of Gondar, Gondar, P. O. Box 196 Ethiopia.

A cross sectional study was conducted from December 2016 to April 2017 to estimate the status of mange infestation in indigenous sheep and goats and identify the major species of mites and potential risk factors in selected districts with different agro-ecological zones of Wag-Himra zone. In addition, a questionnaire survey was conducted to assess the awareness and control practices of livestock owners on mange mite's infestation. From a total of 384 small ruminants (120 sheep and 264 goats), 105 (27.33%) were positive for mange mites infestation on skin scraping examination. *Sarcoptes scabiei* was the only mange mites species identified with a prevalence of 33.3% (n=40) in sheep and 24.6% (n=65) in goats. Host factors such as species, sex, age and body condition were not found as a risk factor of *S. scabiei* infestation in the current study. However, there was a statistical significant (P<0.031) difference in prevalence of *S. scabiei* infestation in small ruminants between the three agro-ecological zones. The pathological lesions (crusts formation and loss of hair) caused by *S. scabiei* were observed on the face, head, ear and tail regions. The result of the questionnaire survey indicated that mange was considered as an important disease by small ruminant holders. From the interviewed livestock owners, 86.27% respondents explained that they use modern acaricides for the treatment of mange. The results of this study indicates that the agro-ecology had effect on the prevalence of *S. scabiei* in sheep and goats in the study area.

Key words: Cross sectional, ectoparasites infestation, small ruminants.

INTRODUCTION

Goats and sheep represent important sources of protein in the world, supplying a good percentage of the daily meat and milk products in urban and rural areas. Small ruminants are important contributors to the economy of Ethiopia (CSA, 2013). They are also important contributors to food production; providing 25% of meat and 14% of milk for domestic consumption (Metaferia et al., 2011). In addition, manure from these animals is very important as source of organic fertilizer from any farming populations in the country. Reports have indicated that

*Corresponding author. E-mail: basaznew2008@yahoo.com.

skin utilization is estimated to be 75% for goat and 97% sheep skin, with expected off-take rate of 33 and 35% for sheep and goat, respectively (Tadesse and Mebrahitu, 2010; Zeryehun and Tadesse, 2012). However, raw skin production from sheep and goats in Ethiopia has faced serious challenges as a result of skin diseases caused by external parasites (Bisrat, 2013). Ectoparasites such as mites, ticks, lice and fleas affect large numbers of sheep and goats in Ethiopia causing a wide range of health problems including mechanical tissue damage, and predispose to myiasis and dermatophilosis. Infestations increase susceptibility to other diseases and create sites for secondary invasion by pathogenic organisms and reduced productivity (Mersha et al., 2010). They have the ability to parasitize wide range of hosts (Sumbria et al., 2016). Though mites are active in keratin layer and causes direct damage to skin, also cause indirect economic loss by decreasing/ceasing reproduction and production performance (Soulsby, 1982).

Mange has been reported as one of the most prevalent and widely distributed skin disease in Ethiopia by degrading skin quality (Yacob, 2013). In Amhara Region mange has been the great threat for the production of small ruminants (Demissie et al., 2000). Despite national and regional efforts and emphasis given to the control programs against parasitic skin diseases, reports have shown that the problem seems to be still alarming (Seid et al., 2014; Yacob, 2014; Bedada et al., 2015).

This study was conducted to isolate and identify mange species and estimate their prevalence and assess their control practices by small ruminant owners in different agro-climatic conditions in the study area.

MATERIALS AND METHODS

Description of study area

This study was carried out in three selected districts (Gazgibla, Sekota and Ziquala) of Wag-Himra administrative zone, Amhara Regional State from November 2016 to April 2017. The districts represent three agro-ecological conditions; highland, midland and lowland, respectively. WagHimra zone is located between 12°C 23' and 13°C 16' north longitudes and 38°C 44' and 39°C 21' east latitudes, in the eastern part of the country. The annual rainfall, which is erratic in distribution, varies between 350 and 650 mm (CSA, 2013).

Study animals

The animals were indigenous breeds of sheep and goats kept in small flocks and managed under extensive farming system in different agro-climates. The sampled sheep and goats were stratified by sex, age and body condition. Animals aged up to one year were classified as young stock while those above two years were categorized as adults (Gatenby, 1991; Steele, 1996).

Study design and sample size determination

A cross-sectional study design was used. Semi-structured questionnaires were used to gather information on the level of awareness of sheep and goat owners about mange and its control practices. Purposive sampling techniques were used to select study districts based on their agro-ecology. In each study site, the farmers were randomly selected from a list prepared from the previous extension activities by the veterinary office. The sample size for the study was determined as described by Thrusfield (2005). Descriptive statistics (percentage, frequency distribution and correlation analysis) were used to determine the prevalence and associated risk factors.

Sample collection and examination

Skin scrapings were collected only from sheep and goats suspected for having clinical sign of mange encountered during field visits. Both superficial and deep skin scrapings were made to diagnose both burrowing and non-burrowing mites.

This was made by clipping the hair around affected areas with scissors, scraping the edges of the lesion with the scalpel blades until capillary blood was evident. The samples were collected in sterile plastic bottles containing 70% alcohol and taken to the parasitology laboratory of College of Veterinary Medicine and Animal Sciences, University of Gondar for proceeding diagnosis. Multiple sites were scrapped to increase the likelihood of mange mites' detection. The scraped material was then treated with 10% KOH solution in the test tubes and centrifuged at 1500 rpm for 5 min (Gupta and Singla 2012). The supernatant was discarded and the sediment was examined under a compound microscope using X10 and X40 magnification. Morpho-anatomical diagnosis keys provided by Soulsby (1982) and Pangui (1994) were used to identify the scabies agents.

Questionnaire survey

Semi-structured questionnaire format were prepared and used to collect information about the general attitude of the individual sheep and goat owners and to assess preventive and control practices against mange and evaluate risk factors on the occurrence of the disease. A total of 153 sheep and goat owners were selected. The information was collected by interviewing randomly selectedsheep and goats owners. The important points included in questionnaire survey were purpose of keeping animals, species of animals (sheep, goats) affected by mange, affected age group (young, adults), seasonality of the disease (wet, dry), effect of the disease on live animals and skin sale and control practices (modern, traditional).

Statistical analysis

Raw data was carefully recorded and stored in Microsoft Excel database system used for data management. Data were analysed using the SPSS for windows, version17.0.Descriptive statistics, percentages and 95% confidence intervals were used to summarize the proportion of infested and non-infested animals. The effects of different environmental and host risk factors were analyzed by using logistic regression and Chi-square test. Statistical significance was set at $p \leq 0.05$.

RESULTS

Questionnaire survey

The result of the questionnaire survey indicated that all

Table 1. Questionnaire survey results.

Focal point	Frequency (n)	Response (%)
Purpose of farming		
For income generation	128	83.66
For home meat and milk consumption	25	16.33
Affected species		
Goat	130	84.9
Sheep	23	15.03
Age group of animals affected		
Adult	123	80.39
Young	30	19.6
Seasonality of mange mites		
Dry season	131	85.62
Wet season	22	14.37
Effects of mange on sale		
Live animal	109	71.2
Skin	44	28.75
External parasite causing skin disease		
Mange mites	136	88.88
Lice	17	11.11
Way of treatment		
Modern	132	86.27
Traditional	21	13.72
Participation of farmers in the control practice		
Yes	149	97.38
No	4	2.61

respondents (153, 100%), practice keeping sheep and goats in the study area. The farmers in those study area keep their animals with the objectives of income generation (85.66%) and home meat and milk consumption (16.33%).

From interviewed respondents, 71.2% replied that mange mite infection had great enforcements to sale their live animals and skins. Concerning the treatment of mange mites, 86.27% of the respondents indicated that mange is more commonly treated using modern acaricides while 13.72% use traditional treatments (ethno-medicines) as well (Table 1).

In addition, 88.8% respondents explained that among external parasites, mange mites and lice infestation are the dominant ones that cause skin diseases and goats are highly affected (84.9%) than sheep's (15.03) by mange mites. Concerning the age groups, 80.39% of the

respondents replied that adults are more affected than young animals. In relation to seasonal variation of mange occurrence, 85.62% of the respondents agreed that the infestation is highly aggravated during the dry or after the rainy season, whereas 14.3% of the respondents replied that mange is a problem during the wet season (Table 1).

Species and characteristics of lesion of mange

In the present study, the only isolated mange mite species affecting both sheep and goats was *S. scabiei*. In sheep and goats, *S. scabieia* affected only the non-woolly areas of the body and lesions were observed mostly around the head, face and ear areas and nodule formation was the characteristics of lesions (Figure 1, A, B, C). The lesions were characterized by loss of hair,

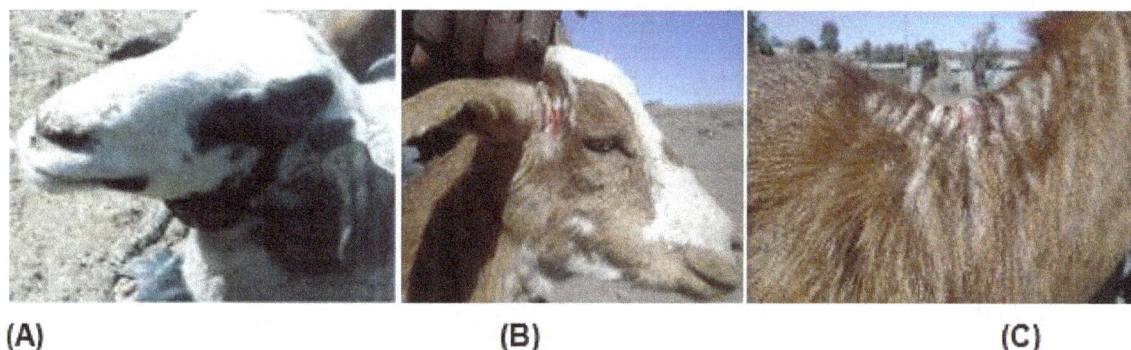

Figure 1. Sheep (A) and Goat (B, C) infested with sarcoptic mange.

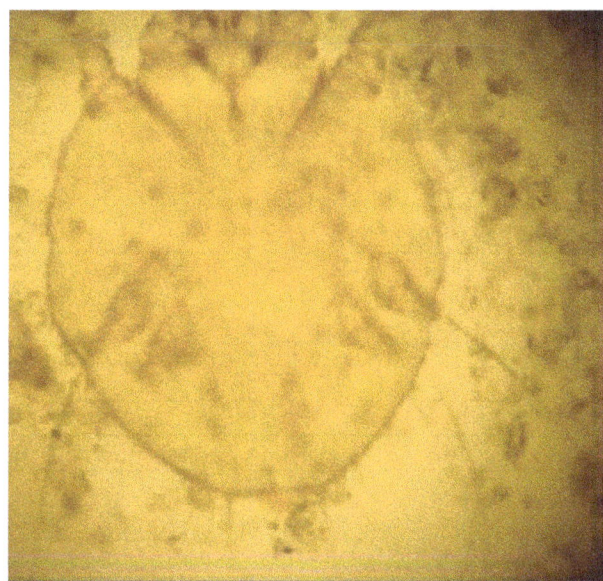

Figure 2. Ventral view of *Sarcoptes* mites.

ragged wool and crust formations and cracking and wrinkling of the skin.

Prevalence of *S. scabiei*

Out of 384 animals (120 sheep and 264 goats) examined, 105 (27. 33%) were found to be infested with *S. scabiei* (Figure 2). Of these, 65 (24.60%) were goats and 40 (33.33%) were sheep. The difference in the prevalence between the two host species was not statistically significant (X^2=3.1519, p=0.076 (Table 2).

In this study, both male and female sheep and goats were infested with *Sarcoptes* mange with an overall prevalence of female and male sheep as 32.55 and 35.29%, respectively while the prevalence in female and male goats was 22.39 and 30.55%, respectively without a statistical difference in prevalence between sex categories in both host species (Table 2).

The overall prevalence of *S.* scabiei in young and adult sheep was 34.28 and 32.94%, respectively (Table 3). The overall prevalence of *Sarcoptes* mite in young and adult goats was 30.43 and 22.5%, respectively. However, there was no statistically significant deference (p>0.05) between the prevalence of age groups in both host species (Table 2).

An overall prevalence of 32.5 and 33.75% *Sarcoptes* mites infestation in sheep and 28.8% and 22.15% in goats was recorded in animals with good and poor body conditions, respectively without any statistical significant difference (p > 0.05) (Table 2).

The prevalence of *S. scabiei* in highland, midland and

Table 2. Prevalence of *Sarcoptes* spp. in sheep and goat based on different risk factors.

Risk factor	Number examined	Prevalence (%)	95%CI	x^2(P-value)
Species				
Sheep	120	40(33.3)	0.24-0.41	
Goat	264	65(24.6)	0.19-0.29	3.1519(0.076)
Female	278	71(25.5)	0.20-0.30	
Male	106	34(32.0)	0.23-0.40	1.6501(0.199)
Age				
Adult	280	72(25.7)	0.20-0.30	
Young	104	33(31.7)	0.22-0.40	1.3817(0.240)
Body condition				
Poor	247	64(25.9)	0.20-0.31	
Good	137	41(29.9)	0.22-0.37	0.7154(0.398)
Agro-ecology				
Lowland	130	26(20)	0.13-0.26	
Midland	172	46(26.7)	0.20-0.33	
Highland	82	33(40.2)	0.29-0.50	10.4280(0.005)
Overall	384	105(27.33)		

Table 3. Prevalence of *Sarcoptes* spp. in sheep and goats in the three agro-ecological zones.

	Goat			Sheep			
	Lowland	Midland	Highland	Lowland	Midland	Highland	x^2(p-value)
	n=111	n=121	n=32	n=19	n=51	n=50	
Sarcoptes	22(19.8)	32(26.4)	11(34.4)	4(21.0)	22(44)		10.4288(0.005)

lowland was 44.0, 27.4 and 21.0% in sheep and 34.3, 26.4 and 19.8% in goats, respectively. The prevalence of *Sarcoptes* spp. in highland, midland and lowland was 44.0, 27.4 and 21.5 % in sheep and 34.3, 26.4 and 19.8 % in goats, respectively. The overall prevalence of *S. scabiei* infestation significantly varied (X^2=10.4288, P=0.005) among the three agroecological zones/ districts (Table 2).

Factors affecting the prevalence of *S. scabiei*

Univariable logistic regression analysis indicated that, agro-ecological variations were the only factors that showed a significant (p<0.031) association in the prevalence of *S. scabiei* infestation between the study populations. A significant association (p<0.031) between *S. scabie* infestation and agro-ecology was observed in which sheep and goats reared in highland areas were1.46 times at risk for sarcoptic mange than those

reared in midland and sheep and goats reared in midland were 0.547 times less likely to be affected than those reared in lowland.

DISCUSSION

In the present study, the only isolated mange mite species affecting both sheep and goats was *S. scabiei* with an overall prevalence of 27.33%. This species was also identified in different agro-ecological areas in Ethiopia (Mulugeta et al., 2010; Fekadu et al., 2013). This value was higher than the prevalence reported by Sertse and Wossene (2007) in Amhara Regional State, and by Beyecha et al. (2014) in central Oromia. The possible explanation for these differences in prevalence among different works could be variations in environmental and host factors, study seasons, control practices and management systems.

In this study, sex was not associated with prevalence of

S. scabiei which was in agreement with the work of Sheferaw et al. (2010) and Enquebaher and Etsay (2010). However, the prevalence was slightly higher in male than female goats in this study. This may be due to frequent contact of male goats at the time of mating and fighting.

The higher prevalence was observed in young animals than adult ones in the present study. This result agreed with the findings of Kasaye and Kebede (2010) and Shiferaw et al. (2010) who reported higher prevalence of *S. scabiei* in young animals than the old age group. It might be related to the degree of movement and frequent contacts of young animals with other flocks. Furthermore, age was reported to have no significant effect on the prevalence of mange mites (Yacob et al., 2008). Mange mite infestation is described to be independent of age and sex (Soulsby, 1982). Therefore, sex and age of the host animals are not contributing factors for the differences in the prevalence of mange in the study area.

In the current study, the highest level of prevalence was observed in animals with good body condition compared to the prevalence in poor body condition. This result disagreed with the findings of Sretse and Wossene (2007a) who reported that poor body conditioned goats were 4.3 times at risk for sarcoptic mange than good body conditioned goats with the explanation that poorly nourished animals appear to be less competent in getting rid of infestation as compared to that of well-managed animals (Sertse and Wossene, 2007).

In the present study, the highest prevalence of *S. scabiei* in goats was observed in highland (40.24%) area than midland (24.74) and lowland (20%) area. This finding disagreed with previous reports of Beyecha et al. (2014). This might be associated with difference in animal population which causes favorable condition for the transmission of mites between animals (Sertse and Wossene, 2007). Therefore, incidence of mange mite is higher in wet, cold areas which are optimum for reproduction, multiplication and mite development favoring its infestation (Olubumni et al., 1995*).

Agro-ecological variations was a factor that yielded significant (p<0.0.31) association to the prevalence of *S. scabiei* infestation among the study population. Goats found in highland areas were 1.46 times at risk of acquiring *S. scabiei* infestation than midland areas. This finding disagreed with those reports by Pangui (1994). The high prevalence of the *S. scabiei* in the highland may be associated with the ideal micro climate environment in these areas which favors the breeding and multiplication of mange mite eggs to their developmental stages (Pangui, 1994).

The result of the questionnaire survey indicated that all respondents (100%) keep sheep and goats in the study area. The farmers in those study area keep their animals with the objectives of income generation and home meat and milk consumption (85.66%). The majority of interviewed respondents (71.2%) replied that mange mite

infestation had great enforcements to sale their live sheep and goats and skins.

From the present study, it is possible to conclude that *Sarcoptesscabiei* is prevalent in sheep and goats in the study area which underlines the need of effective control measures.

CONFLICT OF INTERESTS

The authors have not declared any conflict of interests.

REFERENCES

http://academicjournals.org/articles/view/1009963198B edada H, Terefe G, Hailu Y (2015). Current status of ectoparasites in sheep and management practices against the problem in ectoparasites controlled and uncontrolled areas of Arsi Zone in Oromia Region, Ethiopia. J. Vet. Sci. Technol. S10:002.

Beyecha K, Kumsa B, Beyene D (2014). Beyecha, K., Kumsa, B., & Beyene, D. (2014). Ectoparasites of goats in three agroecologies in central Oromia, Ethiopia. Comp. Clin. Pathol. 23(1):21-28.

Bisrat G (2013). Defect Assessment of Ethiopian Hide and Skin: The Case of Tanneries in Addis Ababa and Modjo, Ethiopia. Glob. Vet. 11(4):395-398.

Central Statistical Agency (CSA) (2013). Agricultural sample survey Statistical bulletin 570, Addis Ababa.

Demissie A, Siraw B, Teferi K, Tsertse T, Mammo G, Mekonnen D, Shimelis S (2000). Mange: a disease of growing threat for the production of small ruminants in the Amhara National Regional State. In The Opportunities and Challenges of Enhancing Goat Production in East Africa. Proceedings of a conference held at Debub, University Awassa, Ethiopia. pp. 80-91.

Enquebaher K, Etsay K (2010). Epidemiological study on menge mite, lice and sheep keds of small ruminants in tigray region, northern Ethiopia. Ethiop. Vet. J. 14(2):51-65.

Fekadu A, Tolosso YH, Ashenafi H (2013). Ectoparasites of small ruminants in three Agro-ecological districts of southern Ethiopia. Afr. J. Basic Appl. Sci. 5(1):47-54.

Gatenby MR (1991). Sheep.12 In: The Tropical Agriculturalist, Coste, R. and J.A. Smith (Eds.). Macmillan and CTA (Waeningen), London, UK. pp. 6-11.

Gupta SK, Singla LD (2012). Diagnostic trends in parasitic diseases of animals. In: Veterinary Diagnostics: Current trends. Gupta RP, Garg SR, Nehra V and Lather D (Eds.), SatishSerial Publishing House, Delhi. pp. 81-112.

Kasaye E, Kebede E (2010). Epidemiological study on mange mite, lice and sheep keds of small suminants in Tigray Region, NorthernEthiopia. Ethiop. Vet. J. 14(2):51-65.

Mersha C, Tamiru N, Asegedech S (2010). Ectoparasites are the Major Causes of Various Types of Skin Lesions in small ruminants in Ethiopia. Trop. Anim. Health Prod. 42:1103-1109.

Metaferia F, Cherenet T, Gelan A, Abnet F, Tesfaye A, Ali JA, Gulilat W (2011). A review to improve estimation of the livestock's contribution to the national GDP.Ministry of Finance and Economic development and Ministry, Addis Abeba, Ethiopia.

Mulugeta Y, Yacob HT, Ashenafi H (2010).Ectoparasites of small ruminants in three selected agro-ecological sites of Tigray Region, Ethiopia. Trop. Anim. Health Prod. 42(6):1219-1224.

Olubumni PA (1995). The prevalence of caprine sarcoptic mange due to Sarcoptes scabiei var capri in Ile-Ife area of Nigeria, its control and management. Bull. Anim. Health Prod.Afr. 43(2):115-120.

Pangui LJ (1994). Mange of domestic animals and methods of control. Rev. Sci. Tech. Off. Intl. Epiz.13:1227-1243.

Seid K, Amare S, Tolossa YH (2016). Mange mites of sheep and goats in selected sites of Eastern Amhara region, Ethiopia. J. Parasite. Dis. 40(1):132-137.

Sertse T, Wossene A (2007). A study on ectoparasites of sheep and goats in eastern part of Amhara region, northeast Ethiopia. Small Ruminant Res. 69(1):62-67.

Sheferaw D, Degefu H, Banteyirgu D (2010) Epidemiological study of small ruminant mange mites in three agro-ecological zones of Wolaita, Southern Ethiopia. Ethiop. Vet. J. 14(1):31-38.

Sheferaw D, Degefu H, Banteyirgu D (2010). Epidemiological study of small ruminant mange mites in three agro-ecological zones of Wolaita, Southern Ethiopia. Ethiop. Vet. J. 14(1):31-38.

Soulsby EJL (1982). Helminthes, Arthropods and protozoa of domestic animals.7th edition. University of Cambridge. Baillie Tindal, London. pp. 321-324.

Steele MR (1996). Goats In: The Tropical Agriculturalist, Coste, R. and J.A. Smith (Eds.). Macmillan and CTA (Waeningen), London, UK. pp. 79-86.

Sumbria D, singla LD, Gupta SK (2016). Arthropod invaders pedestal threats to public vigor: An overview. Asian J. Anim. Vet. Adv. 11: 213-225.

Tadesse A, Mebrahitu K (2010). Study on ectoparasitic defects of processed skins at Sheba Tannery, Tigray, Northern Ethiopia. Trop. Anim. Health Prod. 42:1719-1722.

Thrusfield M (2005). Veterinary Epidemiology, Sampling in Veterinary Epidemiology.3rd edition. UK. Blackwell Science Ltd. pp. 182-198.

Yacob H, Yalew T, Dinka A (2008). Ectoparasite prevalence's in sheep and goats in and around Wolita Soddo, Southern Ethiopia. Rev. Med. Vet. 159:450-454.

Yacob HT (2013). Skin defects in small ruminates and their nature and economic importance: The case of Ethiopia. Glob. Vet. 11(5):107-112.

Yacob HT (2014). Ectoparasitism: Threat to Ethiopian small ruminant population and tanning industry. J. Vet. Med. Anim. Health 6(1):25-33.

Zeryehun T, Tadesse M (2012). Prevalence of mange mite on small Ruminants at Nekemte veterinary clinic, East wollega zone, North west Ethiopia. Middle–East J. Sci. Res. 11(10):1411-1416.

10

Performance, immunology and biochemical parameters of *Moringa oleifera* and/or *Cichorium intybus* addition to broiler chicken ration

M. A. Mousa[1*], A. S. Osman[2] and H. A. M. Abdel Hady[3]

[1]Nutrition and Clinical Nutrition Department, Faculty of Veterinary Medicine, Sohag University, Sohag, Egypt.
[2]Department of Biochemistry, Faculty of Veterinary Medicine, Sohag University, Sohag, Egypt.
[3]Bacteriology Department, Animal Health Research Institute, Egypt.

This study was aimed to evaluate the influence of *Moringa Oleifera* and/or *Cichorium Intybus* powder supplementation on performance, biochemical parameters, immunology and carcass quality of broiler chicks. Two hundred one-day-old chicks (Ross, 308 hybrid) were randomly allotted into four groups. Each group contained 50 chicks with five replicates. Feed was offered *ad libitum* to all groups. Group C were fed basal control diet. Chicks in the group M were fed basal diet supplemented with 1.5% *M. oleifera* and chicks in group CI were fed basal diet supplemented with 1.5% *C. Intybus*, while the chicks of group MC were fed basal diet supplemented with 0.75% *M. oleifera* plus 0.75% *C. Intybus* during experiment time. Body weight and feed amount were recorded every 15 days. Carcass yields were evaluated at the end of the experiment. The results revealed that supplements improved significantly bird weights, whereas the group C has the least mean value among the treatments. Group MC had better weight (239 3±80 g) than other groups (2180±48, 2020.5±97 1893±54 g, respectively for groups CI, M and C). Feed conversion ratio (FCR) was estimated 1.45, 1.48, 1.54 and 1.58 for MC, CI, M and C groups, respectively. Supplements group have lower total cholesterol than control. Finally, the use of a combination of *C. Intybus* and *M. oleifera* was recommended as good feed additives to improve productivity and enhance immunity.

Key words: Broiler, performance, *Moringa Oleifera*, *Cichorium Intybus*, biochemical parameters, immunology, carcass yields.

INTRODUCTION

Poultry health is affected by the surrounding environment. Infectious pathogens such as bacteria, viruses, parasites and fungi can easily infect poultry when its immune system is suppressed, which lead to different complicated infections (Paliwal et al., 2011a; Sandhu et al., 2009). In European Union, from January 2006, antibiotics use is prohibited to avoid antimicrobial- resistance in bacterial strains and antibiotics residues in human food (Catala-

*Corresponding author. E-mail: dr_m_mousa@yahoo.com.

Gregori et al., 2008); nowadays the herbal substitutes to enhance health status and performance is urgently needed (Panagasa et al., 2007; Singla and Gupta 2012). The immunity is challenged by environment and feed habits, with the concept that feed with natural antioxidants and micronutrients can boost the immune response (Paliwal et al., 2011a, b).

Herbs or extracted oils are safe to be fed to livestock with less risk than antibiotics which has harmful side effects and consider the most effective choice (Barrow, 1992), that is why, many types of plants are widely used in alternative medicine (Endo et al., 1999). The benefits of herbs raised the hope of using them instead of antibiotics (Panagasa et al., 2007). Herbs were recommended to enhance metabolic processes and the health condition of livestock (Panagasa et al., 2012). Some herbs can support the digestive enzymes action, improve feed intake, feed conversion ratio (FCR), carcass yields (Pietrzak et al., 2005), whereas, Halle et al. (2004) recorded no positive impact on broilers.

M. oleifera has beneficial anti-inflammatory and antioxidants properties (Yang et al., 2006). Dahot (1988) reported that *Moringa* contains vitamins (A, E, B2, B5, B6, folic acid) and minerals (Ca, Fe). *Moringa* has strong fungicidal and antimicrobial activity (Das et al., 1957). It also has an anti-blood cholesterol effect (Ghasi et al., 2000). Yang et al. (2006) mentioned that *M. oleifera* significantly enhanced immunity and decreased *Escherichia coli* and improved *Lactobacillus* counts in gastrointestinal tract (GIT) of broilers. So *Moringa* improves FCR and enhances immune response of birds. Also, its leaves has natural antioxidant compounds and soluble proteins (Sreelatha and Padma, 2009; Kakengi et al., 2007).

Cichorium intybus (cichory) is considered a good source of fiber that can be utilized by simple stomach livestock; also it is palatable for ruminants (Li and Kemp, 2005). Both inulin and oligofructose are the main constituents of cichory. It was documented that oligofructose improved broilers carcass and breast weights, and decrease abdominal fat percent (Ammermal et al., 1989); these findings is supported by those of Yusrizal and Chen (2003) results in which birds' abdominal fat content decreased. Chicory has essential mineral (Foster, 1988) and uronic acids (15%, DM), considered the main constituent of pectin (Voragen et al., 2001). High growth and improved digestibility of non-starch polysaccharide were observed in swine, besides little adverse influence on organic matter and digestibility with high level (16%) of *C. intybus* (Ivarsson et al., 2011). Prebiotic action of inulin was reported by Castellini et al. (2007), in livestock; also Gibson et al. (2004), observed the selective stimulation of lactobacilli and bifidobacteria, in the large intestine in rodents.

Therefore, the purpose of the study was to declare the benefits of *M. oleifera* and/or *C. intybus* as feed additive on broiler chickens in terms of feed intake (FI), growth

performance, immunology, biochemical parameters, and carcass yields.

MATERIALS AND METHODS

Experimental chicks, housing and management

This study was carried out in accordance with the regulations of the Department of Nutrition and Clinical Nutrition, Faculty of Veterinary Medicine, Sohag University, Egypt. Two-hundred (Ross 308 hybrid) chicks (n = 200) raised with traditional litter system with chopped straw were used as bedding material. Room humidity and temperature were controlled and 24 h of lightening was observed throughout the experimental period. Chicks were fed *ad libitum*, and health status was observed daily. All birds were vaccinated for infectious bronchitis at 7 days old followed by Newcastle (Zoetis, Fort Dodge) and infectious bursal disease (Zoetis, Fort Dodge) at 20 days old.

Experimental design and feeding

Broilers chicks were divided randomly into four groups (50 chicks per each). Each group contained 50 chicks with 5 replicates of 10 birds per pen. The trial lasted 42 days. Chicks in control group (C) were fed *ad libitum* on the basal control diets (starter for first three weeks of age, and grower-finisher for next three weeks); birds of group M received basal diet enriched with *M. oleifera* (1.5%); chicks of group CI were fed basal diet enriched with *C. intybus* (1.5%); birds of group MC were fed basal diet enriched with *M. oleifera* and *C. intybus* (0.75%:0.75%) during experimental period (Table 1). A standard basal diet was formulated to meet the nutrient requirements of broiler (NRC, 1994) as shown in Table 2.

Tested parameters

Performance measurements

Chicks were weighed at the start of the experiment and records were taken every 15 days until the end of the experiment. The feed intake was daily recorded for each of the different experiment groups. The average amount of feed intake of each bird was estimated by dividing the consumed amount by the respective number of birds in each group. Mortality was recorded.

Body weight gain (BWG), feed conversion ratio (FCR) and production efficiency factor (PEF) also known as European Production Efficiency Factor (EPEF) were estimated thus: BWG = average final live body weight (LBW) - average initial LBW at a certain period; FCR = total feed intake / total BW gain, and EPEF = ((Livability × LBW in kg)*100)/age in days × FCR (Mousa et al., 2016).

Carcass yields

At the end of the trial and before slaughter, chicks were given a feed withdrawal period of 12 h. From each group, ten birds were randomly chosen, weighed and slaughtered. Feathers were removed, carcass was eviscerated and carcass yield was calculated. Selected chicks were deboned and breast, thigh, and abdominal fat were weighed.

Blood biochemical parameters

Vein blood samples from ten chicks of each group were collected

Table 1. Herbal plants plan.

Group	Treatment
Control group (C)	Allotted to basal diets without any supplementation
Moringa oleifera group (M)	Allotted to basal diets supplemented with 1.5% *M. oleifera* powder
Cichorium intybus group (CI)	Allotted to basal diets supplemented with 1.5% *C. intybus* powder
M. oleifera plus *C. intybus* group (MC)	Allotted to basal diets supplemented with 0.75% *M. oleifera* plus 0.75% *C. intybus* powder

from the wing. Samples were left to stand for 1 h and centrifuged at 4000 rpm for 15 min. The clear serum was kept in sterilized tubes and stored at -20°C for biochemical analysis. Levels of total proteins, albumin, triglycerides and cholesterol were measured in these samples according to the manufacturer's instruction (Chema Diagnostica, Italy).

Measurement of antibodies (Abs) titers against newcastle disease (ND) and infectious bursal disease (IBD) vaccines

In the collected sera, Abs titer against ND vaccine was measured by haemagglutination inhibition (HI) test according to OIE (2012) and Abs titer against IBD vaccine was measured by enzyme-linked immunosorbent assay (ELISA) test via IBDV ELISA kits (Synbiotics Laboratories, USA) according to the manufacturer's instruction.

Statistical analysis

This data obtain were analyzed with the standard procedures of analysis of variance (ANOVA), using SPSS Statistics 17.0 (Released 23 August 2008). Differences among means were separated using Duncan's multiple range test (Duncan, 1955). Significant difference was identified at a level of $P < 0.05$.

RESULTS AND DISCUSSION

Production performance

The growth data variables are shown in Table 3. The combination of *M. oleifera* (0.75%) and *C. intybus* (0.75%) improved significantly ($P \leq 0.05$) body weight gain along the experimental period, the best body weight gain was obtained by MC group (257±25 g/bird) in comparison with CI group (246±27 g/bird), C group (235±53 g/bird) and M group (216±16 g/bird). When the experiment was ended (after 42 days), the best cumulative LBW and FCR were recorded in the birds in MC group (2393±30 g/bird and 1.45, respectively) followed by broilers in CI group (2180±48 g/bird and 1.48, respectively) and the birds of C group (2020±97 g/bird and 1.54, respectively), but the M group had the lowest values (1893±54 g/bird and 1.58, respectively). Feed intake had the same order of LBW (MC>CI>C>M groups) of 3458, 3216, 3113 and 2996 g/bird, respectively.

European performance efficiency factor index

The EPEF indexes were significantly different between all

the treatments of study, whereas, MC group had better value (385), followed by CI group (344) and C group (293) then M group (279.5). When the EPEF index value is higher, the productive performance is better (Table 3). Health was observed and mortality was recorded throughout the experimental period (Table 3).

The result obtain for chicory as feed additive are in line with that of Yusrizal and Chen (2003) who found that the addition of it significantly improve feed intake, body weight and FCR. These results are supported by those of Ammerman et al. (1989) result, whereas, Waldroup et al. (1995) found no effect. Also, Castellini et al. (2007) found that, green *Cichorium* feeding decreased amount of feed and rabbit weight gain during suckling period. Result shows improvement along the experiment period in contrast with the report of Aghazadeh et al. (2011) who reported no effects during finishing period and explained this with the fact that fructans effects are age dependent, so stimulate microbial population and as a result enhancing performance during starter period.

Indeed, chicory (inulin) feeding to poultry have a good impact on both health status and production (Roberfroid et al., 2010); also absorption was improved via positive changes of the GIT mucosal membrane (Rehman et al., 2007); besides beneficial microflora growth was enhanced while, pathogenic bacteria growth decreased (Sevane et al., 2014). Also, the fat deposition decreased and fat profile improved (Velasco et al., 2010).

Yusrizal and Chen (2003) observed that chicory addition increase length of broilers GIT. When GIT is longer, the digestion and metabolism will be better, and so improve performance. Yeung et al. (2005) suggested that inclusion of chicory improve GIT absorption of Ca, Mg and Fe. Izadi et al. (2013) reported improved productive performance via increase surface of absorption through increase villi length, villi length/crypt depth, and villi number; also the performance improvement of broiler allotted on chicory could be related to insoluble non-starch polysaccharides content, which improve rate of digesta removal, and so enhance feed intake (Kalmendal et al., 2011). Chicory has galacturonic acids, which is the main constituent of pectin, the source of uronic acids that has high digestible values (Voragen et al., 2001).

Cichorium has fructo-oligosaccharides and inulin, which could manipulate intestinal microflora and enhance mucosal integrity (Flickinger et al., 2003); it also contains sucrose, cellulose, protein, esculin, coumarins, flavonoids,

Table 2. Ingredients (kg) and chemical composition of basal and experimental diets for broiler chicks.

Ingredient	Basal diets		Diets supplemented with Moringa		Diets supplemented with chicory		Diets supplemented with Moringa + chicory	
	Starters	Grower-finisher	Starter	Grower-finisher	Starter	Grower-finisher	Starter	Grower-finisher
Corn grain	54.5	62.45	54.5	62.45	54.5	62.45	54.5	62.45
Soy bean meal	28	21	28	21	28	21	28	21
Conc. mixture	10	10	10	10	10	10	10	10
Sunflower oil	2.2	1.6	2.2	1.6	2.2	1.6	2.2	1.6
Di-calcium phosphate	2	1.8	2	1.8	2	1.8	2	1.8
Calcium carbonate	0.8	0.8	0.8	0.8	0.8	0.8	0.8	0.8
Common salt	0.3	0.3	0.3	0.3	0.3	0.3	0.3	0.3
Sodium bicarbonate	0.25	0.1	0.25	0.1	0.25	0.1	0.25	0.1
Minerals-vitamins premix	0.3	0.3	0.3	0.3	0.3	0.3	0.3	0.3
Methionine	0.1	0.1	0.1	0.1	0.1	0.1	0.1	0.1
Lysine	0.05	0.05	0.05	0.05	0.05	0.05	0.05	0.05
Additives tested	1.5 distiller grains	1.5 distiller grains	1.5 Moringa	1.5 Moringa	1.5 chicory	1.5 chicory	1.5 Moringa + chicory	1.5 Moringa + chicory
Sum (kg)	100	100	100	100	100	100	100	100
Estimated analysis								
ME(kcal/kg)	2990	3130	2980	3120	2980	3120	2980	3120
T. P (%)	21.81	19.43	21.8	19.42	21.78	19.41	21.79	19.41
Calcium (%)	1	0.90	1	0.90	1	0.90	1	0.90
phosphorus	0.9	0.8	0.9	0.8	0.9	0.8	0.9	0.8
Lysine (%)	1.4	1.2	1.4	1.2	1.4	1.2	1.4	1.2
Methionine (%)	0.58	0.57	0.58	0.57	0.58	0.57	0.58	0.57

Premix provided the recommended amount of both vitamins and mineral according to NRC (1994).

and vitamins (Meehye and Shin, 1996; Van Loo, 2007). Inulin improves lipid-to-glucose metabolism with potential effects on weight gain, fat deposition and appetite (Urias-Silvas et al., 2007). A beneficial action of chicory (inulin and oligofructose) feeding is decreasing the pH, which could explain thickening of the small intestine wall (Remesy et al., 1992).

Sevane et al. (2014) identified 33 genes associated with protein regulation activity, vital cellular processes, localization and peptidase activity, and so influence productive improvement; 43 genes were also identified that regulate cell division and growth, DNA and RNA synthesis, finally resulting in increasing cellular activity.

Besides, chicory stimulates PPARA, which is a member of peroxisome proliferator-activated receptors, related to energy metabolism regulation, cell growth, dividing and maturation, and in inflammation and immune status (Gervois and Mansouri, 2012).

The result of Moringa is supported by observation of Akhouri et al. (2013), who recorded improved body weight and enhanced FCR of broilers with M. oleifera; it is also in line with the results of Banjo (2012) finding, who reported that supplementation of M. oleifera to diet of broiler

Table 3. Impact of *M. oleifera* and/or *C. intybus* addition to broiler chicken ration on weight gain, feed intake, FCR and EPEF.

Variable		Control group (C)	*Moringa oleifera* group (M)	*Chicory intybus* group (CI)	*M. oleifera* plus *C. intybus* group (MC)
Number of birds		50	50	50	50
Initial body weight		45.3	45.2	45.1	45.2
Body weight (g/bird)	15 days old	216 ± 53^d	235 ± 16^c	246 ± 27^b	257 ± 25^a
	30 days old	1218 ± 145^d	1339 ± 95^c	1397 ± 135^b	1482 ± 62^a
	42 days old	1893 ± 97^d	2020 ± 54^c	2180 ± 48^b	2393 ± 80^a
Feed intake (g/bird)	15 days old	250.2 ± 23^d	266.3 ± 33^c	280.5 ± 24^b	295.5 ± 43^a
	30 days old	1503.7 ± 46^d	1537.5 ± 27^c	1588.5 ± 52^b	1670.6 ± 76^a
	42 days old	1242.3 ± 65^d	1310.1 ± 39^c	1347.4 ± 61^b	1492.3 ± 33^a
Cumulative		2996.2 ± 107^d	3113.9 ± 47^c	3216.4 ± 57^b	3458.4 ± 74^a
FCR		1.58	1.54	1.48	1.45
EPEF		279.5	293.5	344	385
Mortality		3	1	1	1

[a,b,c,d] Means on the same row with different superscripts are significantly different (P<0.05).

Table 4. Antibody titer of broilers chicks against ND and IBD vaccines allotted on *M. oleifera* and/or *C. intybus* supplemented ration at 30 days old.

Group	HI of NDV (log2)	Elisa of IBD
Control group (C)	254.84 ± 70^d	1241 ± 23^d
Group (M)	584.54 ± 59^b	2130 ± 70^b
Group (CI)	296.89 ± 67^c	1802 ± 42^c
Group (MC)	612.23 ± 42^a	2209 ± 34^a

[a,b,c,d] Means on the same column with different superscripts are significantly different (P<0.05).

chicken enhanced weight gain. Nuhu (2010) reported in young rabbits that received diet with *M. oleifera*, improvement in protein digestibility and weight gain, while feed intake, FCR, and carcass yields were not affected. Grubben and Denton (2004) reported higher growth of rabbit as a result of vitamin A and essential elements of *M. oleifera*, that promote health. *M. oleifera* also has antimicrobial ability (Caceres et al., 1990). *M. oleifera* leaves contain 0.1 to 0.23% of tannin (Kakengi et al., 2003, 2007), that decrease protein digestion and absorption while lipids and carbohydrate utilization are less affected (Esonu et al., 2001).

Immunological parameters

An elevation of antibodies titers of both ND and IBD vaccine was found in groups MC, CI, M than group C (Table 4). The titer of IBD and NDV vaccine improved due to the presence of flavonoides, inulin and polyphenolic compound. Result obtained pointed an effect of chicory and *M. oleifera* addition on the improvement of immunity by improving the activity of genes and fastening pathways related to body defense processes, where the addition of chicory (inulin) stimulated various immune pathways. Sevane et al. (2014) identified 20 genes implicated in immune response pathways, antibodies and immune action. Also, chicory has anti-apoptotic activity, via antioxidant activation, which boosts T-helper activity (Wammes et al., 2013) besides activating enzymes which enhance formation of acyl-CoA, ATP and CoA, and so promote mitochondria action (Wammes et al., 2013). Chicory also regulates glutathione metabolism that also enhances antioxidant defense and regulation of cellular metabolism, where its deficiency leads to oxidative stress (Wu et al., 2004).

Oligofructose suppresses challenged infections of broilers (Van Leeuwen et al., 2005). In quails, inclusion of inulin prevents the pathogenic bacteria growth and enhances the activities of microflora, which have a protective role (Catala et al., 1999). Nodular lymphoid tonsils improvement and infiltration of lymphoid cells were recorded with chicory feeding (Spaeth et al., 1990), besides Kelly-Quagliana et al. (2003) described that both inulin and oligofructose triggers immune defense

Table 5. Some blood parameters of broilers chicks received ration supplemented with *M. oleifera* and/or *C. intybus* at 42-days old.

Group	Protein (g/100 ml)	Albumin (g/100 ml)	Globulin (g/100 ml)	Cholesterol (mg/100 ml)	Triglycerides (mg/100 ml)
C	3.84±0.3[d]	1.57±0.13[d]	2.27±0.3[c]	149.8±8[a]	53.73±2.1[a]
M	5.67±0.15[b]	1.68±0.06[c]	3.99±0.2[b]	122.2±9[b]	37.62±1.3[c]
CI	4.25±0.34[c]	1.96±0.08[a]	2.29±0.1[c]	117.6±7[c]	42.71±1.4[b]
MC	5.82±0.52[a]	1.76±0.15[b]	4.06±0.2[a]	106.4±4[d]	41.30±2.3[b]

[a,b,c,d]Means on the same column with different superscripts are significantly different (P<0.05).

mechanism. Without doubt, *M. oleifera* is medicinally used as antioxidants and antifungal (Mohammed and Barhate, 2012; Paliwal et al., 2011a, b), so high-fat foods could be preserved for long time due to potent antioxidants presence such as flavonoids and total phenolic compounds (Doughari et al., 2008; Jain et al., 2010). The leaves are also free of deleterious substances such as tannins and saponins (Celikel and Kavas, 2008).

Antimicrobial activity is the key for the wide use of *M. oleifera* (Suarez et al., 2005). It has immunomodulatory ability in the immune system (Paliwal et al., 2011a). This herb also serves as promoter to immune system and is used to overcome malnutrition (Paliwal et al., 2011b). It was chosen due to its phytochemical compound content, which include saponins, carotenoids, phenolic compounds and flavonoids. Saponin and flavonoid are considered natural immunomodulator because they enhance lymphocyte cells development (Anwar et al., 2007). Lipophilic constituents of *Moringa* explained the antimicrobial activity (Jabeen et al., 2008); *Moringa* also contain antibiotic metabolites and cell wall degrading enzymes (Rachmawati and Rifa'l, 2014).

According to Hefni (2013), aqueous extract of *M. oleifera* increases the number of hematopoietic stem cells, B lymphocytes, naive T cells expression and pro-inflammatory cytokines.

Biochemical parameters

Table 5 show that blood serum total cholesterol values were different (P ≤ 0.05) among the groups, where lower value as well as triglycerides values was recorded in the chicory-*Moringa* (MC) group, followed by CI and M groups, where C group comes last, while there was a significant improvement in total protein and globulin values in both MC and M groups than CI and C groups. The result was similar to those of Yusrizal and Chen (2003) findings that revealed on addition of chicory to broilers diet a decrease in serum cholesterol level and abdominal fat deposition and an increase in cecum weight and GIT length. Also, result of Yusrizal and Chen (2003) showed that inulin decreased cholesterol content in serum. Jeusette et al. (2004) and Diez (1997) observed a decrease in cholesterol and triglyceride values in the

presence of inulin or oligofructose. Delzenne et al. (1995) observe an increase in calcium bioavailability which modifies the bone structure.

The result of the study is similar to the findings of Elson (1995), which recorded that enzyme of synthetic pathway of cholesterol was suppressed by isoprenoids. Moreover, Kim (2000) reported that chicory presence decreased 30% of cholesterol absorption, meanwhile Fremont et al. (2000) recorded that phenolic compounds decrease cholesterol concentration in blood and meat. Similarly, *M. oleifera* extract had hypo-cholesterolemic properties that were explained with low density lipoprotein (LDL) plasma levels due to the presence of B-sitosterol of *Moringa* (Ghasi et al., 2000, Kane and Malloy, 1982). Also, Luqman et al. (2012) confirmed the antioxidant activities as a result of polyphenols and flavonoids found in extract of *M. oleifera*.

The LDL of birds reduced with inclusion of *Moringa* explained by the presence of myriad phytochemicals in *M. Oleifera*. Some compounds present in *Moringa* were reported to have antibacterial and anticancer activity (Fahey, 2005; Mekonnen and Dräger, 2003), as well as antioxidant activity (Win and Jongen, 1996).

Carcass yield

As shown in Table 6 it could be observed that there was a significance difference (P≤0.05) among the groups in dressed carcass % of live body weight, where M (70.3) and MC (86.3) groups are better than CI groups (66.1) and C groups (65.3). Treatments had significant effect on breast, thigh and abdominal fat. Broilers which received diets with M had better carcass weight (%), but not the body weight (MC group). The examined groups had higher breast weight (%) than the control group C (P<0.05).

The study result is in line with the finding of Brunsgaard and Eggum (1995), who reported improving carcass dressing and BW percentage.

The chicory inclusion to broilers improves carcass dressing and BW percentage that could be explained as fiber effect, which is obviously observed through the lower GIT length more than in the upper part (Brunsgaard and Eggum, 1995).

Table 6. Some carcass yield affected by *addition of M. oleifera* and /or *C. intybus* to broiler ration.

Carcass parameter	Control group (C)	Group (M)	Group (CI)	Group (MC)
Dressed carcass (%) of LBW	65.3±2[c]	70.3±1[a]	66.1±3[c]	68.3±2[b]
Breast (%) of carcass	37.3±2[c]	39.8±3[a]	36.5±6[d]	38.9±1[b]
Thigh (%) of carcass	37.1±6[b]	35.3±4[c]	39.1±3[a]	37.3±4[b]
Abdominal fat (%) of LBW	1.9	1.89	1.79	1.77

[a,b,c,d]Means on the same row with different superscripts are significantly different (P<0.05).

These results were confirmed by Yusrizal and Chen (2003) findings, who reported that inclusion of chicory lower the blood cholesterol concentration in broilers chicks, besides increase cecum weight and GIT length, but lowered the abdominal fat. A suggested explanation is diminishing stress condition through the action on immune system.

In rats Jaiswal et al. (2009) recorded that glucose concentration lowered with *M. oleifera* extract addition, that confirm the insulin like action of *Moringa* on body tissues, that might be due to cellular glucose utilization or cease gluconeogenesis. *M. oleifera* has abilities to increase glucose utilization by body tissues (Luqman et al., 2012) via suppress hepatic gluconeogenesis or improve glucose utilization by the body tissues (Desta et al., 2011; Kamanyi et al., 1994). Consequently, this could explain the higher dressed carcass of *Moringa* than other treatments.

Generally, abdominal fat deposition is determined by the amount of fat intake and the amount of fat metabolized and excreted. So, if the fat intake and excreted is equal, decreased body fat accumulation could be due to lipolysis or decreased fatty acid production or to the both mechanisms. In contrary to this, the findings of Sizemore and Siegel (1993), who found no effects of dietary fat amount when the calorie protein ratio remained constant, in broiler diets supplemented with chicory. Similar to the result, Ologhobo et al. (2014) reported better values of carcass weights for birds received diets with *M. oleifera* more than birds received the basal one.

Preston and William (1973) result mentioned that birds with heavier weight have higher dressing percentage and eviscerated yield.

Safa and Tazi (2014) found that feeding *M. oleifera* had fair effect on quality of chicks carcass and increased breast weight of chicks, while Zanu et al. (2012) found that carcass characteristics parameters may not be affected by *Moringa* addition.

Finally, it can be concluded that the use of combination of both *M. oleifera* and *C. intybus* is better than each one alone, due to the beneficial synergistic effect on performance, biochemical parameters and immunology, besides improving carcass quality.

Hence, combination of *M. oleifera* and *C. intybus* was recommended as good feed additives with potential antioxidant ability for broiler chicks.

CONFLICT OF INTERESTS

The authors have not declared any conflict of interests.

REFERENCES

Aghazadeh, AM, Ilkhany F, Allahverdi M (2011). Effect of different levels of chicory and *Satureja hortensis* root powders on performance and carcass characteristics of broilers. J. Agric. Sci. Technol. A1:1261-1264.

Akhouri S, Prasad A, Ganguly S (2013). *Moringa oleifera* leaf extract imposes better feed utilization in broiler chicks. J. Biol. Chem. Res. 30(2):447-450.

Ammermal E, Quarles C, Twining PV (1989). Evaluation of fructooligosaccharides on performance and carcass yield of male broilers. Poult. Sci. 68(Suppl.):167.

Anwar F, Latif S, Ashraf M, Gilani AH (2007). Food Plant with Multiple Medicinal Uses. Phytother. Res. 21(1):17-25.

Banjo OS (2012). Growth and performance as affected by inclusion of Moringa oleifera leaf meal in broiler chicks diet. J. Biol. Agric. Healthcare (9):35-38.

Barrow P (1992). Probiotics for chickens. In: Probiotics, the Scientic Basis (Fuller, R., Ed.). Chapman and Hall, London, UK. pp. 225-257.

Brunsgaard G, Eggum BO (1995). Caecal and colonic tissue structure and proliferation as influenced by adaptation period and indigestible polysaccharides. Comparative Biochemistry and Physiology Part A: Physiology 112(3):573-583.

Caceres A, Cabrera O, Morales O, Mollinedo P, Mendia P (1990). Pharmaceutical properties of Moringa oleifera. Preliminary screening for antimicrobial activity. J. Ethnopharmacol. 33:213-216.

Castellini C, Cardinali R, Rebollar PG, Bosco AD, Jimeno V, Cossu ME (2007). Feeding fresh chicory (*Chicoria intybus*) to young rabbits: performance, development of gastro-intestinal tract and immune functions of appendix and Peyer's patch. Anim. Feed Sci. Technol. 134:56-65.

Catala I, Butel MJ, Bensaada M, Popot F, Tessedre AC, Rimbault A, Szylit O (1999). Oligofructose contributes to the protective role of bifidobacteria in experimental necrotising enterocolitis in quails. J. Med. Microbiol. 48:89-94.

Catala-Gregori P, Mallet S, Travel A, Lessire M (2008). Efficiency of a prebiotic and a plant extract on broiler performance and intestinal physiology. 16th European Symposium on Poultry Nutrition, World Poultry Science Association, Strasbourg, France.

Celikel N, Kavas G (2008). Antimicrobial properties of some essential oils against some pathogenic microorganisms. Czech J. Food Sci. 26(3):174-81.

Dahot MU (1988). Vitamin contents of flowers and seeds of Moringa oleifera. Biochemistry pp. 2122-2124.

Das BR, Kurup PA, Rao PLN (1957). Antibiotic principle from Moringa pterygosperma: VII. Antibacterial activity and chemical structure of compounds related to pterygospermin. India J. Med. Res. 45:191-196.

Delzenne N, Aertssens J, Verplaetse H, Roccaro M, Roberfroid M (1995). Effect of fermentable fructo-oligosaccharides on mineral, nitrogen and energy digestive balance in the rats. Life Sci. 57:1579-1587.

Desta G, Yalemtsehay M, Girmai G, Wondwossen E, Kahsay H (2011).

The effects of Moringa stenopetala on blood parameters and histopathology of liver and kidney in mice. Ethiop. J. Health Dev. 25(1):52-57.

Diez M (1997). Influence of a blend of fructo-oligosaccharides and sugar beet fiber on nutrient digestibility and plasma metabolite concentrations in healthy Beagles. Am. J. Vet. Res. 58:1238-1242.

Doughari JH, El-mahmood AM, Tyoyina I (2008). Antimicrobial activity of leaf extracts of Senna obtusifolia (L). Afr. J. Pharm Pharmacol. 2(1):7-13.

Duncan DB (1955). Multiple range and multiple F-Test. Biometrics 11:1-42.

Elson CE (1995). Suppression of mevalonate pathway activities by dietary isoprenoids: protective roles in cancer and cardio-vascular disease. J. Nutr. 125:1666-1672.

Endo T, Nakano M, Shimizu S, Fukushima M, Miyoshi S (1999). Effect of a probiotic on the lipid metabolism of cocks fed on cholesterol-enriched diet. Biosci. Biotechnol. Biochem. 63:1569-1575.

Esonu BO, Emenalom, OO, Udedibie ABI, Herbert U, Ekpor CF, Okolie IC, Iheukwumere FC (2001). Performance and blood chemistry of weaner pigs fed raw mucuna (velvet bean). Trop. Anim. Prod. Investig. 4:49-54.

Fahey JW (2005). Moringa oleifera: A review of the Medical Evidence for Its Nutritional, Therapeutic, and Prophylactic Properties, Part 1. Trees Life J. 1:5.

Fermont L, Gozzelino MT, Linard A (2000). Response of plasma lipids to dietary cholesterol and wine polyphenols in rats fed polyunsaturated fat diets. Lipids 35:991.

Flickinger EA, Van Loo J, Fahey GC (2003). Nutritional responses to the presence of inulin and oligofructose in the diets of domesticated animals: a review. Crit. Rev. Food Sci. Nutr.43:19-60.

Foster L (1988). Herbs in pasture, development and research in Britain 1850-1984. Biol. Agric. Horticult. 5:97-133.

Gervois P, Mansouri RM (2012). PPARa as a therapeutic target in inflammation associated diseases. Expert Opin. Ther. Targets 16:1113-1125.

Ghasi S, Nwobodo E, Ofilis JO (2000). Hypocholesterolemic effects of crude extract of the leafs of Moringa oleifera Lam. in high-fat diet fed Wistar rats, J. Ethno-Pharmacol. 69:21-25.

Gibson GR, Probert HM, Loo JV, Rastall RA, Roberfroid MB (2004). Dietary modulation of the human colonic microbiota: updating the concept of prebiotics. Nutr. Res. Rev. 17:259-275.

Grubben GJH, Denton OA (2004). Plant Resources of Tropical Africa 2. Vegetables. Wageningen, the Netherlands: PROTA Foundation.

Halle I, Thomann R, Bauermann U, Henning M, Kohler P (2004). Effects of a graded supplementation of herbs and essential oils in broiler feed on growth and carcass traits. Landbauforshung Volkenrode. 54:219-229.

Hefni M (2013). Imunomodulator activity of aqueous extract of M. oleifera Lam on immunity response of mice (Mus musculus) which infected with Salmonella typhi. Master Thesis. University of Brawijaya. Malang.

Ivarsson E, Frankow-Lindberg BE, Andersson HK, Lindberg JE (2011). Growth performance, digestibility and faecal coliform bacteria in weaned piglets fed a cereal-based diet including either chicory (Cichorium intybus L) or ribwort (Plantago lanceolata L) forage. Animal 5:558-564.

Izadi H, Arshami J, Golian A, Raji MR (2013). Effects of chicory root powder on growth performance and histomorphometry of jejunum in broiler chicks. Vet. Res. Forum 4 (3):169-174.

Jabeen R, Shahid M, Jamil A, Ashraf M (2008). Microscopic evaluation of the antimicrobial activity of seed extracts of Moringa oleifera. Pak. J. Bot. 40:1349-1358.

Jain PG, Patil SD, Haswani NG, Girase MV, Surana SJ, Patel RC (2010). Hypolipidemic activity of Moringa oleifera Lam Moringaeceae on high fat diet induced hyperlipidemia in albino rats. Braz. J. Pharmacogn. 20(6):969-973.

Jaiswal D, Kumar Rai P, Kumar A, Mehta S, Watal G (2009). Effect of Moringa oleifera Lam. leaves aqueous extract therapy on hyperglycemic rats. J. Ethnopharmacol. 123(3):392-396.

Jeusette I, Grauwels M, Cuvelier C, Tonglet C, Istasse L, Diez M(2004). Hypercholesterolaemia in a family of rough collie dogs. J. Small Anim. Pract. 45:319-324.

Kakengi AMV, Kaijage JT, Sarwatt SV, Mutayoba SK, Shem MN, Fujihara T (2007). Effect of Moringa oleifera leaf meal as a substitute for sunflower seed meal on performance of laying hens in Tanzania. Livest. Res. Rural Dev. 19:8.

Kakengi AMV, Shen MN, Sarwart SV, Fujihara T (2003). Can Moringa oleifera be used as protein supplement to ruminant diet? Asian-Australian J. Anim. Sci. 18(1):42-47.

Kalmendal R, Elwinger K, Holm L, Tauson R (2011). High fiber sunflower cake affects small intestinal digestion and health in broiler chickens. Br. Poult. Sci. 52:86-96.

Kamanyi A, Djamen D, Nkeh B (1994). Hypoglycemic properties of the aqueous root extracts of Morinda lucida (Rubiaceae) study in the mouse. Phytother. Res. 8:369-371.

Kane JP, Malloy MJ (1982). Treatment of hypercholesterolemia. Med. Clin. North America. 66:537-550.

Kelly-Quagliana KA, Nelsona PD, Buddingtona RK (2003). Dietary oligofructose and inulin modulate immune functions in mice. Nutr. Res. 23:257-267.

Kim M (2000).The water-soluble extract of chicory reduces cho-lesterol uptake in gut-perfused rats. Nutr. Res. 20(7):1017-1026.

Li GD, Kemp PD (2005). Forage chicory (Cichorium intybus L.). A review of its agronomy and animal production. Adv. Agron. 88:187-222.

Luqman S, Srivastava S, Kumar R, Maurya AK, Chanda D (2012). Experimental assessment of Moringa oleifera leaf and fruit for its antistress, antioxidant, and scavenging potential using in vitro and in vivo assays. Evid. Based Complement. Alternat. Med. 519084.

Meehye K, Shin HK (1996). The water-soluble extract of chicory reduces glucose uptake from the perfused jejunum in rats. J. Nutr. 126:2236-2242.

Mekonnen Y, Dräger B (2003). Glucosinolates in Moringa stenopetala. Planta Med. 69:380-382.

Mohammed R, Barhate SD (2012). Phytochemical investigation and study of Anti-inflammatory activity of Moringa oleifera Lam. Intl. J. Pharm. Res. Dev. 3(11):114-119.

Mousa MA, Sayed HH, Osman AS (2016).The impact of palm pollen and ginkgo biloba supplementation on performance, biochemical parameters and immune response of broilers. J. Intl. Acad. Res. Multidiscip. 4(10):236-251.

Nuhu F (2010). Effect of Moringa leaf meal (MOLM) on nutrient digestibility, growth, carcass and blood indices of weaner rabbits. MSc, Faculty of Agriculture and Natural Resources, Kwame Nkrumah University of Science and Technology, Kumasi, Ghana.

Nutrient Requirements of Poultry (NRC) (1994). National Academic Science, 9th ed., Washington, D.C. USA.

OIE (2012). Manual of Diagnostic Tests and Vaccines for Terrestrial Animals: Mammals, Birds and Bees, Biological Standards Commission. World Organization for Animal Health, Paris. pp. 1-19.

Ologhobo AD, Akangbe EI, Adejumo IO, Adeleye O (2014). Effect of Moringa oleifera leaf meal as replacement for oxytetracycline on carcass characteristics of the diets of broiler chickens. Annu. Res. Rev. Biol. 4(2):423-431.

Paliwal R, Sharma V, Pracheta (2011a). A review on horse radish tree (Moringa oleifera) A multipurpose tree with high economic and commercial importance. Asian J. Biotechnol. 3(4):317-28.

Paliwal R, Sharma V, Pracheta, Sharma S (2011b). Elucidation of free radical scavenging and antioxidant activity of aqueous and hydro-ethanolic extracts of Moringa oleifera pods. Asian J. Biotechnol. 4(4):566-571.

Panagasa A, Singla LD, Sood N, Singh andJuyal PD (2007). Histopathological evaluation of anticoccidial activity of an ayurvediccoccidiostat, in induced Eimeriatenella infection in chicken. Indian J. Anim. Sci. 77(3):214-216.

Panagasa A,Singla LD, Bansal N andJuyal PD (2012). Enzyme histochemistry of the Eimeriatenellainfected caeca of chicks: A preliminary study. J. Vet. Parasitol. 26(1):77-79.

Pietrzak D, Mroczek J, Antolik A, Michalczuk M, Niemiec J (2005). Influence of growth stimulators added to feed on the quality of meat and fat in broiler chickens. Med. Wet. 61:553-557.

Preston LH, William WM (1973). Eviscerated yield, component parts and meat, skin bone ratios in chicken broiler. Poult. Sci. 52:718-722.

Rachmawati I, Rifa'i M (2014). In vitro Immunomodulatory Activity of

Aqueous Extract of *Moringa oleifera* Lam. Leaf to the CD4 +, CD8+ and B220+ Cells in Mus musculu. J. Exp. Life Sci. 4(1):15-20.

Rehman H, Vahjen W, Awad WA, Zentek J (2007). Indigenous bacteria and bacterial metabolic products in the gastrointestinal tract of broilers. Arch. Anim. Nutr. 61:319-335.

Remesy C, Behr SR, Levrat MA (1992). Fiber ferment ability in the rat cecum and its physiological consequences. Nutr. Res. 12:1235-1244.

Roberfroid M, Gibson GR, Hoyles L, McCartney AL, Rastall R (2010). Prebiotic effects: metabolic and health benefits. Br. J. Nutr. 104:S1-S63.

Safa MA, Tazi El (2014). Effect of feeding different levels of *Moringa oleifera* leaf meal on the performance and carcass quality of broiler chicks. Intl. J. Sci. Res. 3(5).

Sevane N, Bialade F, Velasco S, Rebole´ A, Rodrı´guez ML, Cañón J1, Dunner S (2014). Dietary Inulin supplementation modifies significantly the liver transcriptomic profile of broiler chickens. PLoS ONE 9(6):e98942.

Singla LD, Gupta SK (2012). Advances in diagnosis of coccidiosis in poultry. In: Veterinary Diagnostics: Current Trends, Gupta RP, Garg SR, Nehra V and Lather D (Eds), Satish Serial Publishing House, Delhi. pp. 615-628.

Sizemore FG, Siegel HS (1993). Growth, feed conversion and carcass composition in females of four broiler crosses fed starter diets with different energy levels and energy to protein ratios. Poult. Sci. 72:2216-2228.

Spaeth G, Berg RD, Specian RD (1990). Food without fiber promotes bacterial translocation from the gut. Surgery 108:240-247.

Sreelatha S, Padma PR (2009). Antioxidant Activity and Total Phenolic Content of Moringa oleifera Leaves in Two Stages of Maturity Plant Foods Hum. Nutr. 64:303-311.

Suarez M, Haenni M, Canarelli S, Fisch F, Chodanowski P, Servis C, Michelin O, Frietag R, Moreillon P, Mermod N (2005). Structure-Function characterization and optimization of a plant-derived antibacterial peptide. Antimicrob. Agents Chemother. 49:3847-3857.

Urias-Silvas JE, Cani PD, Delmee, Neyrinck A, López MG, Delzenne NM (2007). Physiological effects of dietary fructans extracted from Agaves teq-uilana and Dasylirion spp. Br. J. Nutr. 99:254-261.

Van Leeuwen P, Verdonk JMAJ, Kwakernaak C (2005). Effects of fructo oligo saccharide (OF) inclusion in diets on performance of broiler chickens. Confidential report 05/I00650 to Orafti.

Van Loo J (2007). How chicory fructans contribute to zoo-technical performance and well-being in livestock and companion animals. J. Nutr. 137:2594-2597.

Velasco S, Ortiz LT, Alzueta C, Rebole´ A, Trevin˜o J, Rodríguez ML (2010). Effect of inulin supplementation and dietary fat source on performance, blood serum metabolites, liver lipids, abdominal fat deposition, and tissue fatty acid composition in broiler chickens. Poult. Sci. 89:1651-1662.

Voragen F, Beldman G, Schols H (2001). Chemistry and enzymology of pectins. Advanced Dietary Fibre Technology. B. V. McCleary and L. Prosky, ed. Blackwell Science Ltd., Oxford, UK. pp. 379-398.

Waldroup A, Kaniawty S, Mauromoustaxos A (1995). Performance characteristics and microbiological aspects of broiler fed diets supplemented with organic acids. J. Food Prot. 58(5):482-489.

Wammes LJ, Wiria AE, Toenhake CG, Hamid F, Liu KY, Suryani H, Kaisar MM, Verweij JJ, Sartono E, Supali T, Smits HH, Luty AJ, Yazdanbakhsh M (2013). Asymptomatic plasmodial infection is associated with increased tumor necrosis factor receptor II-expressing regulatory T cells and suppressed type 2 immune responses. J. Infect. Dis. 207:1590-1599.

Win B, Jongen F (1996). Glucosinolates in brassica: occurrence and significance as cancer-modulating agents. Ind. Nutr. J. 55:433-446.

Wu G, Fang YZ, Yang S, Lupton JR, Turner ND (2004). Glutathione metabolism and its implications for health. J. Nutr. 134:489-492.

Yang R, Chang LC, Hsu, JC, Weng BBC, Palada MC, Chadha ML, Levasseur V (2006). Nutritional and functional properties of Moringa leaves -from Germplasm, to plant, to food, to health. Moringa and other highly nutritious plant resources: Strategies, standards and markets for a better impact on nutrition in Africa. Accra, Ghana. Available at: www.treesforlifejournal.org.

Yeung CK, Glahn RP, Welch RM, Miller DD (2005). Prebiotics and iron bioavailability: Is there a connection? J. Food Sci. 70:1288-1292.

Yusrizal C, Chen TC (2003): Effect of adding chicory fructans in feed on broiler growth performance, serum cholesterol, and intestinal length. Intl. J. Poult. Sci. 2:214-219.

Zanu HK, Asiedu P, Tampuori M, Asada M, Asante I (2012). Possibilities of using Moringa (*Moringa oleifera*) leaf meal as a partial substitute for fishmeal in broiler chickens diet. Online J. Anim. Feed Res. 2(1):70-75.

11

A cross sectional study on prevalence of cattle fasciolosis and associated economical losses in cattle slaughtered at Gondar Elfora Abattoir, northwest Ethiopia

Addis Kassahun Gebremeskel[1]*, Abebaw Getachew[2] and Daniel Adamu[2]

[1]School of veterinary Medicine, Hawassa University, Hawassa, Ethiopia.
[2]College of veterinary medicine and animal sciences, University of Gondar, Gondar, Ethiopia.

Fasciolosis is a parasitic disease caused by either *Fasciola hepatica* or *Faciola gigantica*. These parasitic infections are of global significance causing diseases in different mammalian species including humans. In this study, the prevalence and economic significance of Fasciolosis in cattle slaughtered at Gondar Elfora abattoirs was assessed. A total of 400 cattle were examined and 85 cattle (21.2%) were affected by fasciolosis. This findings indicated that, the prevalence of cattle fasiolosis is significantly affected by the age of the animals ($P < 0.05$), where young animals (27.7%) were more affected than the adult ones (17.1%). Body conditions disclosed a significant relation with *Fasciola* infection. Poor body conditioned animals showed the highest prevalence (30.8%) followed by medium (19.5%) and good body conditioned animals (17%). There were statistical significant differences between the different geographical locations. Highest prevalence of fasciolosis was exhibited in animals originated from Dembiya (50%) followed by Debarq (31.6%), Wogera (15%), Gondar zuria (13.5%), Belesa (12.9%), Dansha (11.9%) and Metema (4.7%). As recorded, due to cattle fasciolosis livers were condemned for human consumption. Thus, based on retail value of cattle liver, the direct economic loss from fasciolosis in Gondar Elfora abattoir was estimated to be 63,600 Ethiopian Birr (2316.948 USD) annually. In conclusion, cattle fasciolosis is one of the major parasitic diseases in the study area. Therefore appropriate control measures should be designed and implemented so as to reduce financial losses that may occur from organ condemnation and loss of animals from the disease.

Key words: Cattle, economy, Elfora abattoir, fasciolosis, prevalence.

INTRODUCTION

Ethiopia is rich in livestock and believed to have the largest livestock population in Africa. The central statistical agency report indicated the total cattle population of the country which is estimated to be about

*Corresponding author. E-mail: addisk2013@gmail.com.

59.5 million, female (55.5%) and male (44.5%). The sector has been subsidizing a significant portion to the country economy and still promising to rally round the economic development of the country (CSA, 2017). Despite the presence of this huge livestock population, Ethiopia is not exploiting its livestock resources as expected due to a number of factors such as animal diseases, recurrent drought, infrastructures problem, rampant animal diseases, poor nutrition, poor husbandry practices, shortage of trained man power and lack of government policies for disease prevention and control (ILRI, 2009).

Among the animal diseases that affect animal health, parasitic infections have a great economic impact particularly in developing countries. Fasciolosis is of the parasitic diseases of domestic livestock caused by *Fasciola hepatica* and *Faciola gigantica,* commonly called liver flukes that are the most important trematodes afflicting the global agricultural community (Cwiklinski et al, 2016; Deepak and Singla, 2016; Andrews, 1999). Fasciolosis is a neglected tropical disease having both economy and zoonotic importance usually affects poor people from developing countries (Mas-Coma et al., 2014).

It has been estimated that, at least 2.6 million people are infected with fasciolosis worldwide (Fürst et al., 2012).

In Ethiopia, this disease is endemic in most part of the country long time ago as reported by several workers such as Graber, (1978), Goll and Scott (1978), Fufa et al. (2010), Yilma and Mesfin (2000), and Tolosa and Tigre (2007). Although many surveys were conducted, the case is still economic and public health issue. This study assesses the current status of fasciolosis, economical loss due to liver condemnation and identifies associated risk factors for the occurrence of faciolosis in cattle slaughtered at Elfora abattoir enterprise, Gondar, Ethiopia.

MATERIALS AND METHODS

Description of the study area

This study was carried out on 400 slaughtered cattle at Elfora abattoir; Amhara regional state, Northwest Ethiopia, from November 2016 to May 2017. Gondar town is located 739 Km away from Addis Ababa at an elevation of 2,220 m above sea level. The town is aligned on latitude of 12°36'N 37°28'E and longitude of 12.6°N37.467°E. Rain fall varies from 880 to1172 mm with the average annual temperature of 20.3°C (Shewangzaw and Addis, 2016).

Study animals

This study was conducted on 400 slaughtered male cattle brought from different areas nearby Gondar town. The cattle come mainly from Dembiya, Metema, Debarq, Belesa, Dansha, Gondar zuria and wogera.

Study design and sample size determination

A cross-sectional resarch was done to conduct this study and systematic random sampling technique was used to select appropriate samples. The sample size was determined according to the formula given by Thrusfield (2005). Previous study conducted by Mulat et al. (2012) shown the prevalence rate of 29.75% cattle fasiolosis in the same abattoir.

Hence, using 29.75% as expected prevalence and 5% absolute precision at 95% confidence level, the number of sampled animals needed in the study was 320. However, to increase the level of precision and accuracy of the data, the study was carried out on 400 cattle.

Ante-mortem examination

Ante-mortem examination was conducted in lairage, before slaughtering of animals according to Gracy et al., (1999) recommendation. Risk factors such as age, origin and body condition of individual animal were identified and recorded. Body condition for each cattle was estimated based on Nicholson and Butterworth (1986) ranging from score 1 (emaciated) to 5 (obese).

Therefore, in this study three classes of scoring which include poor (Score 2), medium (Score 3 and 4) and good (score 5) were used. No animals were slaughtered at score 1. The age of the animal was estimated on the basis of dentitions (Cringoli et al., 2002).

Post mortem examination

The liver of each study animal was carefully examined externally for the presence of lesions suggestive of *Fasciola* infection and incised for further confirmation. Liver flukes were detected by cutting the infected liver into fine, approximately 1 cm slices with a sharp knife. Investigation and identification of *Fasciola* species was done according to their distinct morphological characteristics following the standard guidelines given by Urquhart et al. (1996).

Direct economic loss assessment

All fasciola infected livers were considered to be unfit for human consumption and if any liver was infected by *Fasciola* at the Gondar Elfora abattoir, it was totally condemned. Therefore it was analyzed by considering the average number of annually slaughtered cattle in the abattoir from retrospective recorded data, the mean selling price of one liver at Gondar town and the prevalence of fasciolosis in the present study (21.2%).

The average market price of one liver at Gondar town was taken as 50 Ethiopian birr. The mean number of cattle slaughtered in this municipal abattoir was 6000 per year which depends on two years recorded data economic losses, calculated based on condemned livers due to fasciolosis. The estimated annual loss from condemned liver was calculated according to mathematical computation using the formula set by Ogunrinade and Adegoke (1982).

$$ALC = CSR \times LC \times P$$

$$=6000*50*21.2\%=63,600 \text{ Ethiopian birr}$$

Where:
ALC = Annual loss from liver condemnation,
CSR = mean annual cattle slaughtered at Gondar Elfora abattoir,
LC = mean cost of one liver in Gondar town and,
P = Prevalence of bovine fasciolosis at Gondar Elfora abattoir.

Table 1. Total number of animal examined and expected prevalence from November 2016 to May 2017.

Total samples	Infected animals	Prevalence (%)
400	85	21.25%

Table 2. Prevalence of cattle fasiolosis based on origin of animals from November 2016 to May 2017.

Origin	Prevalence (%)	X^2 (P-value)
Metema (n=64)	4.7	
Dembiya (n=72)	50	
Debarq (n=57)	31.6	57.218 (0.000)
Dansha (n=42)	11.9	
Belesa (n=31)	12.9	
G/zuria (n=74)	13.5	
Wogera (n=60)	15	

Table 3. Prevalence based on body condition from November 2016 to May 2017

Body condition	Prevalence (%)	X^2	P- value
Good (n=135)	17		
Medium (n=174)	19.5	6.663	0.036
Poor (n=91)	30.8		

Data management and analysis

All data collected was stored in Microsoft excel spreadsheet for statistical analysis and was analyzed using statically package of social science (SPSS) software version (20.0), to determine the prevalence of cattle fasiolosis and significance of associated risk factors. Association between the variable and the distribution of observed lesion in slaughtered cattle was determined using Chi-square test at critical probability value of $p<0.05$.

RESULTS

Overall prevalence of fasciolosis

As shown in Table 1, A total of 400 cattle were examined for the occurrence of fasciolosis out of which, 85 (21.25%) were found infected with facsiola.

Prevalence cattle fasciolosis based on origin of cattle

Statistical significant differences were recorded among animal origins (X^2 = 57.218 P= 0.000). As denoted by Table 2, the highest prevalence of fasciolosis was obtained from Dembiya (50%) followed by Debarq (31.6%), Wogera (15%), Gondar zuria (13.5%), Belesa (12.9%), Dansha (11.9%) and Metema (4.7%).

Prevalence based on body condition

As indicated by Table 3, poor body conditioned animals were mostly affected by cattle fasiolosis compared to medium and good body conditioned animals and shown a high statistical significant differences (P=0.036).

Prevalence based on age

Young cattle were highly affected (27.7%) by cattle fasciolosis. As presented in Table 4, there was a statistical differences between young and adult cattle (P=0.012).

DISCUSSION

Fasciolosis is an important zoonotic disease that is responsible for a significant loss in food resource and animal productivity (Jaja et al., 2017). Cattle are less

Table 4. Prevalence based on age groups.

Age	Prevalence (%)	X^2	P-value
Adult (n=245)	42(17.1)		
Young (n=155)	43(27.7)	6.373	0.012

susceptible to showing clinical signs of fasciolosis as compared to small ruminants (Stella et al., 2017). Therefore, cattle fasciolosis mainly exhibits as a subclinical chronic disease, associated with hepatic damage and blood loss caused by parasites in the bile ducts (Kaplan, 2001). Hence, cattle fasciolosis is of significant economic importance as the resultant liver condemnations need serious consideration in abattoir industries (Abunna, 2010).

The results of the present study publicized that; origin, body condition and age of the animals have significant effect on the prevalence of cattle fasciolosis. The overall prevalence of bovine fasciolosis (21.25%) in the current study was supported by other abattoir-based studies conducted in different parts of Ethiopia such as Alemu and Mekonnen (2013) (22.14%) from Dangila municipal abattoir, Asressa (2011) (24%) from Andassa livestock research center and Berhe et al. (2009) (24.3%) from Mekelle. In contrast to studies such as Mulat Nega et al. (2012), 29.75% was reported from Gondar Elfora abattoir and Yilma and Mesfin (2000) (90.7%) was conducted in Gondar Municipal abattoir; the overall prevalence record in this study was lower.

In the current study, the variations in prevalence rate which based on the origin of animals were probably due to epidemiological factors such as snail population, as a result of favorable conditions. For instance, the occurrence of bovine fasciolosis in Dembiya was the highest and this might be due to the availability of more appropriate environmental conditions such as watershed areas, slowly flowing waterways and lakes like Lake Tana. These factors will create ideal conditions for the occurrence of fasciola infection.

The statistical significance difference between the age groups in this study might be the fact that, young animals are more susceptible to different disease because of poor immunity development and lack of adaptation (Gebremeskel et al., 2017). In this study, the prevalence rate was higher in poor body conditioned cattle than other body condition scores. Different studies revealed the relationship between body conditions and fasciolosis has shown that there is a positive association between fasciolosis and cattle weight loss (Jaja et al., 2017). It is known that animals in good intensive management systems and with adequate veterinary care should be in better body condition than cattle extensively managed with little veterinary services (Jaja et al., 2017). Therefore, types of management system and veterinary services correlate with cattle fasciolosis.

The direct economic loss due to liver condemnation in Gondar Elfora abattoir was closely related with the earlier records of Bekele et al. (2010) (57,960.00 Ethiopian birr) (ETB)) from Adwa and Bekele et al. (2014) (88,806.85 ETB) from Hosanna. These variations in financial loss due to liver condemnation might be as a result of difference in the prevalence of fasciolosis among different study site, period and price of a liver.

Conclusion

Fasciolosis is one of major problem for livestock development in the study area by inflicting direct economic losses and its occurrence closely linked to the presence of environment suitable to the development of snail intermediate host. As reported by the current study, there was a high cattle fasciolosis in the study area. Statistical significant differences were recorded between the risk factors investigated.

Therefore, based on the findings we recommend integrated approach with a combination of chemotherapy. Vector control should be considered more practically and economically, control strategies targeted on the parasite and the intermediate hosts as well as implementation of appropriate grazing management in the study area are warranted due to, the reduction in the risk of infection by planned grazing management especially during high outbreak months by the application of zero grazing (Cut and carry). Farmers who rear cattle should be aware of how to improve feeds to their animals so that the animal can have good body condition that confers some level of resistance against fasciolosis.

CONFLICT OF INTERESTS

The authors have not declared any conflict of interests.

REFERENCES

Alemu F, Mekonnen A (2013). An Abattoir survey on the prevalence and monetary loss of fasciolosis among cattle, slaughtered at Dangila municipal abattoir, Ethiopia.J. Vet. Med. Anim. Health 6(12):309-316.

Andrews S (1999). The Life Cycle of Fasciola hepatica: Fasciolosis, Dalton, J.P. CABI Publishing. pp. 1-29.

Asressa Y 2011). Study of prevalence of major bovine fluke infection at Andassa livestock research North West Ethiopia, Gondar, Ethiopia.

Bekele C, Sisay M, Mulugeta D (2014). On farm study of bovine fasciolosis in Lemo district and its economic loss due to liver condemnation at Hosanna municipal abattoir, Southern Ethiopia. Int.

J. Curr. Microbiol. Appl. Sci. (4):1122-1132.

Bekele M, Tesfay H, Getachew Y (2010). Bovine Fasciolosis: Prevalence and its economic loss due to liver condemnation at Adwa Municipal Abattoir, North Ethiopia. Ejast 1:39-47.

Berhe G, Kasahun B, Gebrehiwot T (2009). Prevalence and economic significance of fasciolosis in cattle in Mekelle area of Ethiopia. Trop. Anim. Health Prod. 41(7):1503-1504.

Cwiklinski K, O'Neill SM, Donnelly S, and Dalton JP (2016). A prospective view of animal and human Fasciolosis. Parasite Immunol. 38(9):558-568.

Deepak S, Singla LD (2016) Immunodiagnosis Tools for Parasitic Diseases. J. Microbiol. Biochem. Technol. 8:514-518.

Central Statistical Agency (CSA) (2017). Federal democratic republic of Ethiopia Agricultural sample survey 2016/2017. Report on livestock and livestock characteristics (private peasant holdings) volume II. Addis Ababa 585 statistical bulletins.

Fufa A, Asfaw L, Megersa B, Regassa A (2010). Bovine fasciolosis: coprological, abattoir survey and its economic impact due to liver condemnation at Soddo municipal abattoir, Southern Ethiopia. Trop. Anim. Health Prod. 42(2):289-292.

Fürst T, Keiser J, Utzinger J (2012). Global burden of human food-borne trematodiasis: a systematic review and meta-analysis. Lancet Infect. Dis. 12(3):210-221.

Gebremeskel AK, Simeneh ST, Mekuria SA (2017). Prevalence and Associated Risk Factors of Bovine Schistosomiasis in Northwestern Ethiopia. World 7(1):01-04.

Goll PH, Scott JM (1978). The parthenogenesis of domestic animals in Ethiopia (I-2):17.

Gracy J, Collins O, Huey R (1999). Meat hygiene. 10th ed. London: Bailliere Tindal. pp. 220-260.

International Livestock Research Institute (ILRI) (2009). Management of vertisols in Sub-Saharan Africa, Proceedings of a Conference Post-mortem differential parasite counts FAO corporate document repository. Institute of Breeding and Veterinary Medicine of Tropical Countries.

Graber M (1978). Helminths and helminthiases of domestic and wild animals in Ethiopia.

Jaja IF, Mushonga B, Green E, Muchenje V (2017). Seasonal prevalence, body condition score and risk factors of bovine fasciolosis in South Africa. Vet. Anim. Sci. 4:1-7.

Kaplan RM (2001). Fasciola hepatica: a review of the economic impact in cattle and considerations for control. Vet. Ther. 2(1):40-50.

Mas-Coma S, Bargues M, Valero M (2005). Fasciolasis and other plant borne trematodes Zoonoses. Int. J. Parasitol. 35:1255-1278.

Mulat N, Basazinew B, Mersha C, Achenef M, Tewodros F (2012). Comparison of coprological and postmortem examinations techniques for the determination of prevalence and economic significance of bovine fasciolosis. J. Adv. Vet. Res. 2:18-23.

Nicholson M, Butterworth A (1986). A guide to condition scoring of zebu cattle. ILRI (aka ILCA and ILRAD).

Ogunrinade A, Adegoke G (1982). Bovine fasciolosis in Nigeria, inter current parasitic and bacterial infection. J. Trop. Anim. Health Prod. 14:120-125.

Shewangzaw A, Addis K (2016). Faculty of Sheep Production and Marketing System in North Gondar Zone of Amhara Region, Ethiopia. Adv. Biol. Res. 10(5):304-308.

Thrusfield M (2005). Veterinary Epidemiology. 2nd Ed. Blackwell Science Ltd., Oxford, UK. pp.182-198

Tolosa T, Tigre W (2007). The prevalence and economic significance of bovine fasciolosis at Jimma abattoir, Ethiopia. Internet J. Vet. Med. 3(2).

Urquhart G, Amour J, Dunn A, Jennings F (1996). Veterinary Parasitology 2nd Ed oxford: black well publishing. pp. 103-112.

Yilma J, Mesfin A (2000). Dry season bovine fasciolosis in northwestern part of Ethiopia. Revue Méd. Vét. 151(6):493-500.

12

Gastrointestinal nematodes of small ruminants in Guto Gida District, East Wolloega, Ethiopia

Anteneh Wondimu[1*] and Sagni Gutu[2]

Haramaya University College of Veterinary Medicine, P. O. Box 138, Dire Dawa, Ethiopia.

A study by qualitative fecal examination of 384 fecal samples (201 sheep and 183 goats) was conducted from November 2011 to April 2012 with the objective to determine the major gastrointestinal (GIT) nematodes of small ruminants and their prevalence in sheep and goats in Guto Gida District. The study showed that 186 (92.5%) sheep and 150 (81.97%) goats were found to harbor eggs of GIT nematodes. Both sheep and goats were infected with identical parasites species, but with different level of infection. The six genera of nematodes were identified with prevalence of 21.87, 14.87, 12.5, 10.67, 11.19 and 7.29% for *Haemonchus*, *Trichostrongylus*, *Trichuris*, *Oesophagostomum*, *Bunostumum* and *Strongloides*, respectively. There was a significant difference ($p < 0.05$) in the prevalence of GIT nematodes between sex and species of animals but not for different age group. The study showed that GIT nematodes are major problems of small ruminants in the study area. Therefore, comprehensive study on GIT nematodes, cost effective control strategy and awareness creation to the farmers should be instituted in the area.

Key words: Sheep, goats gastrointestinal nematodes, Guto Gida District, Nekemte.

INTRODUCTION

In Ethiopia, helminth infections in ruminants are characteristically chronic and insidious in nature. The parasites attract very little attention, including research funds, when compared with viral, bacterial and some protozoan diseases. This is despite of the fact that they undoubtedly exert a heavy toll on the health and productivity of a vitally important livestock resource with obvious implications for the rural and national economy of the country. Gastro intestinal parasites are a worldwide problem for small and large scale farmers, and their impact is major for sub-Saharan Africa in general and Ethiopia in particular. This is due to the range of agro-ecological factors suitable for diversified host and parasite species (Regassa et al., 2006). Endoparasites are responsible for the deaths of one third of calves, lambs and goat kids, and considerable production losses due to parts of carcasses, being condemned during meat inspection. It is well recognized that in a resource poor country, helminth infections of sheep and goats are factor responsible for economic losses through reductions in productivity (Abunna et al., 2009, Abouzeid et al., 2010). Although helminth parasites of small ruminants are ubiquitous in the climatic zones of Ethiopia where prevailing weather provides favorable conditions for their

*Corresponding author. E-mail: anteneha7@gmail.com.

survival and development, their presence does not mean that they necessarily cause overt disease (Abunna et al., 2009).

Among the diseases that constrain the survival and productivity of sheep and goats, gastrointestinal nematode infection rank highest on the global scales, with *Haemonchus contortus* recognized as a major parasite for both small and large scale small ruminant production (Abunna et al., 2009). These disease have major impact on morbidity and mortality rates with annual losses as high as 30 to 50% of the total value of livestock production of Ethiopia (Abunna et al., 2009). With little inputs, sheep and goats play an important role in rural economy through the provision of meat, milk, blood and cash, accumulating capital, fulfilling cultural obligations, manure and contribution to the national economy through export of live animals meat and skins (Abunna et al., 2009).

The prevalence of gastro intestinal parasite, the genera of helminthes parasites involved species and the severity of infection also vary considerably depending on local environmental and managements practices (Singla 1995; Taylor et al., 2007). Therefore, the distribution and prevalence of the disease should be represented by geographical areas that could roughly correspond to climatic conditions (Regassa et al., 2006). These, information are important in the formulation of parasites control strategies since the degree of infection varies according to the parasites involved and other factors (Urquhart et al., 1996; Wadhawa et al., 2011). Thus, the study was designed to determine the prevalence the major GIT nematodes of sheep and goat in Guto Gida Woreda to recommend the most effective control strategies.

MATERIALS AND METHODS

The study was conducted from November 2011 to April 2012 in Guto Gida District, East Wollega zone, Oromia regional state. It is located in western part of Oromia at latitude of 09° 04′; 957″N, longitude of 36°, 32′, 928″ E and altitude of 2124 m above sea level. It is located at 331 km far from our capital city Addis Ababa. It is annual rainfall range from 1800 to 2200 mm. The maximum temperature is 25°C and the minimum temperature of the area is about 20°C. The area receives long rainy season from June to September and short rainy season from March to May. The area is rich in natural vegetation that comprised of tropical rain forest trees, all grasses and brushes (data obtained from agricultural office).

Study animals and design

A cross-sectional study was conducted on small ruminants of all age and sex category to determine the prevalence of nematodes parasites by collecting fecal samples from individual grazing animals.

Sample size determination

Simple random sampling strategy was followed to collect feces from

individual animals. The sample size was decided based on the formula described by Thrusfield (2005) with 95% confidence interval at 5% desired absolute precision and by assuming the expected prevalence of 50%. The estimated sample size was calculated by the formula:

$$N = \frac{1.96^2 \, Pexp \, (1-pexp)}{d^2} = 384$$

Where N = required sample size; pexp = expected prevalence; d = desired absolute precision.

Parasitological examination

Laboratory diagnosis using flotation, fecal culture and Baermann technique conducted for the identification of the parasite.

Collection of eggs

Faecal pellets collected from the rectum of sheep and goats were placed in small vial. Warm water was slowly added to the faeces and the pellets stirred until a relatively uniform homogenate was obtained and liquid suspension was obtained. The suspension was filtered through sieve with 3 mm aperture. The resulting suspension was again made to pass through a sieve of 150 µm pore size. The suspension was then poured into 15 ml test tubes and centrifuged for 2 min at 377 g and the supernatant was decanted. The tube was agitated by vortex mixer to loosen the sediment. Saturated sodium chloride was then added to the test tube until the meniscus forms above the test tube on which the cover slip was placed. After 3 to 5 min, the cover slip was carefully taken off the tube and put into microscope slide for observation (Bowman, 1999).

Fecal culturing

The method of incubating fecal samples at room temperature to hatch egg to larvae and development to L3 was followed, so that the larvae hatched can be indentified according to the criteria listed as follows: Taking certain amount of feces in a tray; incubating it under suitable moisture content for 14 to 21 days with continuous moistening at an interval of 3 days. The recovery larvae (L3) were studied and identified and the criteria used for identification were based on shape of larvae, head, number and shapes of gut cells, presence or absence of retractile bodies, larvae sheath coverage and length of sheath tail. Then L3 were harvested using Baerman apparatus after 14 days of incubation and were identified (Annon, 2005).

Data management and analysis

The collected sample was entered into Microsoft excel and analyzed using statistical software packages for social science (SPSS). Descriptive statistics like percentage can be used to determine prevalence of GIT nematode and Chi-square (x^2) used to check the association between prevalence of GIT nematodes and risk factors. In the analysis, confidence level was held at 95% and p<0.05 was set for significance.

RESULTS

The overall prevalence of gastro intestinal nematodes

Table 1. Overall prevalence of gastro intestinal nematodes of sheep and goats.

Species	No. of examined animals	No. of positives	Prevalence (%)
Sheep	201	186	92.5
Caprine	183	150	81.79
Total	384	336	87.5

Chi(χ^2) =9.789; Pr = 0.02.

Table 2. Prevalence of gastro intestinal nematodes in sex.

Sex	No. of examined animals	Sex		No. of positive male and female sheep and goats	
		Male	Female	Male	Female
Sheep	201	103	98		
Caprine	183	89	94	161 (83.86%)	175 (91.14)
Total	384	192	192		

Pearson Chi^2(χ^2) = 4.6667; Pr = 0.031.

infection was 87.5% and the species wise is 92.5 and 81.97% in sheep and goats, respectively, which was a significant difference in infection rate between the two animal species (Table 1). Prevalence of gastro intestinal nematodes of infection of sheep and goats on the basis of sex is shown in Table 2. There is statistical significant difference (P<0.05) in prevalence of gastro intestinal nematodes which was 175 (91.15%) and 161 (83.85%) in female and male, respectively. In this study species, sex and age were considered as a risk factors and revealed significant difference (p<0.05) with variation in species, and sex of animals while in the case of age, there is no significant difference (p>0.05) in sheep and goats but there is higher number of young sheep and goats infected than old age group.

In this study, 6 types of gastro intestinal nematodes were identified during the study period based on their morphology described (Urquart et al., 1996). During the study period, fecal samples were cultured to determine genera prevalent as shown in Table 4. *Haemonchus* (21.87%) were the most frequently identified helminthes followed by *Trichostrongylus, Trichuris* with *Strongloides* been the least (7.29%) identified in the study.

DISCUSSION

In the present study, the prevalence of gastro intestinal nematodes was 87.5% (Table 1) in sheep and goats. This result coincides with the result of Gebreyesus (1986) (96.38%) at Ogaden range lands; Esayas (1988) (90.41 and 82.13%) in sheep and goats in and around Wolayita soddo; Tesfalem (1989) (88.1 and 84.32%) in sheep and goats in and around Mekelle; Melkamu (1991) (91.435%) in sheep in and around kombolcha; Bayou (1992) (90.94 and 94.855%) in sheep and goats of Gonder; Yoseph

(1993) (92.23 and 94.1%) in sheep and goats in Mendayo district of Bale; Genene (1994) (93.22 and 92.24%) in sheep and goats of four Awarajas of Eastern shoa; Getachew (1998) (90.23 and 88.3%) in sheep and goats of Buno province of Iluababor; Tefera et al. (2009) (91.32 and 93.295%) in sheep and goats in and around Bedelle, respectively.

Statistically significant difference (p<0.05) (Table 1) was recorded between sheep and goats with relative lower number of goats infected than sheep which may be due to different habits of grazing by these two species of animals. This study also indicates significant different was observed between sex of animals and females are more infected than male (Table 2). Thus, pregnant or lactating ewes/does become the major source of infection for the new born. In some manner, other studies in Africa have shown that the age and immune status of the host animals have significant influences on the GIT eggs pus (Magona and Musis, 2002). On the contrary, there was no statistical significant difference (p>0.05) recorded in this study between young and adult but relatively higher number of young animals are infected than older once (Table 3). This could be due to equal exposure of both age groups of animals and they are from similar agro-ecological area.

The prevalence of *Haemonchus* species was 21. 87% (Table 4) in sheep and goats in the study area which disagreed with the work of different scholars: Ahmed (1988) (88.23% prevalence in East Wollega zone); Kumsa and Wossene (2006) (95.1% in ogaden region); Naod et al. (2006) (81.18% in Awassa in Hawassa in sheep and goats). The prevalence of *Trichostrongylus* species was 14.8% in sheep and goats. This result is disagreed with Abunna et al. (2009) who reported prevalence of 90.45% in sheep and goats; Tefera et al. (2009) (43.5 and 55% in sheep and goats in and around

Table 3. Prevalence of gastro intestinal nematodes in different age groups.

Age	Results	
	Positive (%)	Negative (%)
Adult	157 (86.74)	24 (13.26)
Young	179 (88.18)	24 (11.82)

Pearson Chi^2(χ^2) = 0.1807; Pr = 0.671.

Table 4. Relative percentage of parasite identified in sheep and goats.

Species of parasites	Frequency	Percentage
Haemonchus species	84	21.87
Trichuris species	48	412.5
Trichostrongylus species	57	14.8
Oesophagostomum species	41	10.67
Bunostomum species	32	8.33
Strongloides species	28	7.29

Bedelle). But, this study is consistent with the finding reported by Sissay et al. (2007), where *Haemonchus contrortus* was the most prevalent parasites of GIN; this could be associated partly with breed susceptibility, biological plasticity and high environmental adaptability.

The prevalence of *Strongloides* species was detected to be 7.49% in sheep and goats in the study area and this is in line with the work of Tefera et al. (2009) (13.04%) in sheep and 20% in goats in Bedelle and the prevalence of *Bunostomum* species was detected to be 8.33% in sheep and goats in the study area and this was in disagreement Tefera et al. (2009) (26.1 and 35% in sheep and goats in and around Bedelle). This difference in the prevalence of parasite in different area might be attributed to the difference in breed of sheep and goats and different agro-ecological zones where the animals are kept.

Conclusion and recommendation

The result of present study showed the high prevalence rate of gastro intestinal nematodes infection in small ruminants in Guto Gida District, East Wolloega. There was highly significant difference in infection level on the basis of sex and species. This shows that the general scientific facts on those bases can be recognized in the study area and the traditional husbandry and animal management have also valuable contribution in the detection of gastro intestinal nematodes. The existence of these parasites has an impact on the productivity and can hamper the sustainability of the revenue generated from small ruminant production by small holder society of East Wollega zone. Therefore, based on the result

obtained the following recommendation are forwarded:

1. To get clear epidemiological picture of GIN parasites, comprehensive study should be launched in the area.
2. Effective utilization of available of feed resource such as agricultural by products, natural pasture and appropriate nutritional supplements program for young and lactating animals.
3. Detail study should be conducted to identify the parasite using more sensitive and specific methods such as postmortem examination.
4. Strategic nematode control practice should be implemented.
5. Field veterinarian should be aware of the importance and burden of GIN in sheep and goats.

CONFLICT OF INTERESTS

The authors declare that they have no conflict of interest.

REFERENCES

Abouzied N, Saalium AM, Heady KEL (2010). The prevalence of gastro intestinal parasite infection sheep zoo garden and sinai district and study the efficacy of ant helminthic drugs in treatment of these parasites. Faculty of veterinary medicine zagazing university, Egypt.

Abunna F, Tsedeke E, Kumsa B, Megersa B, Regessa A, Debala E (2009). Abomsal nematode: prevalence in small ruminants slaughtered at Bishoftu town, Ethiopia. Int. J. Vet. Med. 7:1.

Ahmed N (1988). Prevalence of GIT helminthes and the comparative efficiency test of nematocidal drugs in goats of Wollega administrative region at mechara settlement area. DVM. Thesis Addis Ababa University Faculty of veterinary medicine Ethiopia.

Annon (2005). Small ruminants research strategy. Ethiopian agricultural research organization (EARO), animal science research directorate, Addis Ababa, Ethiopia.

Bayou A (1992). Prevalence of gastro intestinal helminthes of small ruminants in Buno provine Ilubabor administrative region. DVM Thesis Addis Ababa University Faculty of veterinary medicine Ethiopia.

Bowman DD (1999). Georgies parasitology for veterinarians, 7th ed. W.B. Sconders, Philadelphia.

Esayas T (1988). Study on prevalence of GIT helminthes in Ogaden goats. DVM thesis, Faculty of veterinary medicine, Addis Ababa University, Ethiopia.

Gebreyesus M (1986). Prevalence of gastro intestinal helminthes of small ruminants (sheep and goats) in Gonder administrative region. DVM. Thesis, Faculty of veterinary medicine, Addis Ababa, Ethiopia.

Genene R (1994). A study on prevalence of ovine GIT helminthes in and around kombolcha. DVM. Thesis, Faculty of veterinary medicine, Addis Ababa University Ethiopia.

Getachew G (1998). Prevalence of ovine and caprine GIT helminthes in mekelle and its surrounding. DVM Thesis, Faculty of veterinary medicine, Addis Ababa University, Ethiopia.

Kumsa B, Wossene A (2006). Abomsal nematodes of small ruminants of ogaden region, Eastern Ethiopia, prevalence, worm burden and species composition. Revue Med.Vet. 157:12:27-32.

Magona JW, Musis G (2002). Influence of age, grazing system, season and agro climatic zones on the prevalence and intensity of gastro intestinal strongloides in Uganda goats. Small Ruminates Res. 44:285-290

Melkamu T (1991). Prevalence of gastro intestinal helminthes of small ruiminants in four awrajas of Eastern shoa administrative regions, DVM, thesis, AAU, Debrezeit, Ethiopia.

Naod T, Teshale S, Bersisa K (2006). Prevalence of abomsal nematodes and dicytocaulus filarial of sheep and goats slaughtered in Awassa restaurant. AAU, FVM, Ethiopia.

Regassa F, Sori T, Dhuguma R, Kassa Y (2006). Epidemiology of gastro intestinal parasite of Ruminants in Western Oromia, Ethiopia. Int. J. Appl. Res. Vet. Med. 4(1):51.

Singla LD (1995). A note on sub-clinical gastro-intestinal parasitism in sheep and goats in Ludhiana and Faridkot districts of Punjab. Indian. Vet. Med. J. 19:61-62.

Sissay MM, Uggla A, Waller PJ (2007). Epidemiology and seasonal dynamics of gastrointestinal nematode infections of sheep in a semi-arid region of eastern Ethiopia. J. Vet. Parasitol. 143:311-321

Taylor MA, Coop RL, Wall RL (2007). Veterinary Parasitology 3rd ed UK; Black well science.

Tefera M, Batu G, Bitew M (2009). Prevalence of gastro intestinal parasite of sheep and goat in and around Bedele, south Western Ethiopia. Internet J. Vet. Med. 8:2.

Tesfalem T (1989). Prevalence of GIT helminthes of small ruminants in mendayo province Bale administrative region, Ethiopia, DVM thesis AAU, Ethiopia.

Thrusfield M (2005). Veterinary Epidemiology 3rd edition, UK, Black well science.

Urquhart GM, Armour J, Duncan JL, Dunn AM, Jenning FW (1996). Veterinary Parasitology, 2nd, Black well. Science, UK. P 307.

Wadhawa A, Tanwar RK, Singla LD, Eda S, Kumar N, Kumar Y (2011) Prevalence of gastrointestinal helminths in cattle and buffaloes in Bikaner, Rajasthan, Indian. Vet. World 4(9):417-419.

Yoseph S (1993). Prevalence of ovine GI helminthes in and around Asella, Ethiopia. DVM thesis, AAU, Ethiopia.

13

Telediagnosis: Parasitological experiences in wild ruminants of South African preserves

Gianluca Pio Zaffarano[1], Benedetto Morandi[1*], Alessia Menegotto[2], Fabio Ostanello[1] and Giovanni Poglayen[1]

[1]Department of Veterinary Medical Sciences, University of Bologna, Ozzano dell'Emilia (BO), Italy.
[2]Conservation Global Agency for Environmental Gain npc, Company # 2010/018132/08, P.O. Box 2791, Knysna 6570, Garden Route, South Africa.

A survey on wild ruminants' health status of any South African preserves was attempted, assessing body condition score (BCS) through tele-diagnosis. The wildlife BCS was linked to the presence of gastrointestinal parasites that should be recognized, counted and statistically evaluated. For this purpose, we examined 103 faecal samples of wild ruminants from 6 South African preserves. For practical reasons, the animals were divided into two macro-categories: small and large ruminants. The results obtained showed a prevalence of 78.1 and 15.6% in large ruminants for gastrointestinal strongyles (GIS) and coccidian, respectively, while small ruminants showed 92.3% due to GIS and 30.8% for coccidia. No statistically significant difference in the prevalence among the preserves was detected; on the other hand, a low value of BCS corresponds to a greater presence of parasites with statistics difference in the macro-categories (small ruminant x^2=5.238; P=0.020; large ruminant x^2= 15.215; P<0.001) and sex classes (male x^2=5.409; P=0.020; female x^2 =17.350; P<0.001). For these reasons, our results provide a practical feedback for the management preserves. The present paper is fully part of the limited experiences of telediagnosis in a conservation perspective. Based on the results obtained, we decided to organize a project that could limit and assess the risk factors in the management of these activities in the South African context.

Key words: Wild ruminants, telediagnosis, parasites, body condition scores, South African preserves.

INTRODUCTION

In recent past, Veterinary Medicine has focused its interest on involving wild animals not only as single head fenced in captivity and therefore clinically similar to domestic one, but also as free-living populations. All these are meant to protect biodiversity and curtail the possible spread of pathogens, and zoonotic diseases. These preliminary considerations suggest transferring the clinical approach proposed by Bologna Academy (Messieri and Moretti, 1982) and more recently by Cambridge Academy (Jackson and Cockcroft, 2002),

*Corresponding author. E-mail: benedetto.morandi2@unibo.it.

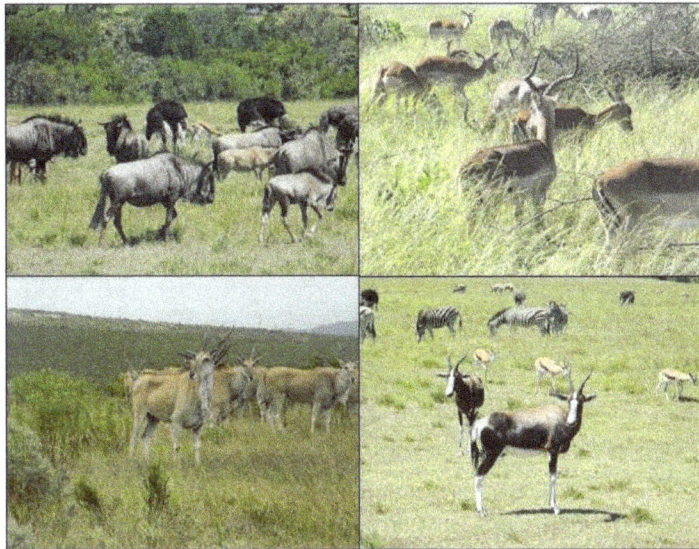

Figure 1. Images of animals and environments in the South African preserves investigated.

simplifying and adapting them to wild ruminants in game preserves of South Africa. These are wild farms suitable for the conservation, including breeding of species of local wildlife particularly valuable, from economic, touristic or endangered point of view. Their management is quite particular: wild ruminants are fenced on many hectares of land and continuously exchanged with other preserves. Considering that from this wild farm parasitological information are lacking and also domestic ruminants are raised close to wild ones, we suggested transferring the clinical approach cited adapting them to wild ruminants by a visual system for scoring body condition (telediagnosis). In the international literature, we have found four specific papers of this non-invasive method to define health status: two in Asian Elephants (*Elephas maximus* L., 1758) (Ramesh et al., 2011; Wijeyamohan et al., 2015) and two on wild ruminants, in particular Bassano et al. (2003) on *Ovis canadensis* (Shaw, 1804) and *Capra ibex* (L., 1758) and Pfeifer (2015) *Cervus elaphus* (L., 1758).

The aim of this study was to survey the health status of wild ruminants by telediagnosis. This was evaluated by scoring body condition. Body condition score (BCS) is a subjective tool to assess the amount of metabolizable energy stored in body fat (primarily subcutaneous) and muscle tissues of a live animal (Edmonson et al., 1989; Burkholder, 2000; Alapati et al., 2010). Body condition is an index of an animal's health (Terranova and Coffman, 1997). An increase or decrease in body condition could mean a change in quality of management or environment in which an animal lives (Figure 1).

The wildlife BCS should be linked to the presence of gastrointestinal parasites that should may be recognized, counted and statistically evaluated.

These described assumptions have had to adapt to the preserves logistical and laboratory requirements provided. Another purpose to study the parasitism of wild ruminants should be to help their management by rangers.

MATERIALS AND METHODS

Study area

Our survey was done in 6 preserves in the Eastern region of Garden Route, Republic of Sud Africa (Figure 2) during February 2016. The area has soil and weather characteristics that allow arid lands mixed with wetlands, characterized by particular kind of bush (named fynbos), especially suitable for game preserve activity aimed to the conservation of autochthonous flora and fauna.

Animals

Overall, we have had the opportunity to work with 103 animals belonging to 15 different ruminant species (Table 1). The adjustment of the clinical procedures applied to domestic animals provides general appearance and physical examination, excluding the medical history, since in wildlife it is impossible to know the history of individuals. The animals were identified through an optical instrument (field glass Olympus 10X50) at dropping time, later they were photographed and then classified according to sex (male, female) and category (small or large ruminants). The sex was determined in 102 animals, 34 males and 68 females, in one instance it was not possible because it was a very young individual and hidden from the herd. BCS was evaluated analysing the ribs, spine, hip bone/rump, tail head and belly, according to the method described by Pfeifer (2015). Randomly, the classification was simplified by grouping the animals into two main categories: emaciated/medium and good/excellent. Faecal samples were collected off the ground, marked with a serial number, scientific and common names of the species. Collected samples were stored in a

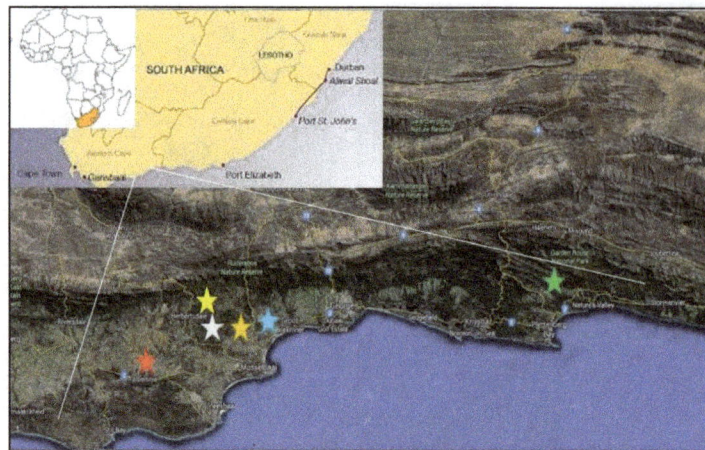

Figure 2. Study area with the six investigated preserves: red star (Garden Route, 34°12'31"S; 21°38'00"E), white (Wolwedans, 34°01'48"S; 21°59'40"E), yellow (Gondwana, 34°04'51"S; 21°54'40"E), orange (Hartenbos, 34°02'41"S; 21°59'41"E), light blue (Bergsig, 34°05'32"S; 22°02'06"E) and green (Plettenberg, 33°56'43"S; 23°21'00"E).

Table 1. Animal species and categories considered.

Category	Species	Number
Large ruminant	Giraffe (*Giraffa camelopardalis* L., 1758)	9
	Blu Wildebeest (*Connochaetes taurinus* Lichtenstein, 1812)	10
	Waterbuck (*Kobus ellipsiprymnus* Ogilby, 1833)	3
	Orix (*Oryx gazzella* L., 1758)	3
	Eland (*Taurotragus oryx* Pallas, 1766)	20
	Buffalo (*Syncerus caffer* Sparrman, 1779)	7
	Kudu (*Tragelaphus strepsiceros* Pallas, 1766)	2
	Sable Antelope (*Hippotragus niger* Harris, 1838)	7
	Black Wildebeest (*Cannochaetes gnou* Zimmermann, 1780)	3
	Total large ruminant	64
Small ruminant	Bontebok (*Damaliscus pygargus* Pallas, 1767)	11
	Gray rhebok (*Pelea capreolus* Forster, 1790)	1
	Red Hartebeest (*Alcelaphus buselaphus* Pallas, 1766)	4
	Impala (*Aepyceros melampus* Lichtenstein, 1812)	16
	Springbok (*Antidorcas marsupialis* Zimmermann, 1780)	6
	Blesbuck (*Damaliscus pygargus phillips* Harper, 1939)	1
	Total small ruminant	39
	Total	103

cooler, transported in a few hours in a refrigerator (+ 4°C), and then in the laboratory examined.

Examined samples

Stool samples were referred for qualitative and quantitative coprological evaluation. It was realized with an alternative tool that stocks parasitic forms without centrifugal step (Mini- FLOTAC, Silva et al., 2013; Godber et al., 2015), using a floatation solution (specific gravity 1.3).

Statistical analysis

The study of prevalence for coccidia and gastrointestinal strongyles

(GIS) was evaluated by comparing the sampling area, sex, and category (small or large ruminants) using chi-square test (χ^2). All statistical analyses were performed using the software SPSS 23.0 (IBM SPSS Statistics, New York, United States).

RESULTS AND DISCUSSION

Qualitative results

Overall, 86 of 103 (83.5%) analysed faecal samples were positive for parasites. Specifically, 86 samples were positive for gastrointestinal strongyles (GIS); and 22

Table 2. Relationship between the four macro-categories considered.

Ruminant	GIS (Prevalence%)	Coccidia (Prevalence%)
Large ruminant	50/64 (78.1%)	10/64 (15.6%)
Small ruminant	36/39 (92.3%)	12/39 (30.8%)

Table 3. Prevalence of the two different parasites categories in the investigated preserves.

Game preserve visited (animals sampled)	GIS (Prevalence %)	Coccidia (Prevalence %)
Bergsig (14)	12 (85.7%)	3 (21.4%)
Garden Route (29)	26 (89.7%)	8 (27.6%)
Gondwana (35)	29 (82.9%)	6 (17.1%)
Hartenbos (9)	7 (77.8%)	Not found
Plettenberg (8)	7 (87.5%)	3 (37.5%)
Wolwedans (8)	5 (62.5%)	2 (25.0%)

Table 4. Statistically significant differences between animal categories related to BCS.

Animal categories	Emaciated/Medium (%)	Good/ Excellent (%)	
Small Ruminant	31 (96.9%)	5 (71.4%)	X^2=5.238; P=0.020
Large Ruminant	33 (97.1%)	17 (56.7%)	X^2= 15.215; P<0.001
Total	64 (97%)	22 (59.5%)	X^2=24.207; P<0.001

Table 5. Statistically significant differences between sex related to BCS.

Sex	Emaciated/Medium (%)	Good/Excellent (%)	
Male	14 (93.3%)	11 (57.9%)	X^2=5.409; P=0.020
Female	49 (98.0%)	11 (61.1%)	X^2=17.350; P<0.001
Total	63 (96.9%)	22 (59.5%)	X^2=23.827; P<0.001

(21.85%) of these were also positive for oocysts of coccidia. Two samples tested positive for whipworm and tapeworm eggs respectively (0.97%). Parasites prevalence was not statistically different (P>0.05) between small ruminants and large ruminants (Table 2).

Statistically significant difference in the prevalence among the preserves was not detected (Table 3). However, there was a lower prevalence, albeit without statistical significance, of GIS in Wolwedans and lack of coccidia in Hartenbos. Even between sexes the parasitism seems to be equal.

Quantitative results

If we take into account the quantitative results, positivity at least one parasite (egg/oocyst), a statistically significant difference emerges for BCS levels and sex (Tables 4 and 5). In one head only positive for GIS we observed diarrhoea.

The lack of previous surveys, the preserves management characteristics and the logistic difficulties led as to modify our initial project. This resulted during data elaboration to consider only the macro categories of ruminants (large and small) and other parasites (GIS and coccidia). For this purpose, it was particularly useful having available a diagnostic tool that allowed a field activity. Both macro categories created reflect the reality of the hosts/parasite/environment situation in the surveyed areas. The absence of the lower category of BCS supports the hypothesis of a natural predation by carnivore. Despite this simplification, our experience allows validating some results by the statistic help, which excludes the results randomness.

Also without the statistic help, the two parasites categories' prevalence in large and small ruminants was higher anyway. This outcome should be justified in that large African ruminants like diet of trees and bushes that do not favor oro-faecal transmission cycle, characteristic of gastrointestinal parasites. According to the preserves' situation, the different parasites' prevalence could depend on Wolwedans in that it is organized like a true breeding unit (few hectares and small yards) with all characteristics management procedures, while the particularly dried environment of Hartenbos could limit the coccidian transmission that needs humidity to reach the infectivity stages. We did not find prevalence differences between sexes, but this was evident in both categories when related to BCS linked parasite prevalence both for GIS and coccidia. The presence of these parasites is significantly associated in both sexes. This data appear particular interesting for the characteristics of the preserves studied; one could benefit from the information relative to the crucial influence of parasites and BCS being able to hypothesize specific control activities.

Conclusion

For this reason, our results although limited in numbers and of simplified approach could have a practical feedback for the preserves management. In fact, if a bad BCS is related to the higher parasites presence same animals should be treated avoiding its loss and at the same time not interfere with the natural distribution of the parasites (Wilson et al., 2002). For a practical purpose, the animals that could benefit from treatment could be those fenced in small pens or captured for transport.

Future updating should reduce the two macro categories correctly recognising the host species and identify parasites found in dead animals. In this regard, it is extremely interesting the experience carried out in the Limpopo National Park (South Africa) by Van Wyk and Boomker, (2011) where it was possible to isolate and identify the parasites species and the conclusions refer to the importance of parasites in the transfer animal, well known at our latitudes (Lanfranchi et al., 2003).

The present paper is full part of the limited experiences of telediagnosis in a conservation perspective. Based on the results obtained, we decided to organize a project that could limit and assess the risk factors in the management of these activities in the South African context.

CONFLICT OF INTERESTS

The authors have not declared any conflict of interests.

ACKNOWLEDGEMENT

The authors would like to thank Natalie Bellet for English language revision.

REFERENCES

Alapati A, Kapa SR, Jeepalyam S, Rangappa SM, Yemireddy KR (2010). Development of the body condition score system in Murrah buffaloes: validation through ultrasonic assessment of body fat reserves. J. Vet. Sci. 11:1-8.

Bassano B, Von Hardenberg A, Pelletier F, Gobbi G (2003). A method to weigh free-ranging ungulates without handling. Wildl. Soc. Bull. 31:1205-1209.

Burkholder WJ (2000). Use of body condition scores in clinical assessment of the provision of optimal nutrition. J. Am. Vet. Med. Assoc. 217:650-654.

Edmonson AJ, Lean IJ, Weaver LD, Farver T, Webster G (1989). A body condition scoring chart for holstein dairy cows. J. Dairy Sci. 72:68-78.

Godber OF, Phythian CJ, Bosco A, Ianniello D, Coles G, Rinaldi L, Cringoli G (2015). A comparison of the FECPAK and Mini-FLOTAC faecal egg counting techniques. Vet. Parasitol. 207:342-345.

Jackson PGG, Cockcroft PD (2002). Clinical examination of farm animals Blackwell Science Ltd, Oxford.

Lanfranchi P, Ferroglio E, Poglayen G, Guberti V (2003). Wildlife Veterinarian, Conservation and Public Health. Vet. Res. Comm. 27:567-574.

Messieri A, Moretti B (1982). Semiologia e Diagnostica medica Veterinaria Libreria Universitaria L. Tinarelli Bologna. (In Italian).

Pfeifer A (2015). Differences in Body Condition of Elk, Cervus elaphus by Location in Yellowstone's Northern Range' Poster produced by University of Washington School of Environmental & Forest Sciences.

Ramesh T, Sankar K, Quereshi Q, Kalle R (2011). Assessment of Wild Asiatic Elephant (Elephas maximus indicus) Body Condition by Simple Scoring Method in a Tropical Deciduous Forest of Western Ghats, Southern India. Wildlife Biol. Pract. 7:47-54.

Silva MR, Vila-Vicosa MJM, Maurelli MP, Morgoglione ME, Cortes HCE, Cringoli G, Rinaldi L (2013). Mini-FLOTAC for the diagnosis of Eimeria infection in goats: An alternative to McMaster. Small Rumin. Res. 114:280-283.

Terranova CJ, Coffma BS, (1997) Body weight of wild and captive lemurs. Zoo Biol.16:17-30.

Van Wyk IC, Boomker J (2011) Parasites of South African wildlife. XIX. The prevalence of helminths in some common antelopes, warthogs and a bushpig in the Limpopo province, South Africa. Onderstepoort J. Vet. Res. 78(1):1-11.

Wijeyamohan S, Treiber K, Schmitt D, Santiapillai C (2015) A Visual System for Scoring Body Condition of Asian Elephants (Elephas maximus) Zoo Biol. 34:53-59.

Wilson K, Bjornstad ON, Dobson AP, Merler S, Poglayen G, Randolph SE, Read AF, Skorping A (2002). Heterogeneities in macroparasite infectious: patterns and processes. in Hudson PJ, Rizzoli A, Grenfell BT, Heesterbeek H, Dobson AP (eds), "The Ecology of Wildlife Disease", Oxford University Press.

14

Observations of oxytetracycline treatment effects in a contagious bovine pleuropneumonia naturally infected herd in Zambia

Geoffrey Munkombwe Muuka*, Ana Songolo, Swithine Kabilika, Harvey Sikwese, Benson Bowa and Obrien Kabunda

Ministry of Fisheries and Livestock, Central Veterinary Research Institute, Lusaka, Zambia.

An observational study on the effects of oxytetracycline treatment on contagious bovine pleuropneumonia in a naturally infected herd of 500 cattle was conducted. A total of 68 cattle that showed pneumonia-like clinical signs were treated. Treatment was effected the moment an animal showed signs of illness. A total of 429 cattle were slaughtered after diagnosis of contagious bovine pleuropneumonia and at slaughter, 40.8% (175) had lesions compared to 59.2% (254) that did not have lesions. Out of the total cattle that were treated with oxytetracycline, 57.4% (39) died from contagious bovine pleuropneumonia over a period of 9 weeks while 42.6% (29) survived. Of the treatment group that survived, 37.9% (11) had fibrous lesions indicative of healing, while 62.1% (18) had pathological lesions consistent of active contagious bovine pleuropneumonia (CBPP). Categorisation of carcases with pathological lesions within the treatment group showed 66.7% (12) and 33.3% (6) of acute and chronic lesions, respectively. The CBPP causative agent was isolated through culture and confirmed using polymerase chain reaction (PCR). The results obtained suggest that oxytetracycline did not stop the spread or death of cattle in this particular herd with the treatment of a proportion of the herd. However, large scale field trials are needed in order to validate these findings. It is therefore recommended that any antibiotic that will be developed and advocated for use in the treatment of contagious bovine pleuropneumonia should be effective to contain spread within the herd by treating only a proportion showing signs of the disease.

Key words: Contagious bovine pleuropneumonia, antibiotics, lung, lesions, oxytetracyline, treatmen, Zambia.

INTRODUCTION

Contagious bovine pleuropneumonia (CBPP) is a highly infectious disease of cattle caused by a mollicute bacteria *Mycoplasma mycoides* subspecies *mycoides* (*Mmm*) and is characterised by severe fibrinous exudative pneumonia (OIE, 2010; Provost et al., 1987). The disease has been recognised as a major hindrance to increased livestock

*Corresponding author. E-mail: geoffreymuuka@yahoo.co.uk.

production in sub-Saharan Africa causing great economic losses due to cattle mortality and morbidity leading to weakness, emaciation, reduced work ability and reduced fertility in affected herds (Amanfu, 2009). Tambi et al. (2006) described the economic importance due to the high financial and economic losses the disease causes to cattle owners and nations, the associated socio-economic implications of these losses and the economic wide impacts (resulting from reduced export earnings and a decline in economic activity in those industries that depend on cattle and their products).

Although CBPP has been successfully controlled in most developed countries (Scacchia et al., 2011), it has continued to spread and affect new areas in sub-Saharan Africa. The disease in Africa is complicated by the uncontrolled movement of cattle and the availability of chronic carriers that have been implicated in the perpetuation of the disease (Masiga et al., 1986).

The main control method that has been adopted by most countries in sub-Saharan Africa is vaccination using an attenuated live T1/44 vaccine strain. The vaccine confers a short immunity requiring booster vaccinations annually and can also revert to pathogenicity at the injection site that can cause death if not treated with antibiotics (Thiaucourt et al., 2007).

Alternative control of CBPP using antibiotics has officially been discouraged although it has been shown that it is widely practised in many African countries (Mariner and Catley, 2004). Mitchell et al. (2012) have demonstrated the effectiveness of oxytetracycline, danofloxacin and tulathromycin in biological matrices as well as artificial media in inhibiting the growth of Mmm, the causative agent of CBPP and suggested the possible use of the three in the treatment of CBPP. Provost et al. (1987) reported that the use of antibiotics may alleviate the clinical signs but would not inhibit the spread of the disease. Studies by Yaya et al. (2004) showed that in an experimental infection, oxytetracycline was able to reduce the losses due to CBPP but could not prevent the persistence of viable Mmm in the treated animals suggesting that treated animals could still spread the disease to susceptible animals. However, in similar studies of naturally infected cattle, Huebschle et al. (2006) reported success in reducing spread of the disease in a trial using danofloxacin, but failed to reduce clinical effects. In an investigation by Niang et al (2010), it was reported that oxytetracycline failed to induce sequestra formation under experimental conditions demonstrating the probability of cure and not the evolution of the disease to chronicity to the treated group. Nicholas et al. (2012) reported success in treatment and prevention of CBPP spread using danofloxacin in naturally infected herds in Caprivi Strip of Northern Namibia.

In FAO meeting of 2002 in Ghana, the effectiveness of antibiotic therapy was put to scrutiny and it was advocated that further research should be carried out to arrive at informed decisions concerning the use of antibiotics in the treatment of CBPP (FAO, 2003). This paper highlights the failure of long-acting oxytetracyclinein reducing the clinical lesions in individual cattle and in halting the spread of CBPP within a herd of naturally infected cattle that were in quarantine.

MATERIALS AND METHODS

Study site

The study was limited to a commercial farm located in the Copper belt Province of Zambia. The farm is mainly a crop farming enterprise that was diversifying into cattle ranching. The farm imported a 500 herd of cattle from Tanzania as its start-up herd. The cattle under study were the only ones on the premises. The farm is triple fenced with a barbed wire, game fence and an electric fence all around its perimeter. It has additional fences within the farm to divide various areas for different activities.

Study cattle

The study was restricted to heifers that were imported from Tanzania and were in quarantine at the time of the study. The age range of the cattle was from 3 to 18 months.

History of illness and treatment

According to the available records, on the fourth day after arrival, 3 of the heifers died after showing difficulties in breathing. A post-mortem was conducted and lung samples showing pneumonic signs were collected, placed in the mobile car freezer with a temperature of -20°C and submitted to the laboratory. They were not processed as the preservation in transit was not good for bacteriological assessment. However, a tentative diagnosis of Pasteurellosis was made in view of the long distance (over 2,800 km) that the heifers covered. Consequently, medication with oxytetracycline was instituted for those heifers showing respiratory discomfort and thereafter those that develop these signs. This led to a total of 13.6% (68) of the herd being treated. A dosage of 20 mg/kg per day (1 ml/10 kg body mass) was given for five days to each of the sick heifers. The sick cattle were not separated from the herd after institution of treatment. Over a 3 month period, 39 of the treated heifers died. The diagnosis of CBPP was only made 112 days after the initial deaths and by then, 92 were showing overt clinical disease characterised by coughing, dyspnoea, polypnoea, and nasal discharge. On running, these signs were accentuated.

Slaughter and collection of samples from the herd

After confirmation of CBPP on serology using CFT (OIE, 2010) and c-ELISA (Le Goff and Thiaucourt, 1998), the herd was ear marked for slaughter.

Pathology/post-mortem

All the cattle that had remained (n=429) were subjected to post-mortem upon slaughter. On the slaughter line, all the animals were identified according to the mark on the ear tagand thus treated and untreated individuals were recognised. Tissue samples that included lungs, lymph nodes and pleural fluid were collected from

Observations of oxytetracycline treatment effects in a contagious bovine pleuropneumonia naturally infected herd in Zambia

83

Table 1. Various stages of infection in oxytetracycline treated and untreated cattle.

Description	% (n)
Total cattle imported	500
Herd size on slaughter	429
Total mortality	14.0(60)
Untreated	86.4(432)
Treated	13.6(68)
Treated but died	57.4(39)
Treated survived	42.6(29)
Total with lesions at slaughter	40.8(175)
Lesions from treated	16.6(29)
Lesions untreated	83.4(146)
Total acute	52.0(91)
Acute from treated	6.6(6)
Acute from untreated	81.3(74)
Total chronic	52.0(91)
Chronic from treated	6.6(6)
Chronic from untreated	81.3(74)
Total fibrotic lesions	13.7(24)
Fibrotic lesions from treated	45.8(11)
Fibrotic lesions from untreated	52.2(13)
Total treated with active lesions	62.1(18)
Acute of active lesions	66.7(12)
Chronic of active lesions	33.3(6)
Fibrotic lesions treated	37.9(11)
Total untreated with active lesions	91.1(133)
Acute of untreated active lesions	44.4(59)
Chronic of untreated active lesions	55.6(74)
Fibrotic lesions untreated	8.9(13)
Total without lesions at slaughter	59.2(254)

both groups and stored at -20°C until analysis.

Culture and PCR of isolates

A total of 20 tissue samples from both the treated (10) and untreated groups (10) were cultured in PPLO broth and agar medium (Himedia® India) containing 20% Horse serum as described by Razinand Freundt (1984) for 10 days.

DNA was extracted from the broth cultures of *Mmm* and purified using the Maxwell ® DNA purification kit following the manufacturer's instructions. They were subjected to PCR and then restriction enzyme digestion using *AsnI* as described by Bashiruddin et al. (1994), (Figure 1).

RESULTS

Of the total that were treated, 57.4% (n=39) died with CBPP symptoms before the decision to slaughter the

whole herd was made while 42.6% (n=29) survived until the whole herd was slaughtered (Table 1).

A total of 429 cattle were slaughtered and on post-mortem examination of all the carcasses, 40.8% (n=175) had lesions of various stages of disease progression while 59.2% (n=254) did not have any lesions. Of those with lesions, 16.6% (n=29) were those from the treated group while 83.4% (n=146) were of the untreated cattle. There was 13.7% (n=24) carcases with fibrotic lesions with indications of healing. Of these 45.8% (n=11) were from the treated group while 52.2% (n=13) were from the untreated group. When the carcasses with lesions and those showing signs of recovery were compared in the treated group, it was found that 37.9% (n=11) had lesions in the lungs showing signs of recovery, while 62.1% (n=18) had classical lesions of clinical CBPP. Those from the untreated group showed 8.9% (n=13) with signs of lesions of CBPP. When the carcasses with classical

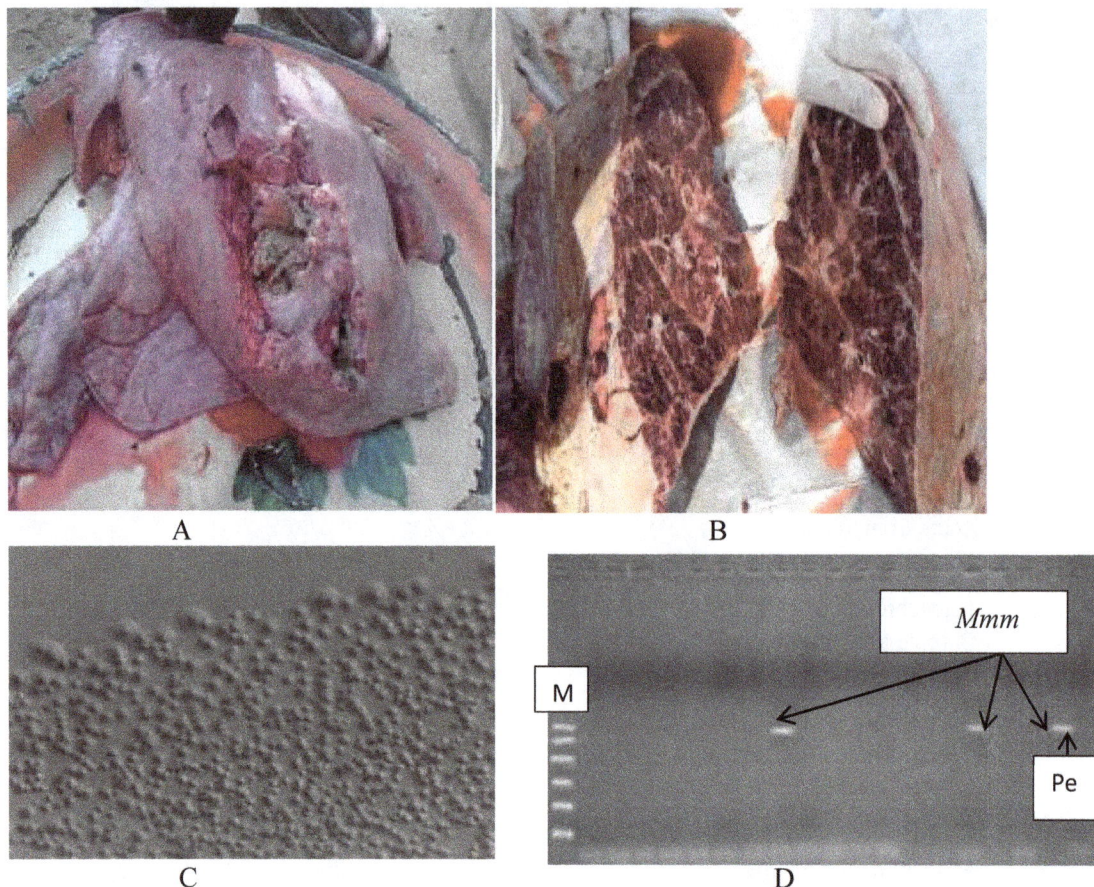

Figure 1. (A) Sequestra in one of the animals; (B) Lesions with typical marbling and consolidation characterstic of acute CBPP in one of the animals; (C) Colonies of *Mycoplasma mycoides* subsp. *Mycoides* as obtained on a plate X 3.2; (D) Gel electrophoresis results from PCR products of samples showing, the 574 bpamplicons of *Mmm* obtained using the Bashirrudin et al. (1994) method. M = Molecular weight markers, *Mmm* at 574 bp; and Pe = T1/44 positive control (*Mmm*) at 574 bp.

healing compared to 91.1% (n=133) that had classical lesions from the treated group were further examined, it was observed that 66.7% (n=12) had lesions in the acute phase of CBPP with typical marbled appearance of the lung, various degrees of adhesion to the pleural wall and copious pleural fluid, while 33.3% (n=6) had chronic lesions with sequestra of various sizes. Those from the untreated group showed 44.4% (n=59) in the acute phase of the disease while 55.6% (n=74) had lesions in the chronic phase of the disease.

DISCUSSION

Treatment of cattle infected with CBPP has long raised controversy due to the non-availability of adequate information on the repercussions of such interventions. This study has demonstrated the failure of oxytetracycline therapy in abetting clinical CBPP in a naturally infected herd where only cattle with clinical signs were treated. The proportion of cattle that was treated with the antibiotic

was 13.6% (68) of the whole herd. Considering the population (500) at risk when clinical signs were noticed, this is too low for an infectious disease as CBPP. This augments the point by OIE (2012) which states that in a CBPP infection, the whole herd will need to be treated with antibiotics in order to achieve recovery. Indeed the cost implication of treating the whole herd in such a situation would be very costly and prohibitive to the peasant farmers who are usually the victims of CBPP in sub-Saharan Africa.

The animals were in quarantine from the time they arrived in Zambia to the time of slaughter. They were not in contact with any other animals and as such, the disease was contracted at source in Tanzania. Thus the exact stages of the disease in these animals at commencement of treatment are not known and the time between exposure and transportation was not determined. However, this is the kind of situation faced in the field where treatment is initiated only after exhibition of clinical signs and the time of acquiring the disease is not known. Infected and non-infected cattle in herds usually share pasture and watering points. In an experiment by Niang et al. (2010), it was noted that all the cattle that were subjected to oxytetracycline therapy recovered with the cicatrical lesions found on slaughter. In their study, all the cattle were treated early with the period of infection to therapy clearly outlined. In the current study however, the period between infection and therapy was not known.

It was observed that 57.4% (n=39) of the treated cattle succumbed to CBPP prior to mandatory slaughter of the herd. This is within the mortality rates expected in a CBPP outbreak where it has been shown that an outbreak usually causes mortality rates of 50 to 80% in a herd (Thomson, 2005). These results are also in agreement with studies of Huebschle et al. (2006) who showed that there was no difference between danofloxacin treated and untreated groups in terms of death due to CBPP. However, this is in contrast to reports made by Nicholas et al. (2012) where all the cattle that were treated using danofloxacin survived except for three that died in the first three months.

The lesions seen in the treated group at slaughter showed that 65.5% (n=19) were exhibiting signs of recovery indicated by fibrotic scar lesions while 34.5% (n=10) had lesions typical of active disease at various stages. This study also showed that 34.5% of the treated cattle had lesions of active CBPP. Of these 70% (n=7) had acute CBPP and 30% (n=3) had chronic lesions with sequestra of various sizes. The presence of sequestra indicates the transition of the disease into chronic phase which is known to be the probable cause of perpetuation of the disease where it exists. This finding is in contrast with the findings of Niang et al. (2010) who showed that none of the cattle treated with oxytetracyclinedeveloped sequestra.

The demonstration of *Mmm* colonies in pathological lesions from the treated group and the eventual confirmation using PCR indicate the presence of viable pathogen. This shows that these animals could still transmit the disease to susceptible individuals in the herd. This is in agreement with Yaya et al. (2004) who stated that the presence of *Mmm* in oxytetracycline treated individuals could still pose a risk of disease spread in the herds.

The observation of effective minimum inhibitory concentrations (MIC) by Mitchell et al. (2012) of some antibiotics including oxytetracycline on the growth of *Mmm* in biological matrices demonstrates their chemical effect in *vivo*. In *vitro* however, the concentration of *Mmm* is in many body fluids and tissues and the mycoplasmastatic effect of oxytetracyclinemay possibly not affect all the available pathogens. This could explain the observations made in this particular study.

Conclusion

This observation study has shown that the effects of oxytetracycline treatment of naturally infected CBPP cattle

in a herdis inconclusive and still requires further study. It has however shown that healing in some animals is possible.

CONFLICT OF INTERESTS

The authors have not declared any conflict of interests

ACKNOWLEDGEMENTS

The authors express gratitude to all the personnel in the Ministry of Fisheries and Livestock for facilitating the study. They would also like to thank colleagues from the Department of Veterinary Services (DVS) who toiled to examine and slaughter the infected cattle. Many thanks are also extended to colleagues at IZS Caporale, Teramo, Italy for providing materials to conduct PCR.

REFERENCES

Amanfu W (2009). Contagious Bovine Pleuropneumonia (Lungsickness) in Africa. Onderstepoort J. Vet. Res. 76:14-17.

Bashiruddin BJ, Taylor KT, Gould RA (1994). A PCR based test for the specific identification of *Mycoplasma mycoides* subspecies *mycoides* SC. J.Vet. Diagn. Invest. 6:428-434.

Food and Agriculture Organization FAO (2003). towards sustainable CBPP control programmes in Africa. FAO-OIE-AU/IBAR-IAEA consultative Group on Contagious Bovine Pleuropneumonia Third Meeting, Rome. pp.12-14.

Huebschle BJO, Ayling DR, Godinho K, Lukhele O, Tjipura-Zaire G, Rowan GT, Nicholas RAJR (2006). Danofloxacin (Advocin™) reduces the spread of contagious bovine pleuropneumonia to healthy in-contact cattle. Res. Vet. Sci. 81:304-309.

Le Goff C, Thiaucourt F (1998). A competitive ELISA for the specific diagnosis of contagious bovine pleuropneumonia (CBPP). Vet. Microbiol. 60:179-191.

Mariner J, Catley A, (2004).The dynamics of CBPP endemism and development of effective control strategies.Proceedings of the third FAO-AU/IBAR-IAEA consultative Group meeting on CBPP in Africa. Rome. pp.76-80.

Masiga WN, Domenech J, Windsor RS (1986).Manifestation and epidemiology of contagious bovine pleuropneumonia in Africa. Rev. Sci. Tech.15(4):1283-1308.

Mitchell DJ, McKellar AQ, McKeever JD (2012). Pharmacodynamics of Antimicrobial against *Mycoplasma mycoidesmycoides* Small Colony, the causative agent of Contagious Bovine Pleuropneumonia. PLoS ONE 7(8):e44158.

Niang M, Sery A, Doucoure M, Kone M, N'Diaye M, Amanfu W, Thiaucourt F (2010). Experimental studies on the effect of long-acting oxytetracycline treatment in the development of sequestra in contagious bovine pleuropneumonia-infected cattle. J. Vet. Med. Anim. Health 2(4):35-45.

Nicholas JAR, Ayling DR, Tjipura-Zaire G, Rowan T (2012). Treatment of Contagious Bovine Pleuropneumonia. Vet. Rec. 171:510-511.

Office International des Epizooties (OIE) (2012). Manual of Diagnostic tests and vaccines for Terrestial animals (Mammals, birds and bees). 7:701-716.

Office International des Epizooties (OIE) (2010). Manual of Diagnostic tests and vaccines for Terrestial animals (Mammals, birds and bees). 6:712-724.

Provost A, Perreau P, Breard A, le Goff C, Martel JL,Cottew GS (1987). Contagious Bovine Pleuropneumonia. Rev. Sci. Tech 6:625-679.

Razin S, Freundt EA (1984).The *Mycoplasmas*. In: Krieg NR, Holt JG (eds) 67th Bergey's manual of systematic Bacteriology. 1:740-770.

Scacchia M, Tjipura-Zaire G, Rossella L, Sacchini F,Pini A (2011). Contagious Bovine Pleuropneumonia: humoral and pathological events in cattle infected by endotracheal intubation or by exposure to infected animals. Vet. Ital 47(4):407-413.

Tambi NE, Maina WO,Ndi C (2006). An estimation of economic impact of Contagious Bovine Pleuropneumonia (CBPP) in Africa. Sci. Tech. Rev. 25:999-1011.

Thiaucourt F, Vander Lugt JJ, Provost A (2007).Contagious Bovine Pleuropneumonia. In Coetzer WAJ, Thomson RG, Tustin CR (eds), Infectious Diseases of Livestock with Reference to Southern Africa, rd

3 Edition, Oxford University, Press.

Thomson G (2005). Contagious Bovine Pleuropneumonia and poverty: A strategy for addressing the effects of the disease in sub-Saharan Africa. Research Report DFID Animal Health Programme, Trop. Vet. Med. Uni. Edin. UK.

Yaya A, Wesonga H, Thiaucourt F (2004). Use of long acting tetracyclines for CBPP-preliminary results.Report of the third meeting of the FAO/OIE/OAU-IBAR consultative group on CBPP, FAO, Rome. pp. 112-113.

15

Microbial safety and its public health concern of *E. coli* O157:H7 and *Salmonella* spp. in beef at Dire Dawa administrative city and Haramaya University, Ethiopia

Abayneh Edget*, Daniel Shiferaw and Shimelis Mengistu

College of Veterinary Medicine, Haramaya University, Haramaya, Dire Dawa, Ethiopia.

A cross-sectional study was conducted in Dire Dawa administrative city and Haramaya University (HU) slaughterhouses and retail shops, with the aim to identify *E.coli* O157:H7and *Salmonella,* to assess the microbial safety of beef and identify potential contamination risk factors. A total of 320 samples consisting of beef samples and environmental pooled samples examined for the presence of *E. coli, E. coli* O157:H7and *Salmonella* following standard bacteriological techniques and procedures outlined by the International Organization for Standardization. From a total of 290 beef samples collected, *E. coli* was isolated from 36 (12.41%) and out of these, 6 (2.06%) were confirmed on Sorbitol MacConkey Agar to be *E. coli* O157 H7. 8(2.75%) *Salmonella* spp. was identified by means of culture and biochemical test. The difference in prevalence was statistically significant ($P \leq 0.01$) between slaughterhouses and retail shops in both study areas. There was significant difference in mean Aerobic Plate Counts between Haramaya University slaughterhouse (7.11 log10 cfug^{-1}) and retail shop (2.3 log10 cfug^{-1}). Fecal coliforms counts (FCC) were significantly higher for beef samples from Haramaya University slaughterhouse (7.50 log10 cfug^{-1}) as compared to carcass sample from Haramaya retail shop (4.80 log10 cfug^{-1}). Out of 30 environmental pooled samples, *E. coli, E.coli* O157:H7 and *Salmonella* was present in 7(23.33%), 2(6.66%) and 2(6.66%), respectively in both study areas. A significant difference ($P \leq 0.01$) in the prevalence of *E. coli* between Haramaya University slaughterhouse (35.6%) and Haramaya University retail shop (11.1%) and Dire Dawa slaughterhouse (9%). Visual observations of slaughterhouse design, layout, slaughtering process, hygienic practice employed, sanitary regulatory system and personnel habit were below the minimum standards. Slaughterhouse and all meat contact surfaces might have served as sources of contamination for the product. Therefore, good management practice and good hygienic practice should be introduced in order to enhance the overall safety and hygienic quality of beef and safeguard the consumer from foodborne pathogens.

Key words: Aerobic plate counts (APC), beef, Dire Dawa, *E. coli, E. coli* O157:H7, fecal coliforms counts (FCC), Haramaya University (HU), *Salmonella.*

INTRODUCTION

Foodborne pathogens are one of the leading causes of illness and death in the world. They place heavy burden costing billions of dollars in medical care, social costs and overall economic and infrastructure effects on countries (Fratamico et al., 2005). Centers for Disease Control and Prevention (CDC) reported that of 19,056 people who get sick, more than 4,200 are hospitalized and 80 deaths recorded States of America (USA) (CDC, 2013). It mostly affects developing countries, due to major contributing factors such as from foodborne illness among 48 million (15%) population in United overcrowding, poverty, changes in eating habits, mass catering, complex and lengthy food supply procedures with increased international movement, inadequate sanitary conditions and poor general hygiene practices (Bhandare et al., 2007; Podpecan et al., 2007; Chhabra and Singla, 2009). In developing countries, including Ethiopia, up to 2 million people die per year due to disease of foodborne pathogens (World Health Organization (WHO), 2007).

Over the last 20 years, the emergence of major foodborne pathogens such as Salmonella and Escherichia coli have persisted as a major public health concerns and provide clear examples of the persistence of foodborne pathogens despite considerable efforts aimed at prevention and control (Diane et al., 2010). For this reason, the basic steps in the control of safety and quality of food include analysis of food products for presence of pathogenic microorganisms that cause the majority of alimentary human diseases. Among them are, Salmonella and E. coli O157:H7. These foodborne pathogens have frequently been linked to a number of cases of human illness (Brown et al., 2000).

Trends in foodborne illness in the industrialized and developing countries indicate that the incidence of foodborne illness is increasing (WHO, 2005). It has resulted in significant social and economic impact and that it is likely to remain a threat to public health well into the next century. There are however, substantial gaps in our understanding of this problem. In 2005, the World Health Organization (WHO) reported that 1.8 million people died from diarrheal diseases, largely attributable to contaminated food and drinking water (WHO, 2005). This is not just only an underdeveloped world problem. Meat processing at retail level is likely to contribute to the higher levels of contamination in minced beef as compared to carcasses (Tegegne and Ashenafi, 1998). The presence of even small numbers of pathogens in meat and edible offal may lead to heavy contamination of minced meat when it is cut into pieces and the surface area of the meat increases; as more microorganisms are added to the surfaces of exposed tissue (Ejeta et al.,

2004). Previous studies conducted in many parts of the country indicated the occurrence of pathogens including Salmonella in different food animals, meat and meat products (Haimanot et al., 2010). In addition, outbreaks of infections related with poor hygiene and consumption of contaminated food were reported in Ethiopia (Mache et al., 1997) and some were caused by Salmonella and E. coli (Alemseged et al., 2009).

In Ethiopia, the widespread habit of raw beef consumption is a potential cause for foodborne illnesses besides the common factors such as overcrowding, poverty, inadequate sanitary conditions and poor general hygiene (Haymanot et al., 2010). Raw meat is available in open-air local retail shops without appropriate temperature control and this is purchased by households and also minced meat (Kitfo) is served as raw, slightly-cooked or well-cooked in Dire Dawa administrative city and Haramaya University. Therefore, the main objectives of this study were to determine the microbial safety of beef through isolation and identification of foodborne bacterial pathogens in beef, to identify potential sources of contamination of beef in slaughterhouse and retail meat shops, to determine the hygiene conditions and practices of slaughterhouse and retail meat shops and to determine the hygienic quality of beef from slaughterhouse and retail meat shops.

MATERIALS AND METHODS

Study area and population

The study was conducted at slaughterhouse and ten retails shop in Dire Dawa administrative city and slaughterhouse and one retail meat shop in Haramaya University from May to November, 2014. Dire Dawa lies in the eastern part of the Ethiopia 515 km away from Addis Ababa with latitude 9° 27' to 9° 49' North and longitude 41° 38' East (Center of Stastical Agency (CSA), 2007). The city has a total area of 1,213 km^2 coverage's and elevation of 226 to 950 m above sea level (Center of Stastical Agency, 2007), and Haramaya University (HU) is located in the Eastern Hararghe Zone of the Oromia Region of Ethiopia, which is about 17 km from the city of Harar and 40 km from Dire Dawa and 5 km from Haramaya town at an altitude of 1980 m above sea level between latitude 9° 26" N and longitude 42° 3" E (Asrat, 2008). The mean annual rainfall is 870 mm with a range of 560 to 1260 mm, and the mean maximum and minimum temperatures are 23.4 and 8.25°C, respectively (Asrat, 2008). The study population represents apparently healthy cattle slaughtered in Dire Dawa and HU slaughterhouse, cattle subjected to slaughter brought from Water, Kersa, Hirna, Chalanko and Kulibi in both study areas and in addition from Issa (Somali) in Dire Dawa. Both local and cross breeds cattle are reared in and around the study areas for meat production mostly. There is one municipal

*Corresponding author. E-mail: edgetabayneh@gmail.com.

slaughterhouse in which different species of animal such as cattle, goat, sheep and camel is slaughtered and both over head rail and horizontal slaughtering system is practiced. Over an average of 70 cattle, 20 camel and 55 goat and sheep are slaughtered daily in Dire Dawa slaughterhouse but one slaughterhouse and one beef retail shop is available inside HU and only horizontal slaughtering system is practiced. Over 17 workers in HU slaughterhouse and 5 workers in HU retail shop are working daily on temporary basis and in range of 5 to 20 cattle are slaughtered every day depending on the needs of student cafeteria (main campus and Harer), staff lounge and the days of the week in HU slaughterhouse. The sample included raw beef and environmental pooled samples from slaughterhouses and retail shops in both study areas. The slaughterhouse structure in Dire Dawa was relatively good like there is a clear division of work, vertical line system and separate room for evisceration as compared with HU slaughterhouse.

Study protocol

A cross-sectional study was conducted to determine the microbial safety and hygienic quality of beef samples drawn from municipal slaughterhouse and retail meat shops. In addition, checklist and interviews were made on food handlers working at food establishment, to determine the hygienic status of the premises and safety practices of meat handlers. In the present study, beef samples and environmental pooled samples were collected from slaughterhouses and retails shops in both study areas. The sample size required for this study to identify the microbial safety of foodborne pathogen from beef was determined according to Thrusfield (2007) by taking expected prevalence of 5.6% for Salmonella in Dire Dawa (Bayleyegn et al., 2003) and 3% for E. coli O157:H7 in Haramaya University (Taye et al., 2013) with the consideration of slaughter animal coming from the same origin in both study area and confidence interval of 95% and 5% absolute precision.

The sample size of the present study were calculated and 81 beef samples from Dire Dawa slaughterhouse and 81 from 10 randomly selected retails shop and the selection of retail shop were done based on lottery method from 542 retails shop in Dire Dawa, and to increase the precision 19 beef samples for each sample collection centers were added and a total of 200 beef samples were collected from Dire Dawa administrative city and exactly the calculated number of 45 beef samples from HU slaughterhouse and 45 beef samples from retail shop were also collected due to resource limitation. Beside that, to assess the source of contamination level, only 30 environmental pooled samples were taken from equipment, surface, workers hand, vehicles in both study areas due to the vastness of the work and the availability of resource. Therefore, a total of 290 beef samples and 30 environmental pooled samples were collected from both study areas. The microbial safety and hygiene quality were then assayed by using the methods recommended by International Commission on Microbiological Specifications for Foods (ICMSF) (1986). All the samples were investigated with respect to Salmonella, E. coli and E. coli O157:H7 detection and aerobic plate and fecal coliforms counts.

The slaughterhouse and each retail shops were visited once in a week for consecutive weeks, and in each visit, ten beef samples were taken from the slaughterhouse and ten beef samples from ten retails shops in Dire Dawa town and five beef samples from HU slaughterhouse and five beef samples from HU retail shop every week for nine consecutive weeks. Each carcass is represented by meat pieces collected from different locations such as leg, flank,

inter costal and neck, and pooled together weighing 200 g. Retail meat samples (200 g) were taken simply from different location under aseptic conditions using sterile blades and sterile containers as described by Gill (2007).

For convenience, before the commencement of the sample collection all the respective samples (meat and environmental swab) were labeled with necessary information including date of sampling, code of sample source (beef) and identification of the shop from which the samples were obtained. The live animals were coded with owners name and the same code were followed for the carcass then the meat and samples were taken from the same carcass from those owner retails shops in Dire Dawa and the same procedure was followed in HU. After completion of sampling, all collected samples from Dire Dawa were placed in nutrient broth or Carry Blair Transport medium (Oxoid Ltd, Basingstoke, Hampshire, England) and immediately transported in cold chain using ice box containing ice pack to Veterinary Microbiology Laboratory of Haramaya University, within an hour and samples from Haramaya University were processed immediately upon arrival. The samples were processed up on arrival or stored overnight in a refrigerator at +4°C and the samples were processed in the next day for identification of pathogenic species, according to the standard set by the International Commission on Microbiological Specification for Food (ICMSF, 1986).

A total of thirty pooled environmental samples were collected from slaughterhouse, retail shop and transport vehicles. The pooled environmental sample collections were conducted two times within three months. On each visit to the slaughter house, a total of four pooled swab samples were taken each from cleaned, disinfected and dry surfaces, others from hooks, knives and aprons, the third from personnel's hands who work flaying, evisceration and carcass cutting before the beginning of the work and the fourth from the surface of transporting vehicles by rubbing thoroughly with a moistened swab. In each visit of each retail shops, a total of three pooled swab samples were taken each from cutting boards and meat grinder, others from hooks, knives and protective cloths and the third from personnel's hands (butcher man) before the beginning of work by rubbing thoroughly with a moistened swab. The samples were then returned to a test tube containing 9 ml sterile buffered peptone water (BPW). All samples were transported to the Veterinary Microbiology Laboratory of Haramaya University in an ice box on ice packs and analyzed upon arrival or within 24 h of sampling. The type and the number of samples processed were presented in Table 1.

For isolation and identification of pathogens from meat, 25 g of sample was weighed, cut into small piece with different sterile scalpel blade and placed into sterile stomacher bags, diluted with 225 ml of sterile BPW and homogenized in a stomacher at 230 R for 2 min (ISO TS 11133-1, 2009). For isolation and identification of pathogens from environmental samples, pooled swab samples were placed into a test tube that contained 9 ml sterile BPW. Subsequently, 10-fold serial dilutions were made to 10^{-6} for spread-plating. Samples were analyzed for the presence of E. coli O157:H7 and Salmonella spp. according to published methods as follows:

The E. coli O157:H7 detection was carried out according to the protocol of ISO 16654 (2001) standard. The pre-enriched beef samples were subsequently subcultured onto MacConkey agar (Oxoid, England) for primary screening of E. coli and incubated at 37°C aerobically for 24 h. Suspected colonies of E. coli (pinkish color appearance) were then subcultured onto nutrient agar (HiMedia, India) (non-selective media) and confirmed by triple sugar iron (TSI) (Oxoid, England) and indole, methyl red, Voges-Proskauer and citrate (IMViC) tests on tryptone broth (Oxoid, England), MRVP medium (Oxoid, England) and Simon citrate agar

Table 1. Summary of the type and total amount of sample collected

No	Sample type	Sample collected area	Total sample
1	Raw beef meat	45 from HU slaughter house 45 from HU retail shop 100 from DD slaughter house 100 from DD retail shop	290
2	Environmental sample Equipment Workers hand Contact surface balance Vehicle Cutting board and table	2 from each of the four site 2 from each of the four site 2 from HU slaughter house and 2 from DD slaughter house 2 from HU retail shop 2 from HU and 2 from DD slaughter house 2 from HU and 2 from DD retail	30
3	Respondents	22 respondents from HU 28 respondents from DD	50

HU= Haramaya University; DD= Dire Dawa

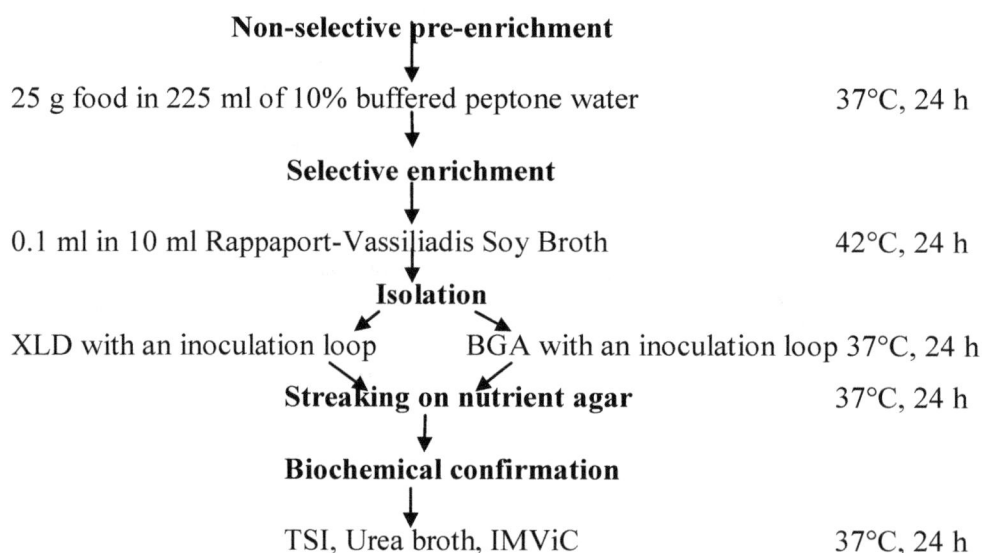

Non-selective pre-enrichment

25 g food in 225 ml of 10% buffered peptone water   37°C, 24 h

Selective enrichment

0.1 ml in 10 ml Rappaport-Vassiliadis Soy Broth   42°C, 24 h

Isolation

XLD with an inoculation loop   BGA with an inoculation loop 37°C, 24 h

Streaking on nutrient agar   37°C, 24 h

Biochemical confirmation

TSI, Urea broth, IMViC   37°C, 24 h

Figure 1. Flow diagram for detection of *Salmonella* (Source, ISO 6579, 2002).

(Oxoid, England), respectively. Then the bacterium that was confirmed as *E. coli* was subcultured onto Sorbitol MacConkey agar (SMA) (Oxoid, England) from nutrient agar (HiMedia, India). SMA (Oxoid, England) plates were incubated at 35°C for 20 to 22 h (Timothy and Smith, 2012). *E. coli* O157:H7 does not ferment sorbitol and therefore, produces colorless colonies. In contrast, most other *E. coli* strains ferment sorbitol and form pink colonies and Latex *E. coli* O157:H7 agglutination test was performed to determine strains.

The procedures for isolation of *Salmonella* from food were based on protocol of the ISO 6579 (2002) standard (Figure 1). To diminish

the risk of obtaining false negative results, a non-selective pre-enrichment of large food sample, followed by two selective enrichments, but due to availability of the resource, used one selective enrichment media which is mandatory and plating on two selective media was performed.

Salmonella was isolated from beef sample (25 g) homogenized in 225 ml of 0.1% buffered peptone water (BPW) (HiMedia, India). Aliquot (1 ml) was added to 10 ml of Rappaport Vassiliadis (Oxoid, England). This was incubated at 41 ± 0.5°C over night. After gentle mixing, a loopful of culture from the enrichment broth was streaked parallely onto Xylose lysine desocholate (XLD) agar (Oxoid,

Table 2. Frequency of bacterial isolate of beef samples from Dire Dawa and HU slaughterhouse and retail shops.

Samples source	Number of samples processed	Bacterial isolates (%)		
		E. coli	*E. coli* O157:H7	*Salmonella* spp.
HU slaughterhouse	45	16 (35.6)	1 (2.2)	3 (6.7)
HU retail shop	45	5 (11.1)	0 (0)	3 (6.7)
DD slaughterhouse	100	9 (9)	4 (4)	1 (1)
DD retail shops	100	6 (6)	1 (1)	1 (1)
Total	290	36 (12.41)	6 (2.06)	8 (2.75)

P≤ 0.01, df= 3 for *E.coli,* P> 0.05, df= 3 for *E.coli* O157:H7 and *Salmonella*

England) and Brilliant green agar (BGA) (Oxoid, England) and incubated at 37°C for 24 to 48 h. Typical *Salmonella* colonies which are pink with or without black centers were isolated from XLD and *Salmonella* colonies grow as red-pink, white opaque colonies surrounded by brilliant red zones in the agar are taken from BGA. The colonies were purified on fresh nutrient agar (HiMedia, India) and then streaked and stabbed into the butt of triple sugar iron (TSI) (Oxoid, England) slants and inoculated into tryptone broth (Oxoid, England), MRVP medium (Oxoid, England) and Simon citrate agar (Oxoid, England) for IMViC test from both selective media. These were incubated at 37°C for 24 h. The test tubes that had alkaline (red) slants and acidic (yellow) butts, with the production of H_2S (blackening) were presumed to be *Salmonella* isolates. Moreover, two or more colonies from pure isolates were inoculated on urea broth (SRL, India) and incubated at 37°C for 24 h. All test tubes that were urease negative were treated as suspects of *Salmonella* (FDA, 1992). In addition, isolate that was Gram-negative rod, oxidase negative, methyl red positive, citrate positive, indole negative, Voges-Proskauer negative and lactose and sucrose non-fermenter were accepted putatively as *Salmonella* (Fawole and Oso, 2001).

Aerobic plate count (APC) were enumerated using plate count agar (APC); twenty five grams of beef sample was weighed and homogenized in 225 ml of 0.1% sterile peptone water using a sterile homogenizer. From the 10-fold dilutions of the homogenates, 0.1 ml of 10^{-4}, 10^{-5} and 10^{-6} dilutions of the homogenates were plated by the spread plate method onto the surface of plate count agar (PCA). Plates were incubated at 35°C for 48 h and plates containing between 30 and 300 colonies were counted (ISO/TS 11133-1, 2009). Fecal coliforms were enumerated using violet red bile agar (VRBL); 25 g of beef sample was weighed and homogenized in 225 ml of 0.1% sterile peptone water using a sterile homogenizer. From the 10-fold dilutions of the homogenates, 0.1 ml of 10^{-4}, 10^{-5} and 10^{-6} dilutions of the homogenates were spread onto agar plates. The VRBL was inoculated with 0.1 ml inoculums after the final incubation at 44 ± 1°C for 24 h, typical and atypical colonies were enumerated. Typical colonies on VRBL medium have fuchsia color with a diameter of approximately 0.5 mm and sometimes surrounded by a reddish-fuchsia zone (1 to 2 mm in diameter) of precipitated bile salts, which reveals lactose degradation in acid. On the VRBL medium, pale colonies with greenish zones reflect lactose fermentation by fecal coliforms, which appear slowly (Marshall, 1993).

Statistical analysis

The data collected through questionnaire survey and laboratory results of the collected samples were entered into databases using Micro-Soft Excel computer program and analyzed using SPSS version-19.0 (SPSS, 2012). Descriptive statistics were used to describe the nature and the characteristics of the questionnaire survey result. The aerobic bacterial and fecal coliform counts were expressed as mean using excel and compared by analysis of variance (ANOVA). A Chi-Square test was applied to examine whether the differences between the values and the level of contamination between slaughterhouse and retail shops and associated risk factor were significant. A p-value of less or equal to 0.05 and chi-square value were considered indicative of a statistically significant difference.

RESULTS

Isolation of bacteria from beef slaughtered and marketed at Dire Dawa city and Haramaya University

Out of 90 beef samples from HU (45 beef samples from slaughterhouse and 45 beef samples from retail shop) examined bacteriologically 21 (23.3%), 1 (1.1%) and 6 (6.7%) had *E. coli, E. coli* O157:H7 and *Salmonella* spp., respectively. None of the 90 beef samples from HU had mixed bacterial contamination. The prevalence of *E. coli, E. coli* O157:H7 and *Salmonella* in HU slaughterhouse and retail shop were presented in Table 2. Out of 200 beef samples from Dire Dawa (100 beef samples from slaughterhouse and 100 from ten randomly selected retail shops) examined bacteriologically, 15 (7.5%), 5 (2.5%) and 2 (1%) had *E. coli, E. coli* O157:H7 and *Salmonella* spp., respectively. One of the 200 samples of beef had yielded both groups of bacteria. The prevalence of *E. coli, E. coli* O157:H7 and *Salmonella* in Dire Dawa slaughterhouse and retail shop were presented in Table 2.

Hygienic quality of beef from Dire Dawa and HU slaughterhouses and retail shops

The results of total aerobic bacteria in beef by using detection methods are summarized in Table 3. This study detected total aerobic bacteria in 27/290 (9.31%) of beef

Table 3. Indicator organisms detected from beef sampled from HU and Dire Dawa slaughterhouse and retail shops.

Sample source	No of sample	Organisms detected	
		No (%) AB	No (%) FCs
HU slaughter house	45	6 (13.33)	8 (17.77)
HU retail shop	45	8 (17.77)	1 (2.2)
DD slaughter house	100	10 (10)	2 (2)
DD retail shops	100	3 (3)	0 (0)
Total	290	27 (9.31)	11 (3.79)

FCs= Fecal coliforms, AB = Aerobic bacteria, $p > 0.05$, df = 1

Table 4. Microbial loads of indicator organisms on beef in HU and Dire Dawa slaughterhouse and retail shops.

Sample source	No of sample	Bacterial colonies log10 cfug^{-1}					
		APCs			FCCs		
		Mean	Min	Max	Mean	Min	Max
HU slaughter house	45	7.11	4.00	8.80	7.50	3.60	9.20
HU retail shop	45	2.30	4.10	8.80	4.80	0.00	5.70
DD slaughter house	100	5.63	0.30	8.80	1.13	0.33	4.89
DD retail shop	100	3.10	6.72	9.73	0.00	0.00	0.00

FCCs= Fecal coliform counts, APCs= Aerobic plate counts. $P \leq 0.01$, df= 1.

samples from slaughter house and retail shops. Results of mean APCs of beef in this study are presented in Table 4. Fecal coliforms count in beef presented in Table 4 indicates the hygienic qualities of meat. In this study, fecal coliforms were detected and enumerated irrespective of pathogencity of the strain to estimate the level of hygiene (Table 3). Out of 290 samples, fecal coliforms were present in 11 (3.79%) samples including HU and Dire Dawa slaughterhouse 8 (17.77%) and 2 (2%), respectively and HU retail shop 1 (2.2%) and Dire Dawa retail shops 0 (0%) (Table 3).

Major source of microbial contamination for beef from slaughterhouse and retail shops

It is generally accepted that microbial loads on surfaces and equipment vary in different food plants depending on the microbial quality of the food (Evans et al., 2004). One of the specific objectives of this study was to examine the sources of microbial contamination of beef intended for human consumption and to determine the acceptability of hygienic levels of slaughterhouse and retail shops. Swab samples were taken from cleaned, disinfected and dry surfaces of slaughterhouse, retail shops facilities and equipment surfaces, and also personnel before the beginning of work by rubbing meat contact surfaces and the hand of meat handler thoroughly with a moistened swab from both sites. All contact surfaces were analyzed for *E. coli* O157:H7 and *Salmonella* spp., detection and enumeration of fecal coliform and aerobic bacteria. Out of 30 environmental pooled samples (8 from HU slaughter house, 8 from HU retail shop, 8 from Dire Dawa slaughterhouse and 6 from Dire Dawa retail shops out of 10 randomly selected retail shops due to the fact that 7 of the selected retail shops could not be voluntary to take swab sample), *E. coli*, *E. coli* O157:H7 and *Salmonella* was present in 7 (23.33%), 2 (6.66%) and 2 (6.66%) samples. The occurrence of *E. coli*, *E. coli* O157:H7 and *Salmonella* spp. in beef contact surfaces from HU and Dire Dawa slaughterhouse and retail shops are summarized in Table 6. Average microbial load for APCs and FCCs in beef contact surfaces at slaughterhouse and retail shops are shown in Table 5. Total aerobic bacteria in different sample groups in retail shop (knives and hooks, cutting boards and personnel hands) were examined.

Fecal coliforms counts in different sample groups in retail shops and slaughterhouse (knives and hooks, cutting boards, personnel hands and transporting vehicle)

Table 5. Microbial loads of indicator organisms on beef contact surfaces from HU and Dire Dawa slaughterhouse and retail shops.

| Sources | No of sample | Enumerated organisms log10 cfu /cm^2 | | | | | |
| | | APCs | | | FCCs | | |
		Mean	Min	Max	Mean	Min	Max
HU slaughterhouse							
Equipments	2	3.05	TFC	6.10	TFC	TFC	TFC
Surfaces	2	TFC	TFC	TFC	TFC	TFC	TFC
Workers hands	2	TFC	TFC	TFC	TFC	TFC	TFC
Vehicle	2	TFC	TFC	TFC	TFC	TFC	TFC
HU Retail shops							
Equipments	2	TFC	TFC	TFC	5.38	5.10	5.67
Cutting boards	2	TFC	TFC	TFC	4.78	4.24	5.33
Workers hands	2	TFC	TFC	TFC	5.06	4.50	5.63
Balance	2	TFC	TFC	TFC	TFC	TFC	TFC
DD slaughterhouse							
Equipment	2	TFC	TFC	TFC	4.43	3.11	5.76
Surface	2	TFC	TFC	TFC	4.42	3.20	5.65
Worker hand	2	TFC	TFC	TFC	4.32	3.32	5.32
Vehicle	2	5.73	4.56	6.91	5.87	4.54	7.20
DD retail shops							
Equipment	2	TFC	TFC	TFC	4.96	4.32	5.61
Cutting board	2	TFC	TFC	TFC	6.26	5.65	6.88
Worker hand	2	TFC	TFC	TFC	5.98	4.87	7.1

TFC= Too Few to Count, P≤ 0.01, df=1.

were examined. The result varied from 3.11 log$_{10}$ cfu/cm^2 to 7.20 log$_{10}$ cfu/cm^2 in knives and hooks, cutting boards, balance, personnel hand and transport vehicle at slaughterhouse and retail shops. The overall mean of coliforms count in retail shops environment was 5.40 log$_{10}$ cfu/cm^2 and 2.38 log$_{10}$ cfu/cm^2 in slaughter house. Furthermore, the result of aerobic plate counts and coliform count were compared by ANOVA and showed that there is significant (P≤ 0.01) variation in the means of fecal coliforms count found in different meat contact surfaces in retail shop and slaughterhouse.

Hygienic practices in Dire Dawa and HU slaughterhouses and retail shops

"Abattoir" in terms of the Republic of South African Meat Safety Act, 2000 (Act 40 of 2000) means a slaughter facility in respect of which a registration certificate has been issued in terms of section 8 (1) and in respect of which a grading has been determined in terms of section 8 (2): (i) A well-designed and constructed structure is needed to systematically process the animal that is slaughtered. According to abattoir, cutting and packing plant standard (ABM, 2008), abattoir wall, floors, ceilings, windows, doors, lighting, air-conditioning/ventilation, services and equipment must be constructed to withstand and facilitate thorough cleaning and minimize contamination of product, either through pests, harboring of dirt or other physical, chemical or microbiological hazards.

In Dire Dawa slaughterhouse except in Muslim slaughter premises, it is a well organized beef slaughter house than Haramaya University slaughter house. In Dire Dawa, slaughterhouse for Christian have clear division of slaughtering process into stunning, bleeding, skinning and evisceration, whereas in Muslim slaughter premises and HU slaughterhouse no clear division existed. In both slaughterhouses, horizontal bleeding on killing floor was conducted, however, only vertical dressing process on

Table 6. Bacterial species detected from beef contact surfaces sampled from HU and Dire Dawa slaughterhouse and retail shops.

Sources	No of sample	Bacterial detected		
		No (%) E. coli	No (%) E.coli O157H7	No (%) Salmonella
HU slaughterhouse				
Equipments	2	2(100)	1(50)	0(0)
Surfaces	2	1(50)	0(0)	0(0)
Workers hands	2	1(50)	0(0)	0(0)
Vehicle	2	0(0)	0(0)	0(0)
HU Retail shops				
Equipments	2	0(0)	0(0)	1(50)
Cutting boards	2	1(50)	0(0)	0(0)
Workers hands	2	0(0)	0(0)	0(0)
Balance	2	0(0)	0(0)	0(0)
DD slaughterhouse				
Equipment	2	1(50)	0(0)	1(50)
Surface	2	0(0)	0(0)	0(0)
Worker hand	2	0(0)	0(0)	0(0)
Vehicle	2	1(50)	1(50)	0(0)
DD retail shops				
Equipment	2	0(0)	0(0)	0(0)
Cutting board	2	0(0)	0(0)	0(0)
Worker hand	2	0(0)	0(0)	0(0)
Total	30	7(23.33)	2(6.66)	2(6.66)

$P > 0.05$, df= 3

overhead rail procedure was conducted in Dire Dawa slaughterhouse. The visual observation result in HU slaughterhouses indicated that the animal brought to slaughterhouse without prior ante-mortem inspection was done and without fasting the animal for 12 to 24 h before slaughter, which increases the micro floral load, and sometimes the animal brought to slaughterhouse immediately after arrival from market results in shading of microorganisms. But in Dire Dawa slaughterhouse, the pre-slaughter procedure was done 12 h before the slaughtering process presided. The animal also encountered stressful handling during riding on foot from the HU farm to HU slaughter house in the night, sometimes they even suffered fracture and excitement. Beside these, stunning process was done by kicking, using the back of axe and most of the time the workers could not make stunning by a single kick rather they kick several times which result the animal to suffering from pain. In general, the pre-slaughtering process in HU

slaughterhouse brought the animal to stress which facilitate the rapid multiplication and shading of *E. coli* O157:H7 and *Salmonella* spp. This could be one of the sources of contamination of meat.

Hands are rarely free from microorganisms. It is of the utmost importance that soap (preferably in a dispenser) and hot running water are used for this purpose, thus aiming to reduce the microbiological load on hands (Desmarchelier et al., 1999). Van Zyl (1995) suggested that soap and hot water, at 45°C, should always be available at the washing-basins. Desmarchelier et al. (1999) recommend that hand-washing alone has no effect on the reduction of bacteria on hands; it depends on the mechanical action, the duration and the type of soap and sanitizers being used. It was important to know the educational background, type and terms of employment in the abattoir, and how the meat handler acquired their skills to establish their knowledge in handling meat safely. The knowledge and educational level of personnel working in both food establishments are summarized in Table 8.

In this study, personnel practices regarding prohibited habits and actions were also assessed. The visual observations indicated that, fraudulent activity and habits like eating, chewing and smoking in the slaughterhouse by the workers were common practices in both slaughterhouses, especially prominent in Dire Dawa slaughterhouse while they were on duty of meat processing. The overall result regarding habit, personnel cloth and cleanness in both slaughterhouses was summarized in Table 9.

DISCUSSION

Food borne illnesses caused by *Salmonella* spp., and *E. coli* O157:H7 represents a major public health problem worldwide. These pathogens are transmitted mainly through consumption of contaminated food and the presence of these organisms in meat animals and in raw meat products has relevant public health implications (Sousa, 2008). The occurrence of *E. coli* in meat samples from HU slaughterhouse in this study was in close agreement with the result of Taye et al. (2013) who isolated *E. coli* in 30.97% of the meat samples studied in the same slaughterhouse. The present result is much lower than the finding of Mekonnen et al. (2012) who isolated *E. coli* in 91.4% of meat samples from abattoir in Mekelle.

Generally, the high prevalence of *E. coli* in the meat samples from HU slaughterhouse indicated the contamination of meat with intestinal content since evisceration take place in the same place. There was a significant difference in the prevalence of *E. coli* between HU slaughterhouse and Dire Dawa slaughterhouse (P ≤ 0.01). This difference could be due to difference in hygienic condition and practice in both slaughterhouses. The prevalence of *E. coli* O157:H7 isolated from beef in HU slaughterhouse (2.2%) and Dire Dawa slaughterhouse (4%) in this study was in agreement with the reported prevalence of 2.60% (Mekonnen et al., 2012) and 2.65% (Taye et al., 2013) in Ethiopia. There was no statistically significant difference in the prevalence of *E. coli* O157:H7 between HU slaughterhouse and Dire Dawa slaughterhouse (P > 0.05).

In comparison to the present study, a higher prevalence of *E. coli* O157:H7 were reported from different countries; 8% in Debre Zeit and Mojo (Hiko et al., 2008) and 8.1% in Mojo, Ethiopia (Mersha et al., 2009), 9% in India (Luga et al., 2007). In the current study, lower prevalence of *E. coli* O157:H7 was also isolated from Dire Dawa retail shop (1%) which is in agreement with the report from America (0.8%)

(Desenclos et al., 1988) and Kenya (0.2%) (Chapman et al., 2000). The frequency of isolation of *Salmonella* spp. in meat samples in this study was 6.7% from both HU slaughter house and retail shop. This result was in agreement with 5.6% prevalence reported from muscle in Addis Ababa, Debre Zeit, Dire Dawa and Jigjiga (Bayleyegn et al., 2003), 8.5% from minced beef in Addis Ababa (Zewdu and Cornelius, 2009) and 4.8% from beef in Bahir Dar (Sefinew and Bayleyegn, 2012).

The detection of 6.7% of *Salmonella* in beef in HU slaughterhouse and retail shop as compared to Dire Dawa slaughterhouse and retail shops (1%) suggests that the process of evisceration could be the main source of carcass contamination in addition to carrier state. Cross-contamination can also occur during the skinning process as a result of poor hygienic conditions. The other probable source of contamination is infected abattoir personnel. When comparing with the present study, a relatively high prevalence of *Salmonella* (14.4%) was reported by Ejeta et al. (2004) from minced beef in Addis Ababa. It was also lower than the 40% prevalence reported by Molla et al. (2000). Similarly, Tegegne and Ashenafi (1998) reported *Salmonella* contamination rate of 42% from minced meat (locally known as «kitfo») samples collected from different hotels, bars and restaurants in Addis Ababa.

The lower prevalence was also revealed in this study from Dire Dawa slaughterhouse (1%) and Dire Dawa retail shops (1%). This result was in agreement with prevalence report of Sibhat et al. (2011) who reported 2% from carcass in Debre Zeit, Ethiopia and Fegan et al. (2004) also reported carcass contamination of 2% from slaughterhouse in Australia. There was no statistically significant difference in the prevalence of *Salmonella* spp. between Haramaya University and Dire Dawa administrative city (P > 0.05). This could be due to unhygienic slaughtering practice in HU slaughterhouse and Dire Dawa halal slaughter house.

Presence of microbes in high numbers (APC > 5 log cfu/cm^2 or g^{-1}) fast tracks the spoilage of the meat. According to the international standard organization (ISO 4833, 2003), APC of 80% of analyzed samples must not exceed 5 log cfug^{-1}or cm^2, whereas 20% of the samples may have counts of up to 5 log cfug^{-1} or cm^2 (Mukhopadhyay et al., 2009). In this study 5.8% of samples had APCs more than 5.00 log$_{10}$ cfug^{-1}, the condition was unacceptable. Lower level of aerobic plate count in this study was much lower than previous studies (Alvarez-Astorga et al., 2002; Bhandare et al., 2007; Haque et al., 2008; Hassan et al., 2010). However, the microbial contamination level of slaughterhouse and retail shops were higher as compared to reports from developed countries and our results do not conform to EU specifications (Gill et al., 2000; Duffy et al., 2001).

The higher aerobic plate count enumerated from HU

slaughterhouse (7.11 $\log_{10}$ cfug^{-1}) suggests an unusual high level of contamination and/or growth which was similar with Gill (2007) report, given the hygienic status of the slaughterhouse and meat processing observed in the slaughterhouse. The result of this study was much lower than the presence of fecal coliforms in meat and meat studied by many researchers (Doyle, 2007; Adu-Gyamfi et al., 2012). Other study results have also been reported for retail chicken (50% incidence of *E. coli*) in Australia (Pointon et al., 2008) which was much higher than the present study. Mean fecal coliforms counts were higher for beef samples from HU slaughterhouse (7.50 $\log_{10}$ cfug^{-1}) as compared to carcass sample from HU retail shop (4.80 $\log_{10}$ cfug^{-1}) and also higher for beef samples from Dire Dawa slaughterhouse (1.13 $\log_{10}$ cfug^{-1}) but there was no fecal coliforms in Dire Dawa retail shops. This difference was statistically significant between both slaughterhouses and retail shops ($p \leq 0.01$).

The prevalence of coliforms was much lower than that of any other microorganism studied. Of the 290 beef samples tested, 11 (3.79%) were positive for FCCs and the microorganism were detected at both processing stage. The concentration of fecal coliforms enumerated from beef (3.57 $\log_{10}$ cfug^{-1}) was higher than established limits (10 to 100 cfug^{-1}) in guidelines (Alvarez-Astorga et al., 2002) which is assumed to be an indicator of fecal contamination. The result showed that only one sample from HU retail shop had count of 6.10 $\log_{10}$ cfu/cm^2 in knives and hooks, while too few to count in cutting boards, balance and personnel hands and 6.91 $\log_{10}$ cfu/cm^2 in vehicle from Dire Dawa slaughterhouse. The overall mean of total aerobic bacteria count in retail shops environment was 3.05 $\log_{10}$ cfu/cm^2 and 5.73 $\log_{10}$ cfu/cm^2 in Dire Dawa slaughterhouse. Furthermore, the result showed that there was significant ($P \leq 0.01$) variation in the means of total aerobic bacteria found in knives and hooks and different meat contact surfaces in retail shops and slaughterhouse.

From the data of retail meats it was evident that the highest FCCs (6.26 $\log_{10}$ cfu/cm^2) levels were found in the cutting boards at Dire Dawa retail shop. Cutting board from HU retail shop got the smallest values of FCCs (4.78 $\log_{10}$ cfu/cm^2) and in HU slaughterhouse was too few to count from knives and hooks, surface, vehicle and workers' hands (Table 5). Based on the data, the highest FCCs (5.87 $\log_{10}$ cfu/cm^2) and APCs (5.73 $\log_{10}$ cfu/cm^2) levels found in the transporting vehicle from Dire Dawa slaughterhouse while the smallest values of FCCs (4.32 $\log_{10}$ cfu/cm^2) found in workers hand in Dire Dawa slaughterhouse and APCs was found too few to count in both slaughterhouses (Table 5). The findings of this study indicated that meat contact surfaces might be real risks associated with the persistence of hazardous organisms. Similar findings were reported by Gill and McGinnis (2004) and Temelli et al. (2006). Based on European

commission standards used in the food processing industry; a standard of less than 1.3 $\log_{10}$ cfu was used for aerobic plate count, less than 1.0 $\log_{10}$ cfu for Enterobacteriaceae count. According to this standard, the results of average mean of APCs and FCCs in our study for food contact surfaces were 4.39 and 5.29 $\log_{10}$ cfu, respectively, which was unacceptable (Sneed et al., 2004).

In the present study, it was found that all of the meat establishments had pathogenic and indicator bacteria. The findings showed the magnitude of contamination at slaughterhouses and retail shops was high. This may contribute to the incidence of food associated illnesses. In this study, the identification of thermo-tolerant *E. coli* showed the presence of recent fecal contamination (Collee and Mackie, 1999). Hence, basic failures occur in the sanitization procedures applied to these utensils, since the establishments were found not to apply the cleaning process on a daily basis. The knives used for filleting and cutting were not sanitized at any of the retail houses visited. Neither the slaughterhouse, nor any of the platforms (bleeding, evisceration and inspection line) adopted the practice of immersing knives in hot water.

In both slaughterhouses, personnel interviewed to assess the hygienic conditions in the slaughterhouse responded that there was adequate potable water supply in the slaughterhouse. However, there is no hot water supply in all meat processing facilities. In both slaughterhouses, there were no facilities for knife sterilization and no rooms for retention of conditionally approved carcasses. Regarding latrine facility, both slaughterhouses had communal latrine which was properly placed but with poor management. There were no enough water supplies as a result, flies infestation of the facilities were observed. Hand washing is an essential component of infection control (Larson et al., 2003). In general, both abattoirs have no mechanism of ensuring sanitation standards, proper waste disposal mechanism and vermin's and scavenger's protection mechanisms. Therefore, there are opportunities of contamination of slaughter facilities which in turn contaminate the exposed tissues of the carcass with microorganisms.

The adequacy of a cleaning program is judged on the basis of the adherence to specified standard operating procedures during the cleaning and disinfection process and the inspection of cleaned facilities and equipment (Gill et al., 1999). Gill et al. (1999) further reports that improperly cleaned equipment have been implicated in outbreaks of foodborne diseases and it is therefore apparent that cleaning and disinfecting processes should fully comply with regulations. Gill and McGinnis (2000) reported that a primary source of *E. coli* deposited on meat during processing appears to be the detritus in equipment which was not removed during daily cleaning.

Assessment on the procedures and frequency of cleaning and disinfection of the equipment in both slaughterhouses are important and the result indicated that, the procedures of cleaning and disinfection of the surface, a notably low percentage (35.7%) in Dire Dawa slaughterhouse and high percentage in HU slaughterhouse (68.2%) of respondents indicated that running water and detergent was used to clean the surfaces. whereas majority of them cleaned their knives whenever they were excessively and visibly soiled with fat or blood before the commencement of work each day. About seventy eight percent of the respondents in Dire Dawa slaughterhouse and ninety five percent in HU slaughterhouse practiced washing their knife with soap and water. The respondents were also questioned on the frequency of cleaning and disinfection of the working surfaces. All (100%) respondents in Dire Dawa and 90.9% in HU slaughterhouse reported that the surfaces were cleaned before the commencement of work each day.

Upon visual observation, the knives used for filleting and cutting were not sanitized at any of the meat retail establishments visited in both study areas. In the slaughterhouse, any of the platforms (bleeding, evisceration and inspection line) did not adopt the practice of immersing knives in hot water. As for the meat hooks for hanging carcasses, most of them were splashing with water and some were not cleaned prior to use and most importantly the floor and surface of transporting vehicles were regularly cleaned with detergent and water but re-contaminated with workers gum boot and in contact with the meat during loading. In both slaughterhouses interview showed that washing of the hand before starting slaughter is not common but after the end of processing hand washing were conducted without the use of hot water and soap. In addition to the frequency, the procedure of hand-washing is also considered important. The proportion of individuals that indicated following the correct procedure of using detergents and water for lathering and rinsing was 96.4% in Dire Dawa slaughterhouse and 77.3% in HU slaughterhouse. Regarding the availability of soap, all of the respondents indicated that soap was not always available.

In the current study, 92.9% of the interviewees in Dire Dawa slaughterhouse and all (100%) of the interviewees in HU slaughterhouse responded that no sanitary regulation system was in place in the slaughterhouse in Table 7. Therefore, effective food safety and quality control programs are essential. The behavior of worker and hygienic practices of retail shop in HU was relatively good as compared to Dire Dawa retails shop, and meat handlers do not have close contact with money and they do so only when cutting and weighing the meat. To get rid of germs and dirt, it is important to wash hands properly and frequently with detergents and warm water. Hands that have long nails are more difficult to clean thoroughly and can collect small pieces of debris and bacteria that do not wash off easily (Trickett, 1997).

All the respondents in both slaughterhouses were employed on a temporary basis which makes it difficult to train the staffs. When assessment on the literacy level, the personnel working on food establishment in both areas, 98% of butcher men attend school and 14% of respondent are obtained their skills from their parents, while 80% of the respondents taught themselves through visual observation and 10.7% of respondent in Dire Dawa gained skill through formal training. Training and education of food handlers regarding the basic concepts and requirements of personal hygiene plays an integral part in ensuring a safe product to the consumer (Adams and Moss, 1997). To ensure this, there should be some form of induction training with regular updating and refresher courses for the food handlers. Meat handlers should furthermore understand the risks associated with contamination of food by microbial agents, and should be trained to avoid the contamination of the meat. A formal employee training and assistance program that describes all the training activities should be made attractive to the meat handlers (CFIA, 1990). Ryser and Marth (1991) conclude that the training and education should be directed towards a thorough understanding of food hygiene, which includes aspects of sanitation.

The result from meat handler indicated that 46.4% in Dire Dawa and 13.6% in HU smoke cigarette when they carry out their task. Smoking inside the slaughterhouse or whenever meat is handled should be prohibited, because whenever a cigarette is handled the fingers come into contact with the lips and saliva, together with microorganisms, may consequently be transferred from the hands to the food (Burton, 1996). Smoking may furthermore cause coughing, thus transferring aerosols containing microorganisms to the food (Gordon-Davis, 1998). Moreover 42% of the respondent in both slaughterhouses had worn jewelry materials. Jewelry is a potential source of microorganisms, because the skin under the jewelry provides a favorable habitat for contaminating microorganisms to proliferate (Trickett, 1997).

Regarding protective cloth, the personnel observation and assessment result in both slaughterhouses indicated that, almost all of the food handlers had a uniform protective cloth. However; minimal personal hygiene was practiced during food preparation. Van Zyl (1995) gave emphasis to protective clothing which should not only be on protection, but also on cleanliness, thus he proposed that the overalls, hairnets (beard nets if applicable), hard hats, gum boots and aprons should at all times be worn by meat handlers. Because the purpose of wearing overalls is to protect both the food product and the meat

Table 7. Hygienic and sanitation practices employed at Dire Dawa and HU slaughterhouses and retail shops.

Practices	Dire Dawa (%)	HU (%)
Cleaning and disinfection of knives and hooks		
Before the commencement of work	28(100)	21(95.5)
When excessively and visibly soiled	-	1(4.5)
Manner of cleaning and disinfection		
Using detergents and water	22(78.6)	21(95.5)
Rinsing with water only	6(21.4)	1 (4.5)
Floor Surface cleaning and disinfection		
Before commencement of work	28(100)	20(90.9)
When excessively and visibly soiled	-	1(4.55)
After commencement of work	-	1(4.55)
Manner of cleaning and disinfection of surface		
Using detergents and water	10(35.7)	15(68.2)
Rinsing with water only	18(64.3)	7(31.8)
Hand washing before starting handling raw meat		
Yes	28(100)	22(100)
Manner of hand washing		
Using detergents and water	27(96.4)	17(77.3)
Rinsing with water only	1(3.6)	5(22.7)
Presence of sanitary regulatory system		
Yes	2(7.1)	0
No	26(92.9)	22(100)

$p \leq 0.01$, df= 1

Table 8. Educational status of meat handler's

Skills	DD slaughterhouse frequency (%)	HU slaughterhouse frequency (%)
Educational status		
None	0	1(4.55)
Elementary/junior	11(39.3)	13(59.1)
High school	12(42.9)	7(31.8)
College	4(14.3)	1(4.55)
Graduate	1(3.6)	
Sources of meat processing skills		
Observation	21(75)	19(86.4)
Parents	4(14.3)	3(13.6)
Formal training	3(10.7)	0

$P \leq 0.001$, df= 4

Table 9. Practices of the meat handlers regarding prohibited habits and actions.

Prohibited habits	Dire Dawa (%)	HU (%)
Jewelry		
Worn	19(67.9)	2(9.1)
Not worn	9(32.1)	20(90.9)
Finger nails		
Short and polished	22(78.6)	15(68.2)
Short/ not polished	6(21.4)	5(22.7)
Long and polished		2(9.1)
Smoking in meat processing plants		
Yes	13(46.4)	3(13.6)
No	15(53.6)	19(86.4)
Hair cover		
Used	24(85.7)	14(63.6)
Not covered	4(14.3)	8(36.4)
Gum boots		
Used	18(64.3)	22(100)
Not used	10(35.7)	0

P ≤ 0.01, df= 1

handler from cross-contamination, overalls should be suitable to wear over other clothing (CFIA, 1990).

The clean gum boots are just as important as clean overalls, because they may also be a source of contamination. Gum boots should therefore be washed at the facility provided (washing-basins supplied with hot and cold water, liquid soap and a brush) before entering the processing room (Van Zyl, 1995). The purpose of hairnets and beard nets is twofold: to prevent loose hairs and dandruff from falling into the food and also to discourage the workers from running their fingers through their hair or scratching their scalps (Educational Foundation, 1992; Pelczar et al., 1993).

CONCLUSION AND RECOMMENDATIONS

The results obtained from this study showed that contamination sources of beef are more likely to be associated with insufficient hygienic practices and improper handling of meat in the slaughterhouse and retail shops. Floor surface, cutting boards, hooks and knives, workers hands and transporting vehicle in slaughterhouses as well as, in retail shops, are potential sources of beef contamination.

The overall prevalence of E. coli, E. coli O157:H7 and Salmonella were 36 (12.4%), 6 (2.06%) and 8 (2.75%) which indicated that slaughterhouses and retail shops in HU and Dire Dawa could be the source of contamination of beef. HU and Dire Dawa slaughterhouses and retail shops are not well structured and the working habits in the slaughterhouse are not good enough to satisfy an acceptable hygienic standard practice for slaughtering and processing of beef for human consumption. The study suggested that beef could be a significant source of foodborne pathogens for people in the study areas.

Based on the findings of the present study, the following recommendations are forwarded in order to guarantee the microbial quality of beef and minimize the risk of E. coli O157:H7 and Salmonellosis outbreak in Dire Dawa and Haramaya University and its surrounding areas.

1. Haramaya University should open the newly constructed slaughterhouses that can improve slaughtering and processing of beef for human consumption and Dire Dawa administrative city authorities should improve their supervision of slaughterhouse workers.
2. Periodic sanitary-hygienic evaluation and inspection of

abattoirs and beef meat retail establishments should be implemented and Health authorities need to enforce legislative requirements and periodic monitoring aimed at insuring the proper slaughtering process and sanitary-hygienic standards. Failure to meet these requirements should result in enforcement action against premises, and this should ultimately lead to prosecution and suspension and/or revocation of their license to operate.

3. Good manufacturing practice and good hygienic practice, together with stringent control of all aspects of meat production, preparation, storage and distribution should be put in place in food establishment in order to reduce contamination of *Salmonella* and other foodborne pathogens to acceptable limit.

4. Training to meat handlers regarding stunning process, food safety and good hygienic practices should be given especially in Haramaya University slaughter house as all workers who had no formal trainings.

CONFLICT OF INTERESTS

The author has not declared any conflict of interest.

ACKNOWLEDGEMENT

We would like to extend our thanks to College of Veterinary Medicine, Haramaya University for all round support.

REFERENCES

Activity Based Management (ABM) (2008). Standards for Abattoir, Cutting and Packing Plant. Version 4.0 January, 2008 Northern Ireland.

Adams MR, Moss MO (1997). Food Microbiol. Cambridge: The R Soc Chem. pp. 200-213.

Adu-Gyamfi A, Torgby-Tetteh W and Appiah V (2012). Microbiological quality of chicken sold in Accra and determination of D10-Value of *E. coli*. Food Nutr. Sci. 3(5):693-698.

Alemseged F, Yami A, Birke W, S/Mariam Z and Worku K (2009). Investigation of Dysentery outbreak and Its causes, Jimma City South west, Ethiopia. Ethiop. J. Health Sci. 19(3):147-154.

Alvarez-Astorga M, Capita R, Alonso-Calleja C, Moreno B, Del M and Garcia-Fernandez C (2002). Microbiological quality of retail chicken by-products in Spain. Meat Sci. 62(1):45-50.

Asrat GT, Berhan T, Solomon M (2008). Inclusion of Different Proportions of Poultry Litter in the Rations of Yearling Hararghe Highland goats. Livest. Res. Rural Dev. 20:48.

Bayleyegn M, Daniel A, Woubit S (2003). Sources and distribution of *Salmonella* serotypes isolated from food animals, slaughterhouse personnel and retail meat products in Ethiopia. Ethiop J. Health Dev. 17:63-70.

Bhandare S, Sherikarv A, Paturkar A, Waskar V, Zende R (2007). A comparison of microbial contamination on sheep/goat carcasses in a modern Indian abattoir and traditional meat shops. Food Control 18:854-868.

Brown MH, Gill CO, Hollingsworth J, Nickelson R, Seward S, Sheridan JJ (2000). The role of microbiological testing in systems for assuring the safety of beef. Int. J. Food Microbiol. 62:7-16.

Burton GR (1996). Microbiology for the health sciences (4th ed.). New York: Lippencott. pp. 234-239.

Canadian Food Inspection Agency (CFIA) (1990). Meat hygiene manual of procedures, Canada. Available at: http://www.inspection.gc.ca/food/meat-and-poultry-products/manual-of-procedures/eng/1300125426052/1300125482318.

Centers for Disease Control and Prevention (CDC) (2013). FoodNet: Incidence and Trends in Foodborne Illness.

Central of Statistics Agency (CSA) (2007). Agricultural sample survey 2006/07(1999 EC). Report on livestock and livestock characteristics (private peasant holdings), CSA, Addis Ababa, Ethiopia.

Chapman PA, Siddons CA, Cerdan Malo AT, Harkin MA (2000). A one year study of *E. coli* O157 in raw beef and lamb products. Epidemiol. Infect. 124:207-213.

Chhabra MB, Singla LD (2009). Food-borne parasitic zoonoses in India: Review of recent reports of human infections. J. Vet. Parasitol. 23(2):103-110.

Collee JG, Mackie TJ (1999). *Practical Medical Microbiology*. 14th ed Churchill living stone. pp 883-884, 898-907.

Desenclos JC, Zergabachew A, Desmoulins B, Chouteau L, Desve G (1988). Clinical, microbiological and antibiotic susceptibility patterns of diarrhoea in Korem, Ethiopia. J. Trop. Med. Hyg. 91:296-301.

Desmarchelier PM, Higgs GM, Mills L, Sullivan AM, Vanderlinde PB (1999). Incidence of coagulase positive *Staphylococcus* on beef carcasses in three Australian abattoirs. Int. J. Food Microbiol. 47:221-229.

Diane GN, Marion K, Linda V, Erwin D, Awa AK, Hein S, Marieke O, Merel L, John T, Flemming S, Koke V-DG, Hild K (2010). Foodborne diseases. Int. J. Food Microbiol. 139:s3-s15.

Doyle ME (2007). Microbial food spoilage – Losses and control strategies, (A brief review of the Literature), FRI Briefings. Available at: www.wisc.edu/fri/

Duffy EA, Belk KE, Sofos JN, LeValley SB, Kain ML, Tatum JD, Smith GC, Kimberling CV (2001). Microbial contamination occurring on lamb carcasses processed in the United States. J. Food Prot. 64 (4):503-508.

Educational Foundation of the National Restaurant Association (1992). Applied food service sanitation (4th ed.). Canada: John Wiley and Sons. pp: 44-45.

Ejeta G, Molla B, Alemayehu D, Muckle A (2004). *Salmonella* serotypes isolated from minced meat beef, mutton and pork in Addis Ababa, Ethiopia. Revue Méd. Vét. 11:547-551.

Evans JA, Russell SL, James C, Corry JE (2004). Microbiological contamination of food refrigeration equipment. J. Food Eng. 62:225-232.

Fawole MO, Oso BA (2001). *Laboratory manual of microbiology*: Revised edition. Ibadan: Spectrum books Ltd. P 127.

FDA (Food and Drug Authority) (1992). Bacteriological Analytical Manual. 7th Ed. AOAC international 2200 Wilson Blvd, Suite 400, Arlington, VA. Available at: ttp://www.fda.gov/Food/FoodScienceResearch/LaboratoryMethods/ucm2006949.htm.

Fegan N, Vanderlinde P, Higgs G, Desmarchelier P (2004). Quantification and prevalence of *Salmonella* in beef cattle presenting at slaughter, J. Appl. Microbiol. 97:892-898.

Fratamico PA, Bhunia AK, Smith JL (2005). Foodborne Pathogens: Microbiology and Molecular Biology, Caister Academic Press, Wymondham, Norfolk, UK. P 273.

Gill CO (2007). Sampling of red meat. In Microbiological Analysis of red meat, poultry and egg, Mead, G.C. (editor). Cambridge, England; Woodhead Publishing Limited. pp. 132-135.

Gill CO, Mcginnis JC (2004). Microbiological conditions of air knives before and after maintenance at a beef packing plant. Meat Sci. 68:333-337.

Gill CO, Badoni M, McGinnis JC (1999). Assessment of the adequacy of cleaning of equipment used for breaking beef carcasses. Int. J. Food

Microbiol. 46:18.

Gill CO, Bryant J, Brereton DA (2000). Microbiological conditions of sheep carcasses from conventional or inverted dressing processes. J. Food Prot. 63(9):1291-1294.

Gordon-Davis L (1998). The hospitality industry handbook on hygiene and safety: for South African students and practitioners. Kenwyn: Juta publication. pp. 49-65

Haque MA, Siddique MP, Habib MA, Sarkar V, Chou KA (2008). Evaluation of sanitary quality of goat meat obtained from slaughter yards and meat stalls at late market hours. Bangl. J. Vet. Med. 6(1):87-92.

Hassan AN, Farooqui A, Khan A, Khan Y, Kazmi SU (2010). Microbial contamination of raw meat and its environment in retail shops in Karachi, Pakistan. J. Infect. Dev. Ctries. 4(6):382-388.

Haymanot T, Alemseged A, Getenet B, Solomon GS (2010). Microbial flora and foodborne pathogens on minced meat and their susceptibility to antimicrobial agents Jimma city, Ethiopia. Ethiop. J. Health Sci. 20(3):137-143.

Hiko A, Asrat D, Zewde G (2008). Occurrence of E. coli O157:H7 in retail raw meat products in Ethiopia. J. Infect Dev. Ctries. 2:389-393.

ICMSF (International Commission on Microbiological Specifications for Foods) (1986). Microorganisms in Foods 2. Sampling for microbiological analysis: Principle and specific application, (2nd ed.) Blackwell Scientific Publications. UK. pp. 132-136.

ISO (International Organization for Standardization)/TS 11133-1 (2009). Microbiology of food and animal feeding stuffs. Guidelines on preparation and production of culture media. Part 1: General guidelines on quality assurance for the preparation of culture media in the laboratory.

ISO (International Organization for Standardization)-16654 (2001). Microbiology of food and animal feeding stuffs. Horizontal method for the detection of E. coli O157:H7.

ISO (International Organization for Standardization)-4333 (2003). A horizontal method for the enumeration of microorganisms by counting the colonies growing in solid medium after aerobic culturing of aerobic bacteria.

ISO (International Organization for Standardization)-6579 (2002). Microbiology-General guidance on methods for the detection of Salmonella, 4rd ed International Organization for Standardization, Geneva.

Larson E, Aiello A, Lee LV, Della-Latta P, Gomez-Duarte C, Lin S (2003). Short and long term effects of hand washing with antimicrobial or plain soap in the community. J. Commun. Health 28(2):139-150.

Luga I, Akombo PM, Kwaga JKP, Umoh VJ and Ajogi I (2007). Sero-prevalence of Faecal Shedding of E. coli O157:H7 from Exotic Dairy Cattle in North-Western Nigeria. Niger. Vet. J. 28:6-11.

Mache A, Mengistu Y, Cowley S (1997). Salmonella sero groups identified from adult diarrheal out-patients in Addis Ababa, Ethiopia: Antibiotic resistance and plasmid profile analysis. East Afr. Med. J. 74:183-187.

Mekonnen H, Habtamu T, Kelali A, Shewit K (2012). Food safety knowledge and practices of abattoir and butchery shops and the microbial profile of meat in Mekelle City, Ethiopia. Asian Pac. J. Trop. Biomed. 12:952-957.

Mersha G, Asrat D, Zewde BM, Kyule M (2009). Occurrence of E. coli O157:H7 in faeces, skin and carcasses from sheep and goats in Ethiopia. Lett. Appl. Microbiol. 50:71-76.

Molla B, Kleer J, Sinell HJ (2000). Occurrence, distribution and level of Salmonella in selected food items in Addis Ababa, Ethiopia. Fleischwirt Int. 4:37-39.

Mukhopadhyay HK, Pillai RM, Pal UK, Kumar VJA (2009). Microbial quality of fresh chevon and beef in retail Outlets of pondicherry. Tamilnadu J. Vet. Anim. Sci. 5 (1):33-36.

Pelczar MJ, Chan ECS, Krieg NR (1993). Microbiology, concepts and applications. New York: McGraw-Hill. pp. 80-100, 158-161, 370.

Podpecan B, Pengov A, Vadnjal S (2007). The source of contamination of ground meat for production of meat products with bacteria Staphylococcus aureus. Slov. Vet. Res. 44:25-30.

Pointon A, Sexton M, Dowsett P, Saputra T, Kiermeier A, Lorimer M, Holds G, Arnold G, Davos D, Combs B, Fabiansson S, Raven G, McKenzie H, Chapman A, Sumner J (2008). A baseline survey of the microbiological quality of chicken portions and carcasses at retail in two Australian states (2005 to 2006). J. Food Prot. 71(6):1123-1134.

Ryser ET, Marth EH (1991). Listeria, Listeriosis, and food safety. New York: Marcel Dekker. pp. 183-189.

Sefinew A, Bayleyegn M (2012). Prevalence and antimicrobial resistance profiles of Salmonella enteric serovars isolated from slaughtered cattle in Bahir Dar, Ethiopia. Trop. Anim. Health Prod. 44:595-600.

Sibhat B, Molla B, Zerihun A, Muckle A, Cole L, Boerlin P, Wilkie E, Perets A, Mistry K, Gebreyes WA (2011). Salmonella serovars and antimicrobial resistance profiles in beef cattle, slaughterhouse personnel and slaughterhouse environment in Ethiopia. Zoonoses Public Health 58:102-109.

Sneed J, Strohbehn C, Gilmore AS, Mendonca A (2004). Microbiological evaluation of food service contact surfaces in Iowa assisted living facilities. J. Am. Diet. Assoc. 104:1722-1724.

Sousa CP (2008). The Impact of Food Manufacturing Practices on Foodborne Diseases. Braz. Arch. Biol. Technol. 51(4):815-823.

Taye M, Berhanu T, Berhanu Y, Tamiru F, Terefe D (2013). Study on carcass contaminating E. coli in apparently healthy slaughtered cattle in Haramaya University slaughter house with special emphasis on E. coli O157:H7, Ethiopia. J. Vet. Sci. Technol. 4:132.

Tegegne M, Ashenafi M (1998). Microbial load and incidence of Salmonella species in kitfo", traditional Ethiopian spiced, minced meat dish. Ethiop. J. Health Dev. 12:135-140.

Temelli S, Dokuzlu C, Cemsen MK (2006). Determination of microbiological contamination sources during frozen snail meat processing stages. Food Control 17:22-29.

Thrusfield M (2007). Veterinary Epidemiology, 3rd Edition. Blackwell Science, UK. P 332.

Timothy M, Smith JR (2012). Isolation, Identification, and Enumeration of Pathogenic Salmonella Serovars from Environmental Waters. J. Food Prot. 76(7):2-251.

Trickett J (1997). Food hygiene for food handlers. London: Macmillan Press. pp. 19-27.

Van Zyl AP (1995). Manual for the abattoir industry (1st ed.). Pretoria: Red Meat Abattoir Association. pp. 123-156.

WHO (World Health Organization) (2007). Food safety and foodborne diseases and value chain management for food safety. "Forging links between Agriculture and Health" CGIAR on Agriculture and Health Meeting in WHO/HQ.

Wilson I (2002). Salmonella and Campylobacter contamination of raw retail chickens from different producers: a six year survey. Epidemiol. Infect. 129:635-645.

Zewdu E, Cornelius P (2009). Antimicrobial resistance pattern of Salmonella serotypes isolated from food items and personnel in Addis Ababa, Ethiopia. Trop. Anim. Health Prod 41:241-249.

16

Review of common causes of abortion in dairy cattle in Ethiopia

Dereje Tulu[1,2*], Benti Deresa[2], Feyisa Begna[2] and Abiy Gojam[2]

[1]Ethiopian Institute of Agricultural Research, Tepi Agricultural Research Center, P. O. Box 34. Tepi, Ethiopia.
[2]School of Veterinary Medicine, College of Agriculture and Veterinary Medicine, Jimma University, P. O. Box 307, Jimma, Ethiopia.

Abortion in dairy cattle may be caused by infectious and non-infectious agents. Infectious causes of abortion in dairy cattle include brucellosis, leptospirosis, listeriosis, Q fever, bovine viral diarrhea, mycotic abortion and neosporosis. Non-infectious causes of abortion in dairy cattle are genetic and non-genetic disorder. Risk factors associated with abortion in dairy cattle are genetic, environmental, management, geographical factors and infectious factors. Abortion in dairy cows brings about breeding and productive damages. Abortions cause significant economic loss to dairy farm. These losses can be attributed to loss of replacement calves, reduced milk production, costs of treatment, feeding of animals and premature culling of productive cows and heifers. Diagnosis of bovine abortion includes the collection of a complete history of the case and relevant epidemiological data and collected sample for analysis. However, determining the cause of bovine abortion is difficult as abortions are caused by numerous infectious and noninfectious factors. Status of abortion and breeds affected by abortion in Ethiopia were also reviewed.

Key words: Causes, abortion, dairy cattle, Ethiopia.

INTRODUCTION

Ethiopia has the largest livestock population in Africa, with a total cattle population of 57.83 million. Out of this total cattle population, the female cattle constitute about 55.38% and the remaining 44.62% are male cattle. At present, about 99% of Ethiopia's national herd is of local breeds managed under extensive farming systems (CSA, 2016). The livestock contributes about 16.5% of the national Gross Domestic Product (GDP) and 35.6% of the agricultural GDP. It also contributes 15% of export earnings and 30% of agricultural employment (Leta and Mesele, 2014). However, the rate of urbanization is high, which places challenges on farmers and government to meet the demand for food (red meat and dairy products) for an increasing population. To increase livestock productivity and satisfy the increasing demand for livestock products, Ethiopia has given more attention to breed improvement, pasture development and animal health (Azage et al., 2001; Shapiro et al., 2015).

*Corresponding author. E-mail: derejetulu5@gmail.com.

Ethiopia has paid considerable attention to livestock productivity (meat and milk) through breeding and health interventions to increase the contribution of livestock to economic growth as well as to meet the increasing local demands. The country has given priority on the development of dairying at farmer's level to increase the supply of milk from smallholder dairy farms (Zegeye, 2003). However, reproductive health problems are becoming the major obstacles hindering this development plan (Adane et al., 2014; Ararsa and Wubshet, 2014). Among these, abortion is the main constraint in sector development plan to achieve its goal. Moreover abortion has direct impacts on reproductive performance of dairy cows (Lobago et al., 2006; Ernest, 2009). Abortion is defined as the termination of pregnancy between 42 and 260 days of gestation (Peter, 2000). The diagnosis of abortions is challenge to the farmers and veterinarian. There is sudden and dramatic increase of abortion in herds over a long period of time (Hossein-Zadeh, 2013).

Bovine abortion has infectious and none infectious causes (Hovingh, 2009). Infectious causes of abortion associated with abortion in cattle include viruses, bacteria, protozoa and fungus. The exact proportion of cases due to infectious agents is not known, but in 90% of cases in which an etiologic diagnosis is achieved, the cause is infectious (Parthiban et al., 2015). These pathogens can result in extensive economic losses, indicating the need for control measures to prevent infection or disease (Givens and Marley, 2008). Non-infectious factors such as genetic and non-genetic disorders have been reported in some investigations. The most important non genetic factors are heat stress, production stress, seasonal effect and seasonal changes (Hansen, 2002; Sani and Amanloo, 2007). The most important genetic disorders include chromosomal and single gene disorders and these disorders result in high abortion rate in cows and increased calf sterility. Cow parity, sire effect, age at conception and abortion history could be some of the non-infectious maternal and paternal factors that cause abortion (Thurmond et al., 2005; Lee and Kim, 2007).

Abortions have a highly negative impact on reproductive efficiency, resulting in significant economic losses for the cattle industry (De Vries, 2006). Spontaneous abortion of dairy cows is the most common problem that contributes substantially to low herd viability and decreasing production potential by reducing the number of potential female herd replacements and lifetime milk production, and by increasing costs associated with breeding and premature culling (Thurmond et al., 2005). The cost of abortion depends mainly on the time of gestation, milk production and time of insemination after parturition, the cost of nutrition, sperm costs, insemination time and labor costs (Rafati et al., 2010). Late term abortions could also result in loss of potential replacement heifers, early culling of productive cows and loss in herd's potential calf production

(Carpenter et al., 2006). The prevalence rate of abortion varies in different production system and from place to place. Prevalence rate of abortion in Ethiopia range from 2.2 to 28.9% (Table 3) (Gizaw et al., 2007; Siyoum et al., 2016). This difference in prevalence rate may be due to variation in cattle breed and husbandry management system. Eshete and Moges (2014) indicated that incidence of abortion of more than 2 to 5% should be viewed seriously, efforts should be made to determine the causes and measures should be taken to control abortion. This paper reviews common cause of abortion, economic important and risk factor of abortion in dairy cattle.

ABORTION IN DAIRY CATTLE

Abortion is the termination of pregnancy at a stage where the expelled fetus is of recognizable size ranging from 45 to 260 days of gestation and not viable (Peter, 2000). Sarder et al. (2010) also defined abortion as a condition in which fetus is delivered live or dead before reaching the stage of viability where the delivered fetus is visible by naked eyes. Some diseases that cause abortion in cattle, such as brucellosis, Leptospirosis are also zoonotic (Levett, 2005; De Vries, 2006). The important infectious agents that have been reported to cause abortion in cattle can be viral, bacterial, protozoa as well as several fungal species among others (Table 1) (Juyal et al., 2011). In addition, any disease causing high fever may also cause abortion (Radostits et al., 2007).

Common infectious causes of bovine abortion

Brucellosis

Brucellosis is an important disease of humans, and domestic and wild animals worldwide and is also a serious zoonosis (Mekonen et al., 2010). In female cattle, the disease is characterized by abortions storms in pregnant cattle, infertility, mastitis, retained placentae and arthritis (Radostits et al., 2007). Infected cow usually abort between the fifth and seventh month of pregnancy. Abortion due to brucellosis commonly occurs during the last trimester of pregnancy (Parthiban et al., 2015). All these manifestations lead to losses in the production system. Several species of the bacterium Brucella can cause brucellosis in cattle; however, Brucella abortus is the primary bovine pathogen (Godfroid et al., 2011). Brucellosis in cattle is spread by ingestion of contaminated pasture, feed and water, licking aborted foetuses or genital exudates from recently aborted cows or carrier cattle that have calved normally. However, with infection through injured/intact skin, the mucosa at the respiratory system and conjunctiva frequently occurs (Acha and Szyfres, 2001; Degefa et al., 2011).

While vaccination of cattle with strains S19 and RB51 has been the cornerstone of brucellosis control programmers in the developed world, adequate information on its occurrence in the developing world is lacking and the adoption of control programmers is still low (Godfroid et al., 2011). Several risk factors for bovine brucellosis have been reported. Among these are increased herd sizes, increased age, sex of the animal, husbandry practices such as animal confinement, contact with wildlife, geographical area and keeping different breeds in a herd (Muma et al., 2007; Tolosa et al., 2010; Matope et al., 2010; Mekonen et al., 2010).

Various techniques have been used to diagnose bovine brucellosis. These include the use of staining techniques, such as modified acid fast staining, culture and molecular techniques, such as polymerase chain reaction. However, in most epidemiological studies, serological tests, such as serum agglutination test (SAT), Rose-Bengal test (RBT), Buffered plate agglutination test (BPAT), fluorescence polarization assay (FPA) and ELISA, are often used. The limitations to the use of serological tests are false positives from vaccinated animals, cross-reactivity with other Gram-negative bacteria, and low sensitivity from tests such as SAT and RBT (OIE, 2009).

Leptospirosis

Leptospirosis is a contagious, bacterial disease of animals and humans. It is a globally important zoonotic disease caused by the pathogenic Gram negative bacteria of the genus, Leptospira (Bharti et al., 2003). The disease occurs worldwide, it is most common in temperate regions in the late summer and early fall and in tropical regions during rainy seasons (Tilahun et al., 2013). Although, the incidence of disease seems to have decreased in developed countries, it is apparently emerging rapidly as a significant public health problem in developing countries (Tangkanakul et al., 2000).

All mammals appear to be susceptible to at least one species of Leptospira. The primary reservoir hosts for most Leptospira serovars are wild mammals, particularly rodents. Reservoir hosts among domestic animals includes cattle, dogs, sheep and pigs and they may act as carriers for several months (temporary carrier) while rodents usually remain carrier throughout their life (permanent carrier) (Sophia, 2013). Rodents are therefore considered as the major reservoir of infection. The specific reservoir hosts vary with the serovar and the geographic region (OIE, 2005). In cattle, leptospirosis has been characterized by a wide variety of conditions including fever, icterus, hemoglobinuria, abortion and death. Cattle are the maintenance hosts for Leptospira serovar hardjo and Leptospira borgpeter-senii serovar hardjo, and incidental hosts for serovar pomona which is maintained in swine (Parthiban et al., 2015).

Leptospirosis can be transmitted either directly between hosts or indirectly in the environment. Leptospira species can be ingested in contaminated food or water, spread in aerosolized urine or water, or transmitted by direct contact with the skin. The organisms usually enter the body through mucous membranes or abraded skin. They may also be able to penetrate intact skin that has been immersed for a long time in water (Sophia et al., 2014). Leptospira species are excreted in the urine and can be found in aborted or stillborn fetuses, as well as in normal fetuses or vaginal discharges after calving (Levett, 2001).

Leptospirosis of animals is investigated by direct and indirect laboratory methods. Direct methods are the isolation of the causative agent and the identification of Leptospira species antigens in tissue and body fluids using methods such as immunofluorescence staining, immunochemistry immune peroxidase staining, silver staining and various methods of polymerase chain reaction (PCR) (WHO, 2006). Direct visualization of leptospirae in blood or urine by dark field microscopic examination has been used for diagnosis. But artefacts are commonly mistaken for leptospirae and the method has both low sensitivity and specificity (Vijayachari et al., 2001). For early diagnosis, serum is the optimal specimen. Urine from severely ill patients is often highly concentrated and contains significant inhibitory activity (Brown et al., 2003). The indirect methods of investigating leptospirosis are based on the detection of specific serum antibodies. These methods are either methods detecting serum antibodies without discriminating serovars, such as various ELISA tests, indirect immunofluorescence, the spot agglutination test or methods reliably identifying the infecting serovars, such as the microscopic agglutination test (MAT). Microscopic agglutination test (MAT) is used as the 'gold standard' serological tests even though the test is very tedious and requires the maintenance of several leptospiral serovars in the laboratory. Also, the test requires the expertise personnel to read the results (Ooteman, 2006).

Understanding the epidemiological features of leptospirosis is a critical step in designing interventions for reducing the risk of the disease transmission (Levett, 2001). Intervention strategies can target many points in the transmission cycle of leptospirosis. Although, little can be done in wild animals, leptospirosis in cattle is controlled through vaccination, prophylactic treatment of exposed cattle with antibiotics, quarantining of newly introduced cattle for at least 4 weeks, rodent control, regular serological testing, improved environmental hygiene, separating young animals from adults and safe artificial insemination (Dhanze et al., 2013).

Leptospirosis could result in a "storm of abortions" causing considerable economic losses from meat and milk reductions. Furthermore, these losses appear as more significant among cattle, because this animal

Table 1. Infectious causes of abortion in dairy cattle in Ethiopia.

Bacteria	Fungal	Protozoan	Viral
Campylobacter fetus	Aspergillus fumigatus	Neospora caninum	Bovine herpesvirus1
Histophilus somni	Mucor spp	Tritrichomanas fetus	Bovine viral diarrhea virus
Ureaplasma spp.	Morteriella wolfii	Toxopllasma gondii	Bluetongue virus
Brucella abortus		Anaplasma marginale	Epizootic bovine abortion
Leptospira spp.			Schmallenberg virus
Listeria monocytogene; Arcanobacterium pyogenes; Chlamydophila spp.; *Salmonella; Coxiella burnetti*			

Source: Givens and Marley, 2008.

species are considered less resistant than small ruminants (Tooloei et al., 2008). Abortion may occur several weeks after infection of the dam and is usually not associated with any obvious illness in the cow. Abortions due to serovar *hardjo* infection tend to occur sporadically. But abortion "storms" may occur as a result of infection with serovars *pomona* or *grippotyphosa*. Abortion storms are more common when the weather is wet and there is standing water that is contaminated with infective organisms (Bharti et al., 2011). Abortion usually occurs during the last trimester of pregnancy but can occur from the 4th month onwards. Infertility and milk drop occurs only in pregnant or lactating cows because *Leptospira* organisms prefer pregnant uterus and lactating mammary gland to proliferate (Yadeta et al., 2016).

Although, there is few documented information so far concerning the occurrence of leptospirosis in animals in Ethiopia, climatologic, socioeconomic and other factors are highly favorable for the occurrence and spread of the disease in the country. In Ethiopia, leptospirosis has been reported to occur in domestic animals working in Ethiopia, with incidences of 70.7% in cows (Yadeta et al., 2016). In the case of human leptospirosis, there is a pilot study in Wonji Hospital. According to Eshetu et al. (2004) from a total of 59 febrile patients attending the outpatient department of Wonji Hospital, 47.5% were positive for leptospirosis and the occurrence of the disease was more common in males than females.

Listeriosis

Listeriosis is an infectious disease of human and animals with a world-wide distribution. It manifests in three major clinical forms, meningoencephalitis, abortion and septicaemia (Hirsh et al., 2004). Listeriosis is caused by a member of the genus Listeria. Majority of the clinical cases are associated with *Listeria monocytogenes* infection. Only a few reported cases have been associated with *L. ivanovii* (Radostits et al., 2007). *Listeria* species are found widely throughout the

environment. *Listeria* can be ingested with poorly preserved silage which is not fermented properly and is not acidic enough to kill the bacteria. It can be ingested via soil on the grass roots and also the placenta and discharges from the infected cow (Aderson, 2007).

Listeria monocytogenes is a well-recognized cause of abortion, encephalitis and septicemia in cattle. *Listeria ivanovii* has also been implicated as a cause of abortion in cattle but occurs less frequently than *L. monocytogenes*. Abortion occurs after ingestion of *L. monocytogenes* contaminated feed and a resultant bacteremia. Experimental studies have shown that after ingestion or parenteral injection of *L. monocytogenes*, the genital organs and foetus are invaded within 24 h of the onset of bacteremia. This results in abortion in 5 to 10 days (Radostits, 2007). *Listeria* infections and abortions usually develop in the late winter or early spring. Abortions are most commonly recognized in the last trimester of pregnancy and abortion storms can occur when all herd eat same batch of contaminated silage at same time (Yaeger et al., 2007).

In abortion, the pathological picture depends on the stage of pregnancy. If it occurs in the early stages of the last trimester, the placenta is quickly invaded by the bacteria and the foetus dies as a result of septicaemia. The dead foetus is expelled within 5 days and by this time autolytic changes cover the minor gross lesions produced by the organism. Metritis usually occurs and results in retention of the foetal membranes. If it occurs at a late stage, the offspring may be born in the normal way but is usually unable to survive. In the aborted foetus the lesions are less severe. Gross lesions are tiny pin-point yellow foci in the liver. Similar foci but visible only microscopically are seen in the lung, myocardium, kidney, spleen and brain. The bacteria can be demonstrated in the center of these focal areas (Thomson, 1988; Quinn et al., 2002).

The organism is sensitive to a wide range of antibiotics. Culling infected animals should be advocated as they secrete the organisms in secretions and excretions, especially in the cases of mastitis. Care in the use and preparation of silage is important as the pathogen grows luxuriantly at a pH greater than 5.5 (Walker, 2007). Farm management practices, such as improvement of nutritional status of animals and better housing conditions, can also be of some value in preventing disease (Dhama et al., 2017).

In Ethiopia, few findings of *L. monocytogenes* have been reported, possibly due to lack of attention or resources (Molla et al., 2004). Study conducted by Seyoum et al. (2015) showed that prevalence of *Listeria* species was 28.4% and specifically that of *L. monocytogenes* was 5.6% from raw bovine milk and milk products from central highlands of Ethiopia. Other study conducted in Gondar on foods of animal origin indicated that 25% were positive for Listeria species and that of *L. monocytogenes* was 6.25% (Garedew et al., 2015)

Mycotic abortions

Mycotic abortion causes great economic losses to the individual farmer and cattle-breeding industry as a whole. Mycotic infection of the placenta is one of the most common causes of sporadic bovine abortion (Ali and Khan, 2006). Mycotic abortion is caused by different species of fungi and yeasts. About 35 different species of fungi have been known to cause abortion, *Aspergillus fumigatus* being the most commonly diagnosed casual organism which accounts for 60 to 80% of abortions. 20 to 35% of abortions have been attributed to fungal causes (Pal, 2015). *Aspergillus fumigatus* is the cause of over 70% mycotic abortions recorded in cattle, around the world (Ali and Khan, 2006)

Abortion occurs when fungal spores enter a pregnant cow's blood stream, settle at the junction of the maternal and foetal placentas, grow and attack the placental tissues (Walker, 2007). In general, fungal spores may be present in cattle feed. However, some feeds such as improperly preserved silage and hay that has been wet, contain many more spores than others. Storm of abortion occur in cattle when feeding with mouldy hay at same time. The mycotic abortions were confirmed by isolation of *Aspergillus fumigatus* fungi from mouldy hay as well as from foetal abomasal contents (Chandranaik et al., 2014).

Pregnancy in a cow with metabolic derangements from stress may predispose the pregnant cow to fungal infection. The incidence of the condition is high in late summer or early autumn, due to the presence of large number of fungal spores in pastures during this period (Ali and Khan, 2006). There is also evidence of a winter rise of disease incidence. The organism may cause abortion from 4 months to term. Other species of molds and yeasts have been associated with abortion (Parthiban et al., 2015).

Any condition that reduces the cow's resistance to infection increases the chances of mycotic abortion. Providing good health (via good management and nutrition) and not feeding moldy feeds can reduce the incidence. When possible, depending on the availability and demand decreases the period of confinement, decrease cow density and improve ventilation (Pal, 2015).

Query fever (Q fever)

Q fever is a zoonosis of worldwide distribution caused by Gram-negative intracellular bacteria *Coxiella burnetii*, which can infect arthropods, birds and animals (Cutler et al., 2007). Currently it is not possible to accurately estimate the true prevalence infection in domestic ruminants, due to lack of well-designed studies. However, there has been detection of *C. burnetii* in all five continents (except in New Zealand being the only country with a reported apparent prevalence of zero), with a wide range, in whatever kind. The apparent prevalence is slightly higher in cattle (20.0 and 37.7%) than in sheep and goats (around 15 to 25%) (Guatteo et al., 2011).

Infections by *C. burnetii* in animal production are mostly asymptomatic, however, may be related to reproductive disorders such as abortion, stillbirths, repetition heat, low birth weight animals and metritis. Nevertheless, latter clinical manifestation appears to be unique in cattle, occurring during first three weeks after birth, with fetid vaginal discharge and/or increase in body temperature (Sheldon et al., 2006).

In most cases, abortion occurs in late pregnancy which range from 3 to 80% with unspecified characteristic clinical signs of infection with *C. burnetii* (Angelakis and Raoult, 2010). Aborted fetuses appear normal but infected placentas exhibit intercotyledonary fibrous thickening and discolored exudates, which are not specific to Q fever (Arricau-Bouvery and Rodolakis, 2005). *Coxiella burnetii* can also be recovered from milk for up to 32 months. Furthermore, there may be shedding bacteria in the urine, semen and vaginal discharge mucus. An important factor related to abortion rates in herds is the temperature, since fewer abortions take place between months of November and December. However, this occurrence increases gradually from January to February, decreasing again in March (Cantas et al., 2011).

A relevant issue is infestation of cattle by ticks during months when temperature is higher. Previous studies have shown that ticks seem to play an important role in the dissemination of bacteria in animals, especially wild, believing it to be an important factor in the transmission to domestic animals (Psaroulaki et al., 2006). On the other hand, a recent study developed in the Netherlands, after three years of an outbreak of Q fever, researchers investigated the role ticks play in the transmission *C. burnetii*, showing that actual risk of this infection by ticks is negligible. Moreover, for future risk assessments, it might be relevant to sample more ticks in the vicinity of previously *C. burnetii* infected goat farms and to assess whether *C. burnetii* can be transmitted transovarially and transstadially in *Ixodus ricinus* ticks (Sprong et al., 2011).

Few studies conducted in Ethiopia indicated that 6.5% seroprevalence of *C. burnetii* was observed in Addis Ababa abattoir workers. Also, the existence of antibody against *C. burnetii* was reported in goats and sheep slaughtered at Addis Ababa abattoir, and its peri-urban zones. A seroprevalence of 31.6% of *C. burnetii* was recorded in cattle in South Eastern Ethiopian pastoral zones of the Somali and Oromia regional states (Gumi et al., 2013).

Bovine viral diarrhea (BVD)

Bovine viral diarrhea is a disease caused by bovine viral diarrhea virus (BVDV). Bovine viral diarrhea is one of the most important diseases of cattle worldwide (Almeida et al., 2010). It is an important cause of diarrhea, reproductive problems and reduced milk yield in affected herds (Lindberg and Houe, 2005). This is a Pestivirus in the family Flaviviridae that is closely related to border disease virus of sheep and classical swine fever virus of pigs (OIE, 2004). The disease occurs worldwide and infections may be subclinical in some animals (Lindberg and Houe, 2005). Bovine viral diarrhea virus can be persistent in infected animal and wild animal asymptomatic while shedding large amount of virus throughout their life time (Nelson et al., 2016).

Bovine viral diarrhea virus is transmitted by direct contact with saliva, faeces, semen, urine, tears and milk of infected cattle, or by in utero infection of fetuses (Radostits et al., 2007). Infection of naive pregnant cows and heifers may lead to abortion and other reproductive disorders, such as early embryonic death (the death of a conceptus within the first 2 months after conception) in the first 45 days, fetal death and mummification (Kabongo and Van Vuuren, 2004). Infection during the first trimester of pregnancy will cause storm of abortions approximately one month prior to parturition. Infection during the second trimester will often lead to a higher risk of birth defects and less abortion, and this is more common in beef cattle than dairy breeds. But in final trimester of pregnancy, there are no more effects (Van Campen, 2010). The other effects of BVDV are birth of calves with congenital defects, calves with poor growth rates, and increased average age at first calving in affected herds (Heuer et al., 2007). The virus has also been shown to depress ovarian function in infected heifers by disrupting gonadal steroidogenesis, and impairing the quality of oocytes produced (Fray et al., 2000; Altamarand et al., 2013). Infection from day 9 to 45 of gestation results in reduced conception rates and infertility, early embryonic death and infertility. From days 45 to 75 of gestation, infection with BVDV will result in abortions, intrauterine growth retardation, and calves with congenital defects especially of the nervous system.

Infection in late gestation (125 to 285) results in birth of normal calves with neutralizing antibodies (Grooms, 2004). This virus has a high affinity for leucocytes and reduces their numbers in infected animals. This immunosuppression potentiates the effects of other pathogens, including abortifacient ones, such as *Neospora caninum* (Bjorkman et al., 2000; Konnai et al., 2008).

Among the risk factors for BVDV infection in cattle are increased age and the origin of the animal (Mainar-Jaime et al., 2001); pasturing and increased herd sizes; and dam factors, such as high BVDV titres at calving and increased parity (Munoz-Zanzi et al., 2003). In addition, the use of artificial insemination breeding technique without the institution of biosecurity measures on the farm has been shown to increase the risk of BVDV spread by 2.8 times, most likely due to contamination of the herd through contaminated insemination equipment and personnel (Almeida et al., 2013).

Several methods have been developed to detect BVDV infection in cattle (OIE, 2008). These include virus isolation in bovine tissue culture (kidney, lung, testis and turbinate cells), immunohistochemistry to detect virus antigen in tissue, nucleic acid detection by polymerase chain reaction, and serological tests, such as virus neutralization and enzyme-linked immune sorbent assay (ELISA). Samples collected for analysis include: bulk milk to determine the herd status, individual milk, serum and plasma samples to determine individual animal sero-status, as well as tissue samples for immunohistochemistry. Serological tests, such as ELISA, are commonly employed in explorative studies since they can be used to determine the sero-status of large numbers of animals sampled in a population (OIE, 2008).

In Ethiopia, few studies conducted on the disease indicated that 9.6, 16.6 and 6.11% seroprevalence of BVDV was reported in dairy cattle herds in Jimma, south western Shoa, and West Shoa, respectively (Nigussie et al., 2010). Seroprevalence of 11.7% of BVDV was also reported in breeding and dairy farms of southern and central Ethiopia (Asmare et al., 2012). There is no study conducted to determine the rate of persistent of infection caused by BVDV in Ethiopia.

Neosporosis

Neosporosis is a disease caused by *Neospora caninum*. This is a protozoan coccidian parasite that structurally resembles and is genetically related to *Toxoplasma gondii* (Silva et al., 2007). There are two species of *Neospora* currently recognized: *N. caninum* which causes clinical disease in dogs, cattle, sheep, equines and many wild animal species, and *Neospora hughesi*, which has been associated with reproductive losses and myoencephalitis in horses. Dogs are the definitive hosts of *N. caninum* and cattle are among the intermediate hosts (Hall et al., 2006; Fernandez et al., 2006).

Cattle become infected by ingestion of feed and water contaminated by oocysts shed in dog faeces, or by congenital infection (Jenkins et al., 2002; Pan et al., 2004). This parasite has been reported to be the most important cause of abortion and neonatal mortality in beef and dairy cattle populations worldwide including Ethiopia (Murray, 2006; Silva et al., 2007; Asmare et al., 2012).

Abortions in cattle due to *N. caninum* occur from 3 months of gestation but are most common from 5 to 6 months of pregnancy. *Neospora* can be associated with sporadic abortions, endemic or abortion storms in cows have been reported. Other signs presented by infected cattle are foetal resorption, mummification, autolysis and stillbirth, and some calves are born alive with neuromuscular defects, while other calves are apparently healthy but persistently infected (Dubey and Schares, 2006). The incidence of abortion is often repeated in subsequent pregnancies, and congenital/vertical transmission from seropositive dams to their offspring is important in the epidemiology of neosporosis (Dubey et al., 2007). Reported risk factors for bovine abortions due to *N. caninum* include geographical location, breed, exposure to dogs or wild carnivores, and pregnant heifers (Dubey and Schares, 2006; Asmare et al., 2013). Various methods have been used to diagnose neosporosis in animals.

These include histopathology of tissues from aborted foetuses and still-births, parasite isolation from sacrificed animals, inoculation in mice, molecular techniques such as polymerase chain reaction, and oocyst recovery from dog faeces. However, serology (ELISA and immuno-fluorescent antibody test [IFAT]) is the most common technique used to diagnose neosporosis since it can be done ante-mortem and postmortem. Serology is useful in epidemiological studies since it can be used to reliably test exposure and infection in large animal populations (Dubey and Schares, 2006; Silva et al., 2007). In Africa, reports on neosporosis are limited; however, the available information is in line with global understanding of the protozoan that underscores the relevance of the *N. caninum* to the dairy sector (Ghalmi et al., 2012). The general seroprevalence of this disease globally ranges from 1.9 to 39.7% (Njiro et al., 2011; Ayinmode and Akanbi, 2013).

Recent studies confirmed that neosporosis is prevailing in dairy cattle of Ethiopia (Asmare et al., 2012; Asmare et al., 2013). However, the available published information comparing different pathogens exposure vis-à-vis reproductive disorders is limited to a single article based on the data from central and southern part of the country (Asmare et al., 2013). Few studies conducted in Ethiopia indicated that seroprevalence of 17.2% of *N. caninum* was reported in breeding and dairy farms of southern and central Ethiopia and 13.3% seroprevalence was also recorded in intensive or semi-intensively managed dairy and breeding cattle of Ethiopia (Asmare et al., 2012,

2013). Neosporosis appears to be a highly prevalent and widely distributed infectious cause of bovine reproductive disorders in urban and peri-urban smallholder farms, commercial dairy farms and breeding cattle in Ethiopia (Asmare et al., 2013). *N. caninum* is common in dairy cattle and is probably a more important cause of abortion in dairy cattle in Ethiopia than other infection cause of abortion (Asmare et al., 2012). The general control and prevention of causes of abortion in dairy cattle summary in Table 2.

Risk factors of abortion

Several causative factors, including external, maternal and genetic factors, have been reported for abortion in dairy cattle. These include heat stress, season, milk production, cow parity, serum progesterone level after conception, the inseminating bull, twin pregnancy and the herd (Lee and Kim, 2007). However, other investigations have reported that milk production and cow parity were not associated with abortion (Moore et al., 2005). Parity status and breed were significant factors affecting the incidence of abortion (Yakubu et al., 2015). However, Haileselassie et al. (2011) reported that parity status had no significant effect on the incidence of abortion. Factors that have been reported to increase the risk of abortion in dairy cattle herds include: being a heifer; being a cow of more than 10 years old; feeding on communal pastures; lack of vaccination against abortifacient diseases, hygiene, animal management and reproductive problems such as retained placentae, dystocia, uterine prolapse and stillbirth in the previous pregnancies (Waldner and Garcia, 2013; Waldner, 2014). Risk factors such as environmental (nutrition, temperature extremes and toxins, among others), management (crowding and use of natural mating), geographical factors and infectious factors, with infections contributing up to 90% of the abortions also reported (Konnai et al., 2008; Mekonen et al., 2010). Environmental high temperature may affect inside-pens temperature and performance of dairy cattle. Omori et al. (2014) reported that hyperthermia during pregnancy causes abortion in dairy cattle. Environmental temperature also affect the level of aflatoxin in the feed given to animals where above tolerable level could be a predisposing stress factor; aflatoxin is more often found in fodder grown in warm and humid climates which support growth of moulds. It has been suggested that aflatoxin lowers resistance to diseases and interferes with vaccine-induced immunity (Diekman and Green, 1992). In another study, third-trimester abortion was reported after cattle consumed mouldy peanuts (Ray et al., 1986).

Normal annual abortion rate were cited to be 3 to 5% once cows are above 42 days of pregnancy (Hovingh, 2009), or similarly, an observable 2 to 5% in most dairies (Kirk, 2003). While some suggest the annual abortion rate should be less than 3% in dairy, others believe this is

Table 2. Summary of common causes of abortion in cattle.

Agent	Abort occur (Trimesters)	Control
Brucella	Second half of gestation (usually around 7th month)	Regulatory program, vaccinate heifers and test/cull
Leptospira spp.	Third Trimesters (*L.pomona*) any time (other Leptospira spp.)	Vaccination and antibiotic
Listeria	2nd or 3rd Trimesters	vaccination and antibiotic treatment
Bovine viral diarrhea (BVD)	1st or 2nd Trimesters	Vaccination of dams, cull PI animals
Mycotoxins	4th and above months	Moldy feed should be avoided
Coxiella burneti	3rd Trimesters	vaccination and antibiotic treatment
Neospore caninum	2nd or 3rd Trimesters	Dog control- fetal tissues' out of feed area

Table 3. Summary of the prevalence rate of abortion in dairy cattle in Ethiopia.

Author	Year	Site	Breed	Prevalence (%)
Haftu and Gashaw	2009	Bako	Cross	6.0
Esheti and Moges	2014	Debre Zeit	Holstein and Borena cross	5.3
Haile et al.	2010	Addis Ababa	Cross	5.9
Dinka	2013	Assella	Local and Cross	14.5
Hadush et al.	2013	Debre Zeit	Cross	6.7
Regassa et al.	2016	Mekelle city	Local and Cross	13.3
Haile et al.	2014	Hossana	Local and Cross	2.6
Bitew and Prased	2011	Bedelle	Local and Cross	13.9
Degefa et al.	2011	Arsi zone	Local and Cross	8.7
Dawit and Ahmed	2013	Kombolcha town	Cross	9.1
Gizaw et al.	2007	Nazareth town	Local and Cross	2.2
Ararsa and Wubishet	2014	Borena zone	Borena	12.2
Enda and Moges	2016	Wolaita Sodo	Jersey and Cross	4.8
Ayana and Gudeta	2015	Bako	Horro and Cross	5.9
Mekonnin et al	2015	Mekelle	Cross	6.4
Wagari and Shiferaw	2016	Horro Guduru	Horro and Cross	4.4
Siyoum et al.	2016	Adea Berga	Jersey	28.9

not typical. This difference may arise from the fact that many abortions may be due to early embryonic death where cows are identified as pregnant and then found to be open without visible signs of an abortion. As a consequence, many early abortions may go undetected or even dismissed as an unsuccessful insemination rather than a failed pregnancy (Carpenter et al., 2006). A low rate of abortions from 2 to 5% per 100 pregnancies per year is usually considered within the expected rate as sporadic abortions occur in any herd. However, occurrence of several abortions in a short period or high rate of abortions warrants investigation to detect the cause and take control measures (Esheti and Moges, 2014; Al Humam, 2014).

ECONOMIC IMPORTANT OF ABORTION IN CATTLE

Abortion is one of the most important major reproductive health disorders of dairy cows in the world including

Ethiopia in terms of economic impact (James and Rushton, 2002; Regassa and Ashebir, 2016). Abortions cause significant economic loss, especially those occurring during late gestation. These losses can be attributed to loss of replacement of calves, reduced milk production, costs of treatment, feeding of animals and premature culling of productive cows and heifers (Carpenter et al., 2006; Abdelhadi et al., 2015). The cost of abortion varies according to effective factors such as the time of gestation, milk production, days in milk, the time of insemination after parturition, the cost of nutrition, sperm costs, insemination time and labor costs, which differ from region to region. Abortions during early pregnancy result in increased days open (De Vries, 2006; Hovingh, 2009). Different values were reported for the cost of abortion ranging from $90 to $2333 based on different studies. These differences are caused by the stage of gestation in which the abortion occurs and by the differences in factors such as predicted cow performance, breeding and replacement decisions, feed and milk price and the stage of lactation (De Vries, 2006; Lee and Kim, 2007; Hovingh, 2009). Estimates of the cost of an abortion to a producer range from $90 to $1,900 (Peter, 2000; Kirk, 2003), depending on when pregnancy and occurred and differences in predicted cow performance, prices, and breeding and replacement decisions. Hanson et al. (2003) stated that losses were $200 million per year in California herds.

Each case of abortion in dairy cattle has been estimated to lead to losses of about US $500 to $900. Per case, the cost of abortion has been estimated at $640 (Thurmond and Picanso, 1990) and from $600 to $800 (Eicker and Fetrow, 2003). Pfeiffer et al. (1997) estimated the cost of an abortion caused by *N. caninum* infections at $624 in New Zealand. Peter (2000) documented a cost of $600 to $1,000 per midterm abortion. Weersink et al. (2002) estimated the cost of an abortion, including reproductive loss and reduced milk yield at $1,286 in Canada. In addition, some of the causes of abortion, such as *Brucella abortus, Toxoplasma* and *Leptospira,* are zoonotic, thus posing a risk to human health (Carpenter et al., 2006; Murray, 2006). However, no reports are available on the estimation of the economic impact of bovine abortion in Ethiopia.

DIAGNOSIS OF ABORTION

General principles in the diagnosis of abortion in dairy animals include the collection of a complete history of the case and relevant epidemiological data, such as recent introductions into the farm, determination of the number of animals affected, examination of the breeding, health and feeding records, careful examination of the affected dam(s), and collection of the expelled fetus and placenta for pathological and microbial examination. Furthermore, samples such as paired serum samples, urine, milk and vaginal swabs can also be collected for analysis. The results are then collated and analyzed to reach a diagnosis (Radostits et al., 2007). However, the diagnostic rate in bovine abortions is very low due to the diverse range of pathogens involved, as well as the fact that factors affecting the dam, fetus and placenta may be involved (Murray, 2006; Ernest, 2009). Abortion also often follows an initial infection which may have occurred for several weeks or months; the etiology often is not detectable by the time the abortion occurs. The high cost of laboratory work to aid in the diagnosis of bovine abortion also compounds the problem (Carpenter et al., 2006; Murray, 2006). Diagnosis of the cause of bovine abortion is difficult as abortions are caused by many infectious and noninfectious factors (Miller, 1987; Jamaluddin et al., 1996). It has been demonstrated in numerous surveys that many abortions occur due to endemic infectious which are normally present in cattle

populations world-wide (Kim et al., 2002). The diagnosis of abortions often presents a challenge to the farm owner and the veterinarian in charge. A sudden and dramatic increase in the abortion rate in a herd is more commonly seen, although a gradual increase may be noted over a long period of time. For this reason, prompt and thorough action is required if abortions occur at any rate. Well-arranged records of a herd is often of benefit during the investigation of abortion problems (Al Humam, 2014). However, it is important to note that the causes of abortion in cattle are numerous and thus, their diagnosis is often challenging (Murray, 2006; Ernest, 2009). Epidemiological tools could help in narrowing down the field of investigation for a better interpretation of laboratory results (Markusfeld, 1997).

Status of abortion in dairy cows in Ethiopia

Ethiopia has various agro ecological zones, which have contributed to the evolution of different agricultural production systems (Beruktayet and Mersha, 2016). Husbandry systems, variation in cattle breed and environmental factors greatly influence the spread of the cause of abortion (Mekonen et al., 2010). Thus, the prevalence of abortion varies in different production system, cattle breed and agro ecological zones (Esheti and Moges, 2014).

Studies on major reproductive problems of cows in different parts of Ethiopia have shown the occurrence of abortion in cattle. Study conducted by Haftu and Gashaw (2009) on major clinical reproductive health problems of dairy cows in and around Bako of West Ethiopia showed that 6.0% (n=217) of dairy cows are affected by abortion. A study of the major reproductive health disorders of dairy cows in ILCA and Almaz dairy farms in Ada'a district, Debre Zeit town in East Shoa showed that 5.3%(n=245) of cows had abortion problem (Esheti and Moges, 2014). Other study conducted in Addis Ababa Milk showed major reproductive disorders in cross breed dairy cows under small holding indicating an overall prevalence of 5.9% (n=384) of abortion problems (Haile et al., 2010). A study conducted by Dinka (2012) showed that 14.6% (n=300) of dairy cattle was affected by abortion based on questionnaire interviews in and around Assella in Central Ethiopia. A retrospective study by Hadush et al. (2013) revealed that 6.7% (n=711) of the cows had abortion problem from dairy cows in three selected farms in Debre Zeit town. Another study conducted using questionnaire and observational survey in urban and peri urban area of Hossana indicated 2.6% (n=390) prevalence of abortion in dairy cattle (Haile et al., 2014). A study in and around Bedelle showed a prevalence of 13.9% (n=302) of abortion in South west Ethiopia (Bitew and Prased, 2011) and 8.7% (n=370) prevalence in selected sites of Arsi zone (Degefa et al., 2011). A prevalence of 9.1% (n=231) abortion was reported at Kombolcha town in north east Ethiopia by Dawit and Ahmed (2013). A study conducted by Gizaw et al. (2007) and Ararsa and Wubishet (2014) also reported 2.2 (n=403) and 12.2% (n=409) in Nazareth town of central Ethiopia and Borena zone in southern Ethiopia, respectively. A prevalence of 6.4% (n=1013) abortion was also recorded in dairy cattle in and around Mekelle, Tigray (Mekonnin et al., 2015) and 5.9% (n=372) of prevalence of abortion was reported in Bako Livestock Research Farm (Ayana and Gudeta, 2015). A study conducted by Regassa et al. (2016) on major factors influencing the reproductive performance of dairy farms in Mekelle city, Tigray reported 13.3% (n=798) prevalence of abortion. Recent reports from Adea Berga (Siyoum et al., 2016), Horro Gudru (Wagari and Shiferaw, 2016) and Wolaita Sodo town (Enda and Moges, 2016) indicated that the prevalence of 28.9 (n=97), 4.4 (n=402) and 4.8% (n=104) of abortion was recorded in cattle, respectively.

The incidence of abortion of more than 2 to 5% should be viewed seriously, and efforts should be made to determine the causes so that proper methods of control can be instituted (Mainar-Jaime et al., 2005; Esheti and Moges, 2014). Abortion problem is the most common in dairy cows (Gizaw et al., 2007). In order to reduce these problems and their risk factors, formulation of strategic control measures including health education on the cause of abortion transmission, treatment and control has to be introduced (Dinka, 2012).

Conclusion

Abortion is one of the most important reproductive health problems of dairy cows in Ethiopia in terms of economic impact. Both infectious and non-infectious agents may cause abortion in cattle. Non-infectious factors are genetic and non-genetic disorders. The non-genetic causes of abortion are heat stress, production stress, seasonal effect and seasonal changes. The common infectious causes of abortion in cattle include brucellosis, leptospirosis, listeriosis, Q fever, bovine viral diarrhea, mycotic abortion and neosporosis. These causes can result in extensive economic losses, showing the need for control measures to prevent abortion. Whereas, the infectious causes of abortion have been a primary focus of attention, and non-infectious cause of abortion is actually more common in endemic situations. Several risk factors associated with abortion are genetic, environmental, management, geographical and infectious factors. Incidence of abortion in Ethiopia ranges from 2.2 to 28.9%, efforts should be made to determine the causes and measures should be taken to control abortion. Prevention should be focused on accurate records keeping and collection of samples for laboratory analysis and using good biosecurity practices that inhibit the introduction and spread of infectious causes of abortion and using vaccination programs could limit abortion occurrence. There should be maintenance of the

general health and immune function of animals by providing a balanced feed, clean water and a clean and dry environment. It was suggested that detail epidemiological study on cause of abortion in cattle should be undertaken.

CONFLICT OF INTERESTS

The authors have not declared any conflict of interests.

REFERENCES

Abdelhadi F, Abdelhadi S, Niar A, Benallou B, Meliani S, Smail N, Mahmoud D (2015). Abortions in cattle on the level of Tiaret Area Algeria. Glob. Vet. 14:638-645.

Acha N, Szyfres B (2001). Brucellosis in zoonosis and communicable diseases common to humans and animals. 3rd Ed., Pan. America Health Organization Washington, D.C., USA. pp. 40-62.

Adane H, Yisehak T, Niguse T (2014). Assessment of major reproductive disorders of dairy cattle in urban and per urban area of Hosanna, Southern Ethiopia. Anim. Vet. Sci. 2:135-141.

Anderson ML (2007). Infectious causes of bovine abortion during mid- to late-gestation. Theriogenology 68:474-486.2007.

Al Humam N (2014). An epidemic of abortion in a commercial dairy farm in the eastern region, kingdom of Saudi Arabia. Glob. J. Dairy Farming Milk Prod. 2(3):074-080.

Ali R, Khan IH (2006). Mycotic abortion in cattle. Pak. Vet. J. 26(1):44-46.

Almeida L, Kaiser GG, Mucci NC, Verna AE, Campero CM, Odeon AC (2013). Effect of bovine viral diarrhoea virus on the ovarian functionality and in-vitro reproductive performance of persistently infected heifers. Vet. Microbiol. 165:326-332.

Almeida L, Miranda IC, Hein HE, Neto WS, Costa EF, Marks FS, Rodenbusch CR, Canal CW, Corbellini LG (2013). Herd-level risk factors for bovine viral diarrhoea virus infection in dairy herds from Southern Brazil. Res.Vet. Sci. 95:901-907.

Altamarand EA, Kaiser GG, Mucci NC, Verna AE, Campero CM, Odeon AC (2013). Effect of bovine viral diarrhoea virus on the ovarian functionality and in-vitro reproductive performance of persistently infected heifers. Vet. Microbiol. 165:326-332.

Angelakis E, Raoult D (2010). Q fever. Vet. Microbiol. 140(4):297-309.

Ararsa DB, Wubishet Z (2014). Major reproductive health problems of indigenous Borena cows in Ethiopia. J. Adv. Vet. Anim. Res. 1(4):182-188.

Arricau-Bouvery N, Rodolakis A (2005). Is Q fever an emerging or reemerging zoonosis? Vet. Res. 36(3):327-349.

Asmare K, Regassa F, Robertson LJ, Martin AD, Skjerve E (2012). Reproductive disorders in relation to Neospora caninum, Brucella spp. and bovine viral diarrhoea virus sero status in breeding and dairy farms of central and southern Ethiopia. Epidemiol. Infect. 141(8):1772-1780.

Asmare K, Regassa F, Robertson LJ Skjerve E (2013). Seroprevalence of Neospora caninum and associated risk factors in intensive or semi-intensively managed dairy and breeding cattle of Ethiopia. Vet. Parasit. 193:85-94.

Ayana T, Gudeta T (2015). Incidence of Major Clinical Reproductive Health Problems of Dairy Cows at Bako Livestock Research Farm over a Two-Year Period (September 2008-December 2010), Ethiopia. Anim. Vet. Sci. 3(6):158-165.

Ayinmode AB, Akanbi IM (2013). First report of antibodies to Neospora caninum in Nigerian cattle. J. Infect. Dev. Countries 7:564-565.

Azage T, Tsehay R, Alemu G, Hizkias K (2001). Milk recording and herd registration in Ethiopia. In Proceedings of the 8 Annual Conference of the Ethiopian Society of Animal Production (ESAP), 24- 26 August 2000, Addis Ababa, Ethiopia. pp. 90-104.

Beruktayet W, Mersha C (2016). Review of Cattle Brucellosis in Ethiopia. Acad. J. Anim. Dis. 5(2):28-39.

Bharti AR, Nally JE, Ricaldi JN, Matthias MA, Diaz MM, Lovett MA (2003). Leptospirosis, a zoonotic disease of global importance. Lancet Infect. Dis. 3:757-771.

Bitew M, Prased S (2011). Study on major reproductive health problems in indigenous and cross breed cow in and around Bedelle, South west Ethiopia. J. Anim. and Vet. Adv. 10:723-727.

Bjorkman C, Alenius S, Manuelson U, Uggla A (2000). *Neospora caninum* and bovine viral diarrhoea virus infections in Swedish dairy cows in relation to abortion. Vet. J. 159:201-206.

Brown PD, Carrington DG, Gravekamp C (2003). Direct detection of leptospiral material in human postmortem samples. Res. Microbiol.154:581-586.

Cantas H, Muwonge A, Sareyyupoglu B, Yardimci H, Skjerve E (2011). Q fever abortions in ruminants and associated on-farm risk factors in northern Cyprus. Vet. Res. 17(1):7-13.

Carpenter TE, Chrie` M, Andersen M, Wulfson L, Jensen A, Houe H, Greiner M (2006). An epidemiologic study of late-term abortions in dairy cattle in Denmark. Prev. Vet. Med. 77:215-229.

Chandranaik BM, Rathnamma D, Earanna N, Shivashankar BP, Kalge RS, Srinvasababu T, Kanaka S, Gangadharaiah HK, Muniyellappa HK, Raveendrahegde P, Venkatesha MD (2014). Abortion Storm in Cattle Due to *Aspergillus Fumigatus* Contaminated Feed in Drought Hit Southern Karnataka. Indian Vet. J. 91(11):82-84.

Central Statistical Agency (CSA) (2016). Livestock and Livestock Characteristics, Agricultural sample Survey. Addis Ababa, Ethiopia. Statistical Bull. 2(583):9-13.

Cutler SJ, Bouzid M, Cutler RR (2007). Q fever. J. Infect. 54(4):313-318.

Dawit T, Ahmed S (2013). Reproductive health problems of cows under different management systems in Kombolcha, North east Ethiopia, Hawassa University, School of Veterinary Medicine, Hawassa, Ethiopia.   Available   at: https://pdfs.semanticscholar.org/6e25/9c1963bbdaf360314631cc8bfb 3709b5cd2d.pdf

De Vries A (2006). Economic value of pregnancy in dairy cattle. J. Dairy Sci. 89: 3876-85.

Degefa T, Duressa A, Duguma R (2011). Brucellosis and some reproductive problems of indigenous Arsi cattle in selected Arsi zones of Oromia Regional State, Ethiopia. Glob. Vet. 7:45-53.

Diekman DA, Green ML (1992). Mycotoxins and reproduction in domestic livestock. J. Anim. Sci. 70:1615-1627.

Dinka H (2012). Reproductive performance of crossbred dairy cows under smallholder condition in Ethiopia. Int. J. Livest. Prod. 3(3):25-28.

Dhama K, Karthik K, Tiwari R, Shabbir MZ, Barbuddhe S, Malik SV, Singh RK (2015). Listeriosis in animals, its public health significance (food-borne zoonosis) and advances in diagnosis and control: a comprehensive review. Vet. Quarterly 35(4):211-235.

Dhanze H, Kumar M, Mane BG (2013). Epidemiology of leptospirosis, An Indian perspective. J. Food Borne Zoonotic Dis. 1(1):6-13.

Dubey JP, Schares G (2006). Diagnosis of bovine neosporosis. Vet. Parasitology. 140:1-34.

Dubey JP, Schares G, Ortega M (2007). Epidemiology and control of neosporosis and Neospora caninum. Clin. Microbiol. Review. 20:323-367.

Eicker S, Fetrow J (2003). Eicker, S., & Fetrow, J. (2003). New tools for deciding when to replace used dairy cows. In Proc. Kentucky Dairy Conf., Cave City, KY. Univ. Kentucky, Lexington. pp. 33-46.

Enda W, Moges N (2016). Major Reproductive Health Problems in Dairy Cows in Wolaita Sodo Town in Selected Farms in Ethiopia. Eur. J. Biol. Sci. 8(3):85-90.

Ernest H (2009). Common Causes of Abortions. Virginia cooperative extension publication. pp. 404-288.

Eshete G, Moges N (2014). Major reproductive health disorders in cross breed dairy cows in Ada'a District, East Shoa, Ethiopia. Glob. Vet. 13(4):444-449.

Eshetu Y, Simone K, Tsehaynesh M, Dawit W, Bethelehem N, Neway G, Belachew D. Eduard J (2004). Human leptospirosis, in Ethiopia: A pilot study in Wonji Hospital, Ethiopia. J. Health Dev. 18:48-51.

Fernandez E, Arna´iz-Seco I, Burgos M, Rodriguez-Bertos A, Aduriz G, Ferna´ndez- Garcı´a A, Ortega-Mora L (2006). Comparison of *Neospora caninum* distribution, parasite loads and lesions between epidemic and endemic bovine abortion cases. Vet. Parasitol. 142:187-191.

Fray MD, Mann GE, Clarke MC, Charleston B (2000). Bovine viral diarrhea virus: Its effect on ovarian function in the cow. Vet. Microbiol. 77:185-194.

Garedew L, Taddese A, Biru T, Nigatu S, Kebede E, Ejo M, Fikru A Birhanu T(2015). Prevalence and antimicrobial susceptibility profile of listeria species from ready-to-eat foods of animal origin in Gondar Town, Ethiopia. BMC Microbiol. 15:100

Givens MD, Marley MS (2008). Infectious causes of embryonic and fetal mortality. Theriogenology pp. 1-16.

Gizaw M, Bekana M, Abayneh T (2007). Major reproductive health problems in smallholder dairy production in and around Nazareth town, Central Ethiopia. J. Vet. Med. Anim. Health 5(4):112-115.

Godfroid J, Scholz HC, Barbier T, Nicolas C, Wattiau P, Fretin D, Whatmore AM, Cloeckaert A, Balsco JM, Moryon I, Saegerman C, Muma JB, Al Dahouk S, Neubauer H, Letesson JJ (2011). Brucellosis at the animal/ecosystem/human interface at the beginning of the 21st century. Prev. Vet. Med. 102:108-113.

Grooms DL (2004). Reproductive consequences of infection with bovine viral diarrhoea virus. Vet. Clin. North Am. Food Anim. Pract. 20:5-19.

Guatteo R, Seegers H, Taurel AF, Joly A, Beaudeau F (2011). Prevalence of *Coxiella burnetii* in domestic ruminants: A critical review. Vet. Microbiol. 149 (2):1-16.

Gumi B, Firdessa R, Yamuah L, Sori, T, Tolosa T, Aseffa A, Zinsstag J, Schelling E (2013). Seroprevalence of Brucellosis and Q-Fever in Southeast Ethiopian Pastoral Livestock. J. Vet. Sci. Med. Diagn. 2:1.

Hadush A, Abdella A, Ragassa F (2013). Major Prepartu and postpartum Reproductive problems of dairy cattle in central Ethiopia. J. Vet. Med. Anim. Health 5: 118-123.

Haftu B, Gashaw A (2009). Major Reproductive Health Problems of Dairy Cows in and around Bako, West Ethiopia. Ethiopian J. Anim. Prod. 9 (1):89-98.

Haile A, Kassa T, Mihret M, Asfaw Y (2010). Major Reproductive Disorders in Crossbred Dairy Cows under Small holding in Addis Ababa Milk shed, Ethiopia. World J. Agric. sci. 6:412-418.

Haile A, Tsegaye Y, Tesfaye N (2014). Assessment of major reproductive isorders of dairy cattle in urban and per urban area of Hosanna, Southern Ethiopia. Anim. Vet. Sci. 2 (5):135-141.

Haileselassie M, Kalayou S, Kyule M Belihu K (2011). Effect of Brucella infection on reproduction conditions of female breeding cattle and its public health significance in Western Tigray, Northern Ethiopia. Vet. Med. Int. 2011: 354943.

Hall CA, Reichel MP, Ellis JT (2006). Performance characteristics and optimisation of cut-off values of two enzyme-linked immunosorbent assays for the detection of antibodies to *Neospora caninum* in the serum of cattle. Vet. Parasitol. 140:61-68.

Hansen PJ (2002). Embryonic mortality in cattle from the embryo's prospective. J. Anim. Sci. 80 (2):33-44.

Heuer C, Healy A, Zerbini C (2007). Economic effects of exposure to bovine viral diarrhoea virus on dairy herds in New Zealand. J. Dairy Sci. 90:5428-5438.

Hirsh DC, Machachlan NJ, Walker RL (2004).Veterinary Microbiology. 2nd ed. Malaysia: Blackwell publishing. pp. 185-189.

Hanson T, Bedrick EJ, Johnson WO, Thurmond MC (2003). A mixture model for bovine abortion and foetal survival. Stat. Med. 22:1725-1739.

Hossein-Zadeh GN (2013). Effects of main reproductive and health problems on the performance of dairy cows: A review. Spanish J. Agric. Res. 11(3):718-735.

Hovingh E (2009). Abortions in dairy cattle. Common causes of abortions. Virginia Coop. Virginia Polytechnic Institute and State University, Blacksburg.

Jamaluddin AA, Case JT, Hird DW, Blanchard PC, Peauroi JR, Anderson ML (1996). Dairy cattle abortion in California: Evaluation of diagnostic laboratory data. J. Vet. Diag. Investig. 8:210-218.

James AD, Rushton J (2002). The economics of foot and Mouth Disease. Rev. Sci. Tech. off. Int. Epiz. 3:637-644.

Jenkins M, Baszler T, Bjo¨rkman C, Schares G, Williams D (2002). Diagnosis and seroepidemiology of *Neospora caninum*-associated bovine abortion. Int. J. Parasitol. 32:631-636.

Juyal PD, Bal MS, Singla LD (2011). Economic impact, diagnostic investigations and management of protozoal abortions in farm animals. In: All India SMVS' Dairy Business Directory 11:39-46.

Kabongo N, Van Vuuren M (2004). Detection of bovine viral diarrhoea virus in specimens from cattle in South Africa and possible association with clinical disease. J. South Afr. Vet. Assoc. 75:90-93.

Kim J, Lee J, Lee B, Park B, Yoo H, Hwang W, Shin N, Kang M, Jean Y, Yoon H, Kang S, Kim D (2002). Diagnostic survey of bovine abortion in Korea: with special emphasis on Neospora caninum. J. Vet. Med. Sci. 64:1123-1127.

Kirk JH (2003). Infectious abortions in dairy cows. Available at: http://www.vetmed.ucdavis.edu/vetext/INF-DA/Abortion.html

Konnai S, Mingal CN, Sato M, Abes NS, Venturina A, Gutierrez CA, Sano T, Omata Y, Cruz CL, Onuma M, Ohashi K (2008). A survey of abortifacient infectious agents in livestock in Luzon, the Philippines, with emphasis on the situation in a cattle herd with abortion problems. Acta Trop. 105:269-273.

Lee J, Kim HI (2007). Pregnancy loss in dairy cows: The contributing factors, effect on reproductive performance and the economic impact. J. Vet. Sci. 8(3):283-288.

Leta S, Mesele F (2014). Spatial analysis of cattle and shoat population in Ethiopia: growth trend, distribution and market access. Springer Plus 3:310.

Levett PN (2001). Leptospirosis, Clin. Microbiol. Rev. 14(2):296-326.

Levett PN (2005). Leptospirosis. In: Principles and Practice of Infectious Diseases. Eds., G. Mandell, J. Bennett and R. Dolin. pp. 2789-2794.

Lindberg A, Houe H (2005). Characteristics in the epidemiology of bovine viral diarrhea virus (BVDV) of relevance to control. Prev. Vet. Med. 72:55-73.

Lobago F, Bekana M, Gustafsson H, Kindahl H (2006). Reproductive performances of dairy cows in small holder production system in Selalle, Central Ethiopia. Trop. Anim. Health Prod. 38:333-342.

Mainar-Jaime RC, Berzal-Hervanz B, Arias P, Rojo-Va'zquez FA (2001). Epidemiological pattern and risk factors associated with bovine viral diarrhea virus in a non-vaccinated dairy cattle population from the Astorias region of Spain. Prev. Vet. Med. 52:63-73.

Mainar-Jaime RC, Muñoz PM, de Miguel MJ, Grilló MJ, Marin CM, Moriyón I, Blasco JM, (2005). Specificity dependence between serological tests for diagnosing bovine brucellosis in Brucella-free farms showing false positive serological reactions due to Yersinia enterocolitica O9. Canadian Vet. J. 46:193-196.

Markusfeld NO (1997). Epidemiology of bovine abortions in Israeli dairy herds. Prev. Vet. Med. 31:245-255.

Matope G, Bhebe E, Muma JB, Lund A, Skjerve E (2010). Herd level factors for Brucella seropositivity in cattle reared in smallholder dairy farms in Zimbabwe. Prev. Vet. Med. 94:213-221.

Mekonen H, Kalayou S, Kyule M (2010). Serological survey of bovine brucellosis in Barka and Orado breeds (Bos indicus) of western Tigray, Ethiopia. Prev. Vet. Med. 94:28-35.

Mekonnin AB, Harlow C, Gidey G, Tadesse D, Desta G, Gugssa T, Riley S (2015). Assessment of Reproductive Performance and Problems in Crossbred (Holstein Friesian X Zebu) Dairy Cattle in and Around Mekelle, Tigray, Ethiopia. Anim. Vet. Sci. 3(3):94-101.

Miller R (1987). Diagnosing the cause of bovine abortion. Bovine Practitioner 22:98-101.

Molla B, Yilma R, Alemayehu D (2004) Listeria monocytogenes and other Listeria species in retail meat and milk products in Addis Ababa, Ethiopia. Ethiop. J. Health Dev. 18:131-212.

Moore DA, Overton MW, Chebel RC, Truscott ML, BonDurant RH (2005). Evaluation of factors that affect embryonic loss in dairy cattle. J. Am. Vet. Med. Assoc. 226:1112-1118.

Muma JB, Samui KL, oloya J, Munyeme M, Skjerve E (2007). Risk factors of brucellosis in indigenous cattle reared in in livestock-wildlife interface area in Zambia. Prev. Vet. Med. 80:306-317.

Munoz-Zanzi CA, Hietala SK, Thurmond MC, Johnson WO (2003). Quantification, risk factors and health impact of natural congenital infection with bovine viral diarrhoea virus in dairy calves. Am. J. Vet. Res. 64:358-365.

Murray RD (2006). Practical approach to infectious bovine abortion diagnosis. In: Proceedings of the 24th World Buiatrics Conference, Nice, France.

Nelson DD, Duprau JL, Wolff PL, Evermann JF (2016).Persistent bovine viral diarrhea virus infection in domestic and wild small

ruminants and camelids including the mountain goat (Oreamnos americanus). Frontiers Microbial. 6:1415.

Njiro SM, Kidanemariam AG, Tsotets AM, Katsande TC, Mnisi M, Lubisi BA, Patts AD, Baloyi F, Moyo G, Mpofu J, Kalake A, Williams R (2011). A study of some infectious causes of reproductive disorders in cattle owned by resource poor farmers in Gauteng Province, South Africa. J. South Afr. Vet. Assoc. 82:213-218.

Nigussie Z, Tariku M, Tefera S, Tadele T, Fekadu R (2010). Seroepidemiological study of bovine viral diarrhea (BVD) in three agroecological zones in Ethiopia. Trop. Anim. Health Prod. 42(3):319-321.

OIE (Office International des Epizooties), (2005). Institute for International Cooperation in Animal Biology. Iowa State University, College of Veterinary Medicine, Available at: http://www.cfsph.iastate.edu/IICAB/.

OIE (World Organization of Animal Health), (2008). Manual of diagnostic tests and vaccines for terrestrial animals. pp. 698-711.

OIE (World Organization of Animal Health), (2009). Manual of diagnostic tests and vaccines for terrestrial animals. 2-14:5-35

Omori H, Otsu M, Suzuki A, Nakayama T, Akama K, Watanabe M ,Inoue N (2014). Effects of heat shock on survival, proliferation and differentiation of mouse neural stem cells. Neurosci Res. 79:13-21.

Ooteman M, Vago A, Koury M (2006). Evaluation of MAT, IgM ELISA and PCR methods for the diagnosis of human leptospirosis. J. Microbiol. Method 65:247-257.

Pal M (2015). Growing Role of Fungi in Mycotic Abortion of Domestic Animal. J. Bacteriol. Mycol. 2(1):1009.

Pan Y, Jansen GB, Duffield TF, Hietala S, Kelton D, Lin CY, Peregrine AS (2004). Genetic susceptibility to Neospora caninum infection in Holstein cattle in Ontario. J. Dairy Sci. 87:3967-3975.

Parthiban S, Malmarugan S, Murugan M, Johnson S, Rajeswar J, Pothiappan P (2015). Review on Emerging and Reemerging Microbial Causes in Bovine Abortion. Int. J. Nutr. Food Sci. 4(4-1):1-6.

Peter AT (2000). Abortions in dairy cows: New insights and economic impact. Adv. Dairy Technol. 12:233

Pfeiffer DU (2002). Basic concepts of Veterinary epidemiology, evidence-based Veterinary Medicine. Veterinary epidemiology-an introduction. P 4.

Psaroulaki A, Hadjichristoudoulou C, Loukaides F, Soteriades E, Konstantinidis A, papastergiou P, ioannidou M C, Tselentis Y (2006). Epidemiological study of Q fever in humans, ruminant animals, and ticks in Cyprus using a geographical information system. Euro. J. Clin. microbial. Infect. Dis. 25(9):576-586.

Quinn PJ, Carter ME, Markey BK, Donnelly DJC, Leonard FC (2002). Veterinary Microbiology and Microbial Diseases USA: Blackwell science. pp. 72-75.

Radostits OM, Gay CC, Hinchcliff KW, Constable PD (2007). Veterinary Medicine. A Text book of Diseases of Cattle, Sheep, Pigs, Goats and Horses, 10th Ed. W.B., Saunders, London. pp. 963-985.

Rafati N, Mehrabani Y, Hansonb TE (2010). Risk factors for abortion in dairy cows from commercial Holstein dairy herds in the Tehran region. Prev. Vet. Med. 96:170-178.

Ray AC, Abbitt B, Cotter SR, Murphy MJ, Reagor JC, Robinson RM, West JE, Whitford HW (1986). Bovine abortion and death associated with consumption of aflatoxin-contaminated peanuts. J. Am. Vet. Med. Assoc. 188(10):1187-1188.

Regassa T, Ashebir G (2016). Major Factors Influencing the Reproductive Performance of Dairy Farms in Mekelle City, Tigray, Ethiopia. J. Dairy Vet. Anim. Res. 3(4):88.

Sani MB, Amanloo H (2007). Heat stress effect on open days in Holstein dairy cattle in Yazd province, Iran. 3rd Cong of Animal Science, Mashhad, Iran. P 85.

Sarder MJ, Moni MI, Aktar S (2010). Prevalence of reproductive disorders of cross breed cows in the Rajshahi district of Bangladesh. J. Agric. 8:65-75.

Seyoum T, Woldetsadik A, Mekonen K, Gezahegn A, Gebreyes A (2015). Prevalence of Listeria monocytogenes in raw bovine milk and milk products from central highlands of Ethiopia. J. Infect. Dev. Ctries 9(11):1204-1209.

Shapiro BI, Gebru G, Desta S, Negassa A, Nigussie K, Aboset G, Mechal H (2015). Ethiopia livestock master plan. ILRI Project Report.

Nairobi, Kenya: International Livestock Research Institute (ILRI).

Sheldon IM, Lewis GS, LeBlanc S, Gilbert RO (2006). Defining postpartum uterine disease in cattle. Theriogenology 65(8):1516-1530.

Silva D, Lobato J, Mineo T, Mineo J (2007). Evaluation of serological tests for the diagnosis of Neospora caninum infection in dogs: Optimization of cut off titers and inhibition studies of cross-reactivity with Toxoplasma gondii. Vet. Parasitol. 143:234-244.

Siyoum T, Yohannes A, Shiferaw Y, Asefa Z, Eshete M (2016). Major reproductive disorders on Jersey breed dairy cattle at Adea Berga dairy farm, West Shewa Zone, Oromia Region, Ethiopia. Ethiop. Vet. J. 20(1):91-103.

Sophia H (2013). Leptospirosis in dogs in Lima, Peru. Description of changes in serology, hematology, blood chemistry and urinalysis before and after one month of treatment. Available at: http://epsilon.slu.se.

Sprong H, Tijsse-Klasen E, Langelaar M, De Bruin A, Fonville M, Gassner F, Takken W, Van Wieren S, Nijhof A, Jongejan F, Maassen B, Scholt J, Hovius W, Hemil Hovius K, Spiltalská E, van Duynhoven T (2011). Prevalence of Coxiella burnetii in ticks after a large outbreak of Q fever. Zoon. Public Health 58(4):1-7.

Tangkanakul W, Tharmaphornpil P, Plikaytis BD, Bragg S, Poonsuksombat D, Choomkasien P, (2000). Risk factors associated with leptospirosis in Northeastern Thailand, Am. J. Trop. Med. Hyg. 63:204-208.

Thurmond MC, Branscum AJ, Johnson WO, Bedrick EJ, Hanson TE (2005). Predicting the probability of abortion in dairy cows: a hierarchical Bayesian logistic-survival model using sequential pregnancy data. Prev. Vet. Med. 68:223-239.

Tolosa T, Bezabih D, Regassa F (2010). Study on seroprevalence of bovine brucellosis, and abortion and associated risk factor. Bull. Anim. Health Prod. Afr. 58:236-247.

Tooloei M, Abdollapour G, Karimi H, Hasanpor A (2008). Prevalence of serum antibodies against six leptospira serovars in sheep in Tabriz, North-western Iran. J. Anim. Vet. Adv. 7:450-455.

Van Campen H (2010). Epidemiology and control of BVD in the U.S. Vet. Microbiol. 142(1-2):94-98.

Vijayachari P, Sugunan AP, Umapathi T (2001). Evaluation of darkground microscopy as a rapid diagnostic procedure in leptospirosis. Indian J. Med. Res. 114:54-58.

Wagari A, Shiferaw J (2015). Major Reproductive Health Problems of Dairy Cows at Horro Guduru Animal Breeding and Research Center, Horro Guduru Wollega Zone, Ethiopia. Available at: http://article.sciencepublishinggroup.com/pdf/10.11648.j.ijbbmb.2016 0101.13.pdf

Waldner CL (2014). Cow attributes, herd management, and reproductive history events associated with abortion in cow-calf herds from Western Canada. Theriogenology 81(6):840-848.

Waldner CL, García G (2013). Cow attributes, herd management, and reproductive history events associated with the risk of non-pregnancy in cow-calf herds in Western Canada. Theriogenology 79(7):1083-1094.

Walker RL (2007). Mycotic bovine abortion. Current therapy in large animal theriogenology.2nd ed., St. Louis: Elsevier. pp. 417-419.

World Health Organization (WHO) (2006). Guidelines for the prevention and control of leptospirosis.Zoonosis Division, National Institute of Communicable Diseases, 22-Sham Nath Marg, Dehli.

World Organization of Animal Health (OIE) (2009). Manual of diagnostic tests and vaccines for terrestrial animals. 2(14):5-35.

World Organization of Animal Health (OIE) (2004). Manual of Diagnostic Tests and Vaccines for Terrestrial Animals. www.oie.int.

World Organization of Animal Health, (OIE) (2008). Manual of diagnostic tests and vaccines for terrestrial animals. pp. 698-711.

Yadeta W, Bashahun GM, Abdela N (2016). Leptospirosis in Animal and its Public Health Implications: A Review. World Appl. Sci. J. 34(6):845-853.

Yaeger MJ, Holler LD (2007). Bacterial causes of bovine infertility and abortion. In: Youngquist RS, Threlfall WR, editors. Current therapy in large animal Theriogenology. 2nd ed., St. Louis: Elsevier. pp:389-399.

Yakubu A, Awuje AD, Omeje JN (2015). Omparison of multivariate logistic regression and classification tree to assess factors influencing prevalence of abortion in Nigerian cattle breeds. Plant Sci. 25(6):1520-1526.

Zegeye Y (2003).Challenges and opportunities of livestock marketing in Ethiopia. In: Proceedings of the 10th annual conference of Ethiopian Society of Animal Production (ESAP), 22- 24 August 2002 held in Addis Ababa, Ethiopia, 7:47-54.

17

Seroprevalence of chlamydial abortion and Q fever in ewes aborted in the North-West of Algeria

Karim Abdelkadir[1,2]*, Ait Oudia Khatima[1] and Khelef Djamel[1]

[1]National Veterinary Higher School of Algiers, Rue Issad Abbes, Oued Smar- Alger, Algeria.
[2]Laboratory of Research, Food Hygiene and Quality Assurance System (HASAQ), High National Veterinary School of Algiers, Algeria.

Very little information is available in Algeria on Q fever and chlamydial abortion sheep, two zoonosis caused by *Coxiella burnetii* and *Chlamydophila abortus* and their main reservoirs are domestic ruminants. This study aimed at investigating the seroprevalence of these two diseases in sheep flocks from six Daïra (Telagh, Tanira, Moulay Slissen, Marhoum, Ras Elma and Merine). A serological survey was conducted in 39 flocks with a history of abortions, which were classified by size. A total 180 sera were collected from the aborted ewes. Q fever indirect ELISA kit and *C. abortus* indirect ELISA kit (ID Screen®) kits were used to know the percent prevalence in sheep. The results showed that 28% (N = 50/180) of sheep were seropositive for Q fever and 31% (N = 55/180) of sheep were seropositive for chlamydial abortion. Twenty eight herds (72%) showed at least one seropositive animal for Q fever and 29 herds (74%) showed at least one seropositive animal for chlamydial abortion. Larger herds led to more infected herds of small and medium for Q fever. These results showed that infection with Q fever and chlamydial abortion were common in the study area, therefore encouraging efforts are needed to propose measures to reduce the spread and zoonotic risk.

Key words: Q fever, chlamydial abortion, seroprevalence, enzyme-linked immunosorbent assay (ELISA), zoonosis.

INTRODUCTION

Chlamydial abortion and Q fever are two zoonoses caused by two small obligate intracellular Gram-negative bacteria, *Chlamydophila abortus* and *Coxiella burnetii* (Maurin and Raoult, 1999; Rodolakis, 2006: Aitken and Longbottom, 2007) which grow in the cytoplasm of eukaryotic cells. They are the most important causes of reproductive failure in sheep and goats (Berri et al., 2001, 2005; Arricau-Bouvery and Rodolakis, 2005). These infections cause abortion, stillbirth, delivery of weak offspring and infertility in the small ruminant (Rodolakis et

*Corresponding author. E-mail: karimeabdelkadir@gmail.com.

al., 2004; Agerholm, 2013). The losses caused by these two agents evaluated on several levels. In economic terms, the non-sale of the product (lamb or goat), the non-renewal of young breeding (antenaise or goat) and decreased milk production (dairy farming) are the most negative impact on the scale of livestock. In health terms, the main concerns are the risk of contamination of several lots on livestock, as well as professional zoonotic transmission. Both agents were the subject of increasing research from the years 2002 in small ruminants, due to their proven implication in human focus (Wallenstein et al., 2010).

The present study attempted to investigate the prevalence of chlamydial abortion and Q fever at the level of district Sidi Belabbes through sero-prevalence studies in flocks that have experienced abortions and correlate its possible association with managerial (flock size, region, type of farming, and contact with other flocks) risk factors. In conjunction, the study try to clarify the interpretation of complementary investigations required by veterinary practitioners by confirming diagnostic tools available for both agents searched.

MATERIALS AND METHODS

Animals and blood sampling

This study was carried out from September to December 2013 (season of lambing); this study was based on the declaration of 1, 2 or 5 abortions on a period less than or equal to 4 weeks as equivalent to an abortion episode. While those with two reported abortions at 5 weeks of interval were eliminated from this study.

From 39 sheep flocks, a total of 180 blood samples were collected by jugular venous puncture in 4 ml sterile vacutainer tubes using Tubes BD Vacutainer® secs "BD, France" from aborted ewes aged between 1 and 6 years. After storage at room temperature for 1 h, blood samples were centrifuged at 3000 rpm for 5 min at room temperature. Sera were carefully harvested and stored at -20°C until assayed. Selected flocks ranged in size from 42 to 450 sheep. Flocks sizes were <100, 100-200 and >200 sheep for 6, 22 and 11 flocks, respectively, in order to establish the sero-prevalence of chlamydial abortion and Q fever via an indirect diagnosis. All flocks visited only once, no vaccine against chlamydial abortion or Q fever used.

Serological techniques

For the detection of antibodies against C. burnetii and C. abortus, two different ELISAs were used. For Q fever, indirect ELISA kit and C. abortus indirect ELISA kit (ID Screen® France) were used. Positive and negative control provided by the manufacturer and an internal positive laboratory reference was included in each test. Results were expressed as a percentage of the optical density reading of the test sample (% OD) calculated as % = 100 × OD sample / OD positive control. Recommended readings OD%<40 as negative, OD%>40, OD%<50 as doubtful, OD%>50<80% as positive and OD>80 highly positive for C. burnetii, and OD%<50 as negative, OD%>50<60 as doubtful, and OD%>60 as positive for C. abortus.

Statistical analysis

All data were entered and validated using a Microsoft Excel package. To bring out the association between a supposed risk factor and the disease, the odds ratio (OR) and relative risk (RR) were calculated.

The odds ratio is the probability of having the disease according to the presence or absence of risk factors and allows for addition to the degree of significance of the association, the direction and strength of the association.

RESULTS

According to the experimental design, all 39 flocks studied had a history of abortions and stillbirths, 180 aborted ewes belonging to these 39 flocks were examined for antibodies against C. abortus and C. Burnetii. The seropositivity results towards for these two bacteria obtained in aborted sheep at individual and flock levels were summarized in the Table 1.

At the farm level, 74% (29/39, 95% CI: 58 to 86) of farms had at least one seropositive sheep to C. abortus and 72% (28/39, 95% CI: 55-84) of farms had at least one seropositive sheep to C. burnetii. The seroprevalence of C. abortus infection in ewes is not associated (P > 0.05) with the three flocks size groups, it was the same for C burnetii. The seroprevalence rate ranged from 29 to 88% and from 45 to 95% for C. abortus and C burnetii, respectively.

Overall, the sheep level seroprevalence was 31% (55/180, 95% CI: 23, 92 -37, 84) for C. abortus and was 28% (50/180, 95% CI: 21, 37 -34, 93) for C. burnetii. In sheep level, there was significant difference (P < 0.05) between the seroprevalence of chlamydial infection and the location (Table 2). The highest prevalence rate (46.67%) of chlamydial infection was observed in Telagh area, while the lowest rate (17, 65%) was observed in Tanira area.

DISCUSSION

Exposure of sheep to C. abortus and C. burnetii was evaluated by testing for the presence of antibodies with an indirect ELISA test. The detected antibodies in this study imply a natural response to exposure to the microorganisms because there is no vaccination program against ruminant chlamydiosis or Q fever in Algeria before. The survey design provided data on seroprevalence at the flock and the animal level in this area. Results of the present study revealed an animal-level seroprevalence to C. abortus of 31% and to C. burnetii of 28% in Sidi Bel Abbes region, Algeria. This figure is higher than that reported from other Algerians regions (Khaled et al., 2016; Hireche et al., 2014;

Table 1. Seroprevalence of *Chlamydophila abortus* and *Coxiella burnetii* infection in sheep according to flock size in Wilaya of SIDI BEL ABBES west of Algeria (2013).

Parameter		Flock size			Total
		<100	[100 - 200]	>200	
Number of flocks		6	22	11	39
Aborted sheep		27	178	153	358
Aborted sheep taken		17	90	73	180
Chlamydial abortion	Number of seropositives sheeps[a] (%)	7/17 (41%)	34/90 (38%)	14/73 (19%)	55 (31%)
	Number of seropositives flocks[b] (%)	5/6 (83%)	18/22 (82%)	6/11 (56%)	29 (74%)
	Range of seropositives flocks (%)	57%-88%	60%-94%	29%-83%	58%-86%
Q fever	Number of seropositives sheeps[a] (%)	6/17 (35%)	31/90 (34%)	13/73 (18%)	50 (28%)
	Number of seropositives flocks[b] (%)	3/6 (50%)	15/22 (68%)	10/11 (91%)	28 (72%)
	Range of seropositives flocks (%)	45%-88%	45%-86%	57%-94%	55%-85%

[a]Animal is considered positive if serum is positive (%DO > 40 by ELISA). [b]Flock is considered positive if at least one animal serum is positive.*x^2 test: $p < 0.05$.

Table 2. Seroprevalence of Q fever and chlamydial abortion depending on the region.

Area	Sera	Sera (+) for FQ	Seroprevalence (%)	Sera (+) for CH	Seroprevalence (%)
Telagh	30	7	23.23	14	46.67*
Ras Elma	30	7	23.23	15	50.00
Tanira	34	17	50	6	17.65*
M.slissen	40	8	20	9	22.50
Merine	27	8	29.63	7	25.93
Marhoum	19	3	15.79	4	21.05
Total	**180**	**50**	**27.78**	**55**	**30.56**

Sera (+) for QF: Sera positive for Q fever ; Sera (+) for CH: sera positives for chlamydial abortion. *Significant difference ($P < 0.05$) between areas by chi-square test.

Merdja et al., 2014). Also, several authors had previously reported high prevalence in Maghreb countries such as Marocco (El Jai et al., 2003), Tunisia (Russo et al., 2005), Egypt (Abdel-Moein and Hamza, 2017) and in world countries such as Turkey (Kennerman et al., 2010), Italy (Francesca et al., 2016), Slovakia (Trävnicek et al., 2001), Spain (Mainar-Jaime et al., 1998) and Jordan (Al-Qudah et al., 2004). The overall seroprevalence rate at the flock level in our survey was 74% to chlamydial abortion and 72% to Q fever. These rates are higher than those reported by Francesca Rizzo et al. (2016) in flocks 38% in Italy and Angela et al. (2012) with 28% in Germany. However, due to numerous parameters such as differences in study design and inclusion criteria (e.g. high abortion rates), flock size and management, prevalence of other abortifacient agents (e.g. Brucellae, Salmonellae, Toxoplasma, Chlamydia, Campylobacter) it is virtually impossible to compare the present study's prevalence findings with the aforementioned studies

(Masala et al., 2004).

A higher prevalence rate was revealed for flocks with more than 200 animals compared with that of small flocks (91 and 50%, respectively) for Q fever, while, no significant correlation was revealed between flock size and the rate of seroprevalence for chlamydial abortion. The difference rate of seroprevalence revealed for the flock high size for Q fever might be that due to animal overcrowding in livestock buildings. Also may be related to the high number of lambing at lambing season, which increases the total population at risk and, subsequently, the risk of pathogen introduction and transmission, where high density may influence animal welfare and the occurrence of infectious diseases. The study showed that there is a significant difference ($P < 0.05$) between chlamydial infection in sheep and areas of northwest of Algeria (Table 2). Tanira and Ras Elma areas having the highest rate of chlamydial infection in sheep may be explained by the behavior of these species breeding in these sites (frequency of herding group belonging to several farmers in the same village). These factors favor the rapid spread of infection.

Conclusions

The geographic distribution of *C. burnetii* and *C. abortus* indicate that both pathogens are present throughout the district of Sidi Bel Abbes. The highest percentage of positive samples was found for chlamydial abortion in Ras Elma (50%), and for Q fever in Tanira (50%). It seems that abortions in sheep following infection with *C. burnetii* and *C. abortus* have a higher frequency, even in young animals. Q fever and chlamydial abortion are a public health problem in Algeria. To for better control both in animals and humans, veterinary and public health sector should strengthen their collaboration for the establishment of a national program to fight against the major zoonoses in general and against Q fever and chlamydial abortion in particular.

CONFLICT OF INTERESTS

The authors have not declared any conflict of interests.

REFERENCES

Abdel-Moein KA, Hamza DA (2017). The burden of Coxiella burnetii among aborted dairy animals in Egypt and its public health. acta tropica.166:92-95.

Agerholm JS (2013). Coxiella burnetii associated reproductive disorders in domestic animals- a critical review. Acta Vet. Scand. 55(1):13.

Aitken ID, Longbottom D (2007). Chlamydial abortion. In: Aitken, I. (Ed.), Diseases of Sheep. Blackwell Publishing Ltd., Oxford. pp. 105-112.

Al-Qudah KM, Sharif LA, Raouf RY, Hailat NQ, Al-Domy FM (2004). Seroprevalence of antibodies to *Chlamydophila abortus* shown in Awassi sheep and local goats in Jordan. Vet. Med.-Czech 12:460-466.

Angela H, Gernot S, Hannah L, Udo M, Roland D, Andreas F, Lothar H, Steffen H, Michael E, Herbert T, Klaus H, Heinrich N, Lisa DS (2012). Prevalence of Coxiella burnetii in clinically healthy German sheep flocks. BMC Research Notes. 5(1):152.

Arricau-Bouvery N, Rodolakis A (2005). Is Q fever an emerging or reemerging zoonosis? Vet. Res. 36:327-349.

Berri M, Crochet D, Santiago S, Rodolakis A (2005). Spread of Coxiella burnetii infection in a flock of sheep after an episode of Q fever. Vet. Rec. 157(23):737-740.

Berri M, Souriau A, Crosby M, Crochet D, Lechopier P, Rodolakis A (2001). Relationships between the shedding of Coxiella burnetii, clinical signs and serological responses of 34 sheep. Vet. Rec. 148 :502-505.

El Jai S, Bouslikhane M, El Idrissi AH (2003). Suivi épidémiologique des avortements de petits ruminants dans les zones pastorales du Maroc. Revue Marocaine des Sciences Agronomiques et Vétérinaires 23(2):95-100.

Francesca R, Nicoletta V, Marco B, Vitaliano B, Camilla L, Laura C, Maria LM (2016). Q fever seroprevalence and risk factors in sheep and goats in northwest Italy. Prev. Vet. Med. 130:10-17.

Hireche S, Bouaziz O, Djennad D, Boussen S, Imgur R, Kabouia R, Bererhi E (2014). Seroprevalence and risk factors associated with Chlamydophila spp. infection in ewes in the northeast of Algeria. Trop. Anim. Health Prod. 46:476-473.

Kennerman E, Rousset E, Gölcü E, Dufour P (2010). Seroprevalence of Q fever (coxiellosis) in sheep from the Southern Marmara Region, Turkey. Comp. Immunol. Microbiol. Infect. Dis. 33(1):37-45.

Khaled K, Sidi-Boumedine H, Merdja S, Dufour P, Dahmani A, Thiéry R Rousset E, Bouyoucef A (2016). Serological and molecular evidence of Q fever among small ruminant flocks in Algeria. Comp. Immunol. Microbiol. Infect. Dis. 47:19-25.

Mainar-Jaime RC, De La Cruz C, Vázquez-Boland JA (1998). Epidemiologic study of chlamydial infection in sheep farms in Madrid, Spain. Small Rumin. Res. 28:131-138.

Masala G, Porcu R, Sanna G, Chessa G, Cillara G, Chisu V, Tola S (2004). Occurrence, distribution, and role in abortion of Coxiella burnetii in sheep and goats in Sardinia, Italy Vet. Microbiol. 99:301-305.

Maurin M, Raoult D (1999). Q fever. Clin. Microbiol. Rev. 12:518-553.

Merdja S-E, Khalid H, Dahmani A, Bouyoucef A (2015). Chlamydial abortion in algerian small ruminants. Bulletin of University of Agricultural Sciences and Veterinary Medicine Cluj-Napoca. Vet. Med. 72(1):23-26.

Rodolakis A (2006). Chlamydiosis and Q fever, similarity and difference between these two zoonoses. Renc. Rech. Ruminants, 13:365-401. Available at : http://journees3r.fr/IMG/pdf/2006_12_zoonoses_securite_01_Rodolakis.pdf

Rodolakis A, Berri M, Rekiki A (2004). Le point sur le diagnostic et la prevention de la chlamydiose et la fièvre Q Journée nationales GTV, Tours, 751-754.

Russo PS, Pepin M, Rodolakis A, Hammami S (2005). Enquête sérologique sur les principales causes d'avortements infectieux chez les petits ruminants en Tunisie. Revue Méd. Vét. 156(7):395-401.

Trävnicek M, Kovacova D, Zlbricky P, Cislakova L (2001). Serosurvey of sheep and goats to Chlamydia psittaci in Slovakia during the years 1996-2000. Vet. Med. -Czech 46:281-285.

Wallenstein A, Moore P, Webster H, Johnson C, Van derburgt G, Pritchard G, Ellis J, Oliver I (2010). Q fever outbreak in Cheltenham, United Kingdom, in 2007 and the use of dispersion modelling to investigate the possibility of airborne spread. Euro. Surveill. 15(12):19521.

18

Sonographic evidence of follicle development in a fixed time AI synchronization protocol involving ovatide in Bunaji cows

Ubah Simon Azubuike[1]*, Rekwot Peter Ibrahim[2], Adewuyi Abdulmujeeb Bode[2], Ababa James Andrew[3] and Mustapha Rashidah Abimbola[4]

[1]Department of Theriogenology, Faculty of Veterinary Medicine, University of Abuja, Nigeria.
[2]Artificial Insemination Unit, National Animal Production Research Institute, Shika, Zaria, Kaduna State, Nigeria.
[3]Veterinary Teaching Hospital, Ahmadu Bello University Zaria, Kaduna State, Nigeria.
[4]Department of Theriogenology and Production, Ahmadu Bello University, Zaria, Kaduna State, Nigeria.

An investigation was done to observe follicle development and ovulation by ultrasound in a synchronization protocol in Bunaji cows using ovatide. Cows (n=16), aged 4 to 6 years with average body condition scores of 2.5 to 3.5 and weighing between 250 and 350 kg were used. They were managed according to the routine management practice of the Diary Research Programme NAPRI. Only cycling cows at 75 days post-partum with palpable CL were included in the study. Cows were randomly assigned to 1 or 2 treatment groups for synchronization of ovulation. Treatment group 1 comprising Bunaji (n=8) received 50 µg of GnRH and 25 mg of $PGF_{2\alpha}$. While, treatment group 2 comprising Bunaji (n=8) received 50 µg of ovatide and 25 mg of $PGF_{2\alpha}$. The treatment was as follows: Group 1: (Day 0, 50 µg GnRH; Day 7, 25 mg $PGF_{2\alpha}$ and day 9, 50 µg GnRH), group 2: (Day 0, 50 µg ovatide, Day 7, 25 mg $PGF_{2\alpha}$ and Day 9, 50 µg ovatide). Ultrasound examinations were conducted. Examinations were conducted at the time of second gonadotropin injections, to determine presence of one or more antral follicles > 10 mm in diameter and at 48h after second gonadotropin injections, to determine absence of 1 (single – ovulation) or 2 (double – ovulation) of those earlier antral follicles. Results showed synchronization rate for ovatide was 75%, while that of GnRH (Cystorellin) was 62.5% (p>0.05). Double ovulation rate for both groups was 0%. It was concluded that 50 µg Ovatide in Ovsynh protocol has synchronization potentials in Bunaji cows. Further studies on gonadotropins of fish origin are recommended.

Key words: Ovatide, follicle, sonographic, synchronization, Bunaji, cows.

INTRODUCTION

Ovatide is an indigenous, cost-effective and new hormonal formulation for induced breeding of fishes. It is also effective in breeding major carps. The dosages for females are 0.20 to 0.40 ml/kg for rohu and mrigal, 0.40 to 0.50 ml/kg for catla, silver carp and grass carp, the dosages for males are 0.10 to 0.20 ml/kg for rohu, mrigal, 0.20 to 0.30 ml/ kg for catla and 0.20 to 0.25 ml/kg for silver carp and grass carp (Naipagropediaraichur, 2012). It is a new, highly potent and ready to use injectable formulation containing a synthetic peptide analogous to the naturally occurring hormone, salmon GnRH. The formulation also contains a dopamine antagonist, whereas the GnRH analogue stimulates the pituitary to release gonadotropins and trigger the process of reproduction, the dopamine antagonist inhibits the release of dopamine and makes sure that the secretion of gonadotropins is not inhibited. The use of Ovatide, thus constitutes the latest and the most advanced technology employed for induced breeding of fishes and production of high quality fish seed. It is composed of Gonadorelin A (GnRH A) 20 mcg, Domperidone BP 10 mg and benzyl alcohol IP 1.5% v/v (HemoPharma, 2014).

Gonadotropic releasing hormone (GnRH) is labeled for treating follicular cysts in cows at a dosage of 100 µg (Merial Animal Health, Duluth, GA) in the United States. This is why the Ovsynch protocol utilizes a 100 µg dose. Administration of 100 µg GnRH after $PGF_{2\alpha}$ injection increases the rate of synchronized ovulation in bovines (Pursley et al., 1995). A study by Navanukraw et al., (2002) reported a 37.5% pregnancy rate at 42 post AI using Ovsynch with two half dose of GnRH. Also, Fricke et al., (2003) found similar pregnancy rates using half dose Ovysynch on second service animals.

Another study conducted using Holstein Friesian cows in Wisconsin compared 100 µg dose of GnRH to lower 50 µg dose and reported no statistical difference between treatment groups (Fricke et al., 1998). Thus, 50 µg dose of GnRH decrease total hormone cost from $16. 10 to $9.70 and the total cost per pregnancy was reduced from $47.88 to $27.61, making it comparable to the cost of $PGF_{2\alpha}$ only program (Fricke et al., 1998). Because of the increasing demand for the application of AI in Nigeria's indigenous cattle breeds and the need for fixed timed AI, the cost of using conventional hormones plays a negative role in disseminating the technology and making it available to poor farmers. The application of ovatide, which is a synthetic analogue of GnRH of fish (Salmon) origin in a synchronization protocol in bovines, may be a potential relief from the exorbitant cost of imported hormones. If cows respond to ovatide well in a synchronization protocol, there will be hope that the hormone extracted from live catfish can replace the expensive analogues. The pituitary of live catfish can be harvested from fish processing plants, currently the bye products of such processing plants are being wasted in our society. This work is designed to investigate follicle development and ovulation by ultrasound in a synchronization protocol in Bunaji cows using ovatide.

MATERIALS AND METHODS

Study location

This study was carried out at the cattle farm of Diary Research Programme (DRP) of the National Animal Production Research Institute (NAPRI), Shika, Ahmadu Bello University, Zaria. Shika is situated in the Nothern Guinea Savannah between Latitudes 11°

and 12° and Longtitudes 7° and 8° E at elevation of 659 m above sea level with an average annual maximum and minimum temperature of 31.0± 3.2 and 18.0±3.7°C, respectively. It has two distinct seasons: dry season (November to April) with mean daily temperature ranging from 15 – 36°C and rainy season (May to October) with average annual rainfall of 1100 mm and mean relative humidity of 72% (Rekwot et al., 1998).

Research animals and management

The animal experiments followed the principles of the laboratory animal care (CACC, 1993). Bunaji cows (n=16) aged 4 to 6 years and weighing between 250 to 350 kg were used. Selected cows with average body condition scores (BCS) of 2.5 to 3.5 using 0 to 5 scale from the most emaciated to the fattest (Pullman, 1978). Cows were identified by means of plastic ear tags. They were managed according to the routine management practice of the Diary Research Programme. Two transrectal examinations a month apart were carried out to ensure cyclicity of the cows before commencement of the study. Only cycling cows at 75 days post-partum with palpable CL were included in the study.

Experimental design

Cows were randomly assigned to 1 or 2 treatment groups for synchronization of ovulation. Treatment group 1 comprising Bunaji (n=8) received 50 µg of GnRH (Cystorellin; Nerial, Ltd., Iselin, NJ) and 25 mg of $PGF_{2\alpha}$ (Lutalysethe Pharmacia – Upjohn Co., Kalamazoo, MI). While, treatment group 2 comprising Bunaji (n=8) received 50 µg of ovatide (Hemo Pharm. PVT Ltd., Mahalaxmi, Mumbai) and 25 mg of $PGF_{2\alpha}$. The treatment is as illustrated below.

Treatment Group 1

Day 0, 50 µg GnRH; Day 7, 25 mg $PGF_{2\alpha}$ and day 9, 50 µg GnRH. Bunaji cows administered first injection of 50 µg of GnRH on the day 0, followed by 25 mg of $PGF_{2\alpha}$ 7 days later and a second injection of 50 µg GnRH 48 h after $PGF_{2\alpha}$ administration (Figure 1).

Treatment group 2

Day 0, 50 µg Ovatide; Day 7, 25 mg $PGF_{2\alpha}$ and Day 9, 50 µg ovatide. These cows were administered first injection of 50 µg ovatide on day 0, followed by 25 mg of $PGF_{2\alpha}$ 7 days later and a second injection of 50 µg ovatide 48 h after $PGF_{2\alpha}$ administration (Figure 2)

Ultrasonography and rectal palpation

Ultrasound examinations were conducted using ultrasound machine equipped with a transrectal 7.5 MHz linear – array transducer (Aloka 500v; Corometrics Medical Systems, Inc., Willing Ford, (CT). Examinations were conducted at the time of second GnRH injection, to determine presence of one or more antral follicles > 10 mm, in diameter and at 48 h after second GnRH injection, to determine absence of 1, (single – ovulation) or 2 (double –

*Corresponding author. E-mail: drubah2000@yahoo.com.

GnRH	PGF$_{2\alpha}$	GnRH
50 µg	25 mg	50 µg
1 ml	5 ml	

Day 0   day 7   day 9 at 6 pm

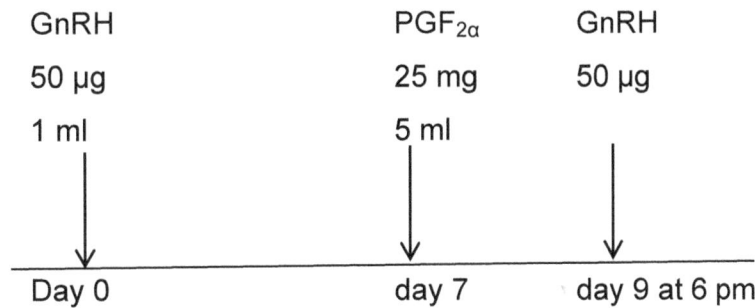

Figure 1. Treatment days and doses with Cystorelin and PGF2α.

ovulation) of those earlier antral follicles.

Transrectal palpation was conducted twice at a month interval to select cycling cows within 5 to 12 days of the estrous cycle before initiating Ovsynch protocol (Voh, 1997).

Fertility rates

Synchronization rate

Synchronization rate was calculated as the number of cows that ovulated at least 1 follicle within 48 h of the second GnRH injection, expressed as a percentage of the total number of cows that received the Ovsynch protocol.

Double ovulation rate

Double- ovulation rate was calculated as the number of cows that ovulated 2 follicles within 48 h of the second GnRH injection, expressed as a percentage of synchronized cows.

Statistical analysis

Data obtained on follicle development, synchronization rate, double ovulation rate were expressed in percentages and represented in charts. Differences in the parameters between treatment groups were analyzed using Chi-squares test. Values of P <0.05 were considered significant. A data analysis was carried out using Statistical Package for Social Sciences (SPSS) Version 17.0.0 (SPSS Inc. Chicago IL, USA).

RESULTS

Synchronization rate (SR)

SR = No. of ovulations 48 h after 2ndGnRH/total no. of animals that received the treatment.
Ovatide = 6/8 x100 = 75%; GnRH = 5/8 X100 = 62.5%; P = 1.00, O.R = 1.80.

Double ovulation rate (DR)

DR = No. of cows that ovulated 2 follicles within 48 h of the 2ndGnRH injection divided by the number of synchronized cows. Ovatide = 0.6 x100 = 0%; GnRH =

0.5 x100 = 0%.

DISCUSSION

The use of 50 µg of ovatide in the fixed time artificial insemination synchronization protocol showed that there was adequate follicular development (Figure 4 and Plate 1). The GnRH (Cystorelin) at 50 µg also showed adequate follicular development by day nine just before the 2nd gonadotropin injections (Figure 4 and Plate 2). This means that the bunaji cows responded equally to both treatments in respect of follicle development. This response may be complementary to prostaglandin injections on day seven. Subsequently, the number of cows that ovulated 48 h following 2nd gonadotropin injections did not differ significantly between the two groups (P>0.05), this means that both treatments were capable of luteinizing the developed follicles at the treatment doses of 50 µg. A synchronization rate of 75% was recorded for the ovatide while 62.5% was recorded for the GnRH (Cystorelin) (Figure 3). Synchronization rate between the two groups did not differ significantly. The implication of this is that ovatide has synchronization potentials in the Bunaji cows just like Cystorelin.

The emergence of a new follicular wave is synchronized only when GnRH treatment causes ovulation (Martinez et al., 1999). If the first GnRH does not synchronize follicular wave emergence, ovulation following the second GnRH may be poorly synchronized (Martínez et al., 2002a), resulting in disappointing pregnancy rates following TAI (Martínez et al., 2002b). The ovatide showed a higher value of synchronization rate (75%) as compared to Cystorelin (62.5%), this may be attributed to factors such as poor compliance and dose.

Anytime you add another cow handling to a program, you are likely increase the probability that not every cow will be treated with the right product at the right time. Keeping things simple and understandable for everyone involved in the breeding program is priority. Knowing the difference between products to be used, using proper syringe and needle sizes (18 g, 1.5 inch), and following

Chart Title

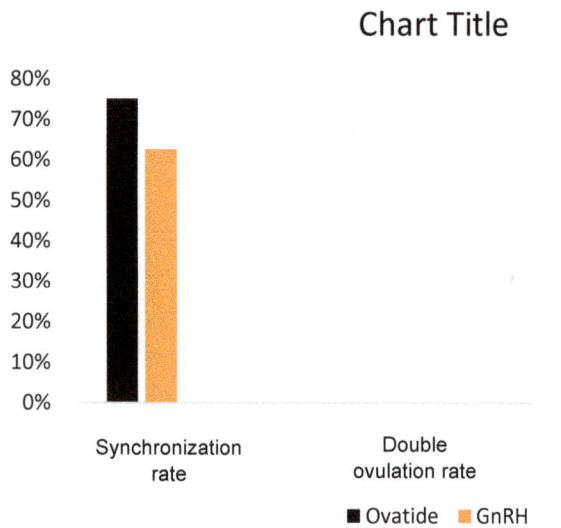

Figure 3. Synchronization and double ovulation rates of ovatide and GnRH (Cystorelin) following the Ovsynch protocol.

Chart Title

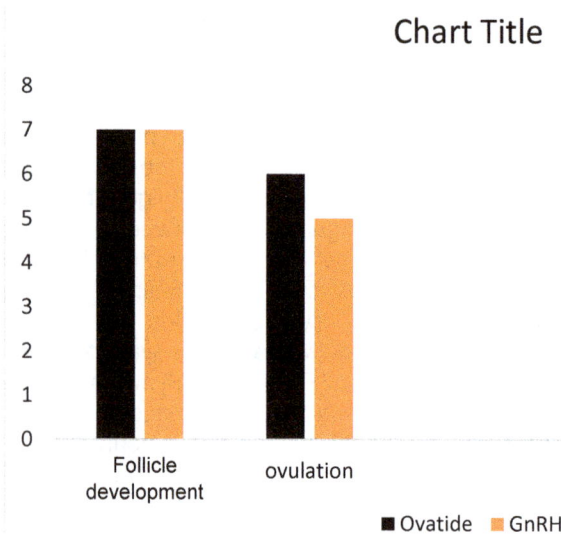

Figure 4. Parameters measured following treatment and sonography. P=1.00, O.R= 0.4286;   P=1.00, O.R =1.80; O.R = Odds ratio.

instructions are key to a high rate of compliance and good AI conception rates (Jeff, 2016). The recommended dose of Cystorelin for cows is 100 μg. In this study, using 50 μg may have contributed to the lower synchronization rate of 62.5% as compared to 75% of ovatide. It has been reported that the dose of ovatide used in fish affects fertility parameters in fish. A study was conducted to evaluate ovatide doses (0.6, 0.8 and 1.0 ml/kg body weight of female) on breeding performance of *Clarias batrachus* in the subtropical region of Hisar. The breeding

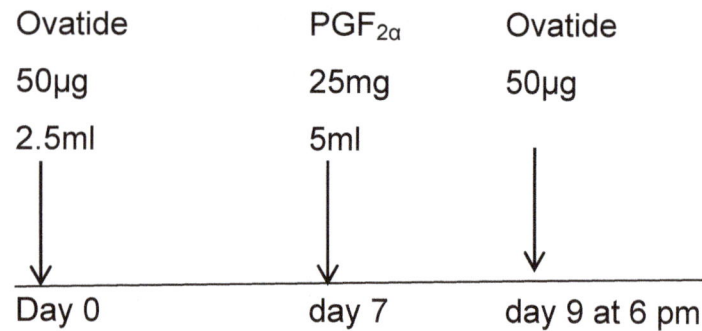

Figure 2. Treatment days and doses with Ovatide and PGF2α.

performance was judged on the basis of the total weight of stripped eggs, net fecundity, fertilization, hatching and survival. To judge the egg quality, the per cent fertilization, hatching and survival of fry were considered. The results indicated that the total weight of stripped eggs and spawning fecundity were the highest ($p < 0.05$) when females were injected with 1 ml of ovatide per kg body weight (BW) as compared to those injected with other dose levels. The lowest stripping response was observed with injection of 0.6 ml ovatide per kg BW of female brood fish. At the 1 ml dose, the percentages of total fertilized egg and hatching were 82.33 and 55.35% respectively, which were the highest ($p < 0.05$) among all treatments. The net survival of fry was found to be 98.52% at 1 ml ovatide per kg BW. Therefore, it has been recommended that 1 ml of ovatide per kg BW of female brood fish was found optimum among the three experimental doses for best breeding performance and egg quality in *C. batrachus* (Sharm et al., 2010). Similarly, GnRH is recommended for treatment of follicular cysts at 100 μg. This report means that there is an optimum dose of gonadotropin (Ovatide or Cystorelin) that is required for ovulation to occur in a particular species as reflected in the total number of stripped eggs in fish.

Conclusions

Both ovatide and GnRH (Cystorelin) showed sonographic evidence of follicular development on day nine of the treatments, before the 2nd gonadotropin injections. Ovulations occurred in both treatment groups which were not significantly different. A synchronization rate of 75 and 62.5% were recorded for ovatide and GnRH (Cystorelin), respectively. It was concluded that treatment of bunaji cows with 50 μg ovatide in Ovsynh protocol has synchronization potentials. Based on the outcome of this study, it was recommended that further studies be carried out using pituitary extract of *C. gariepinus* (African catfish) in a fixed time AI synchronization protocol in bunaji cows.

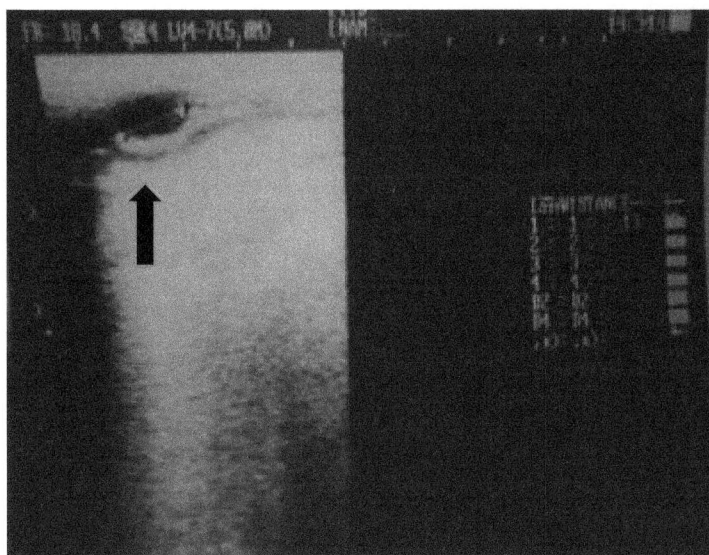

Plate 1. Sonographic evidence of antral follicle on the ovaries before 2nd ovatide injection.

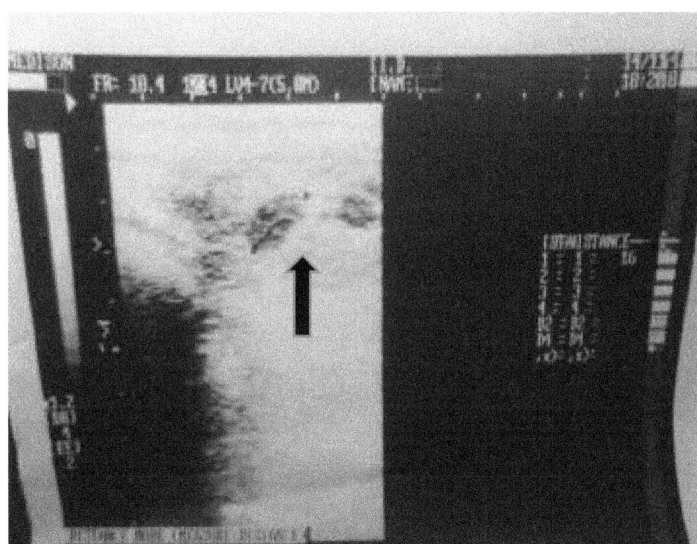

Plate 2. Sonographic evidence of antral follicle on the ovaries before 2nd GnRH (Cystorelin) injection.

CONFLICT OF INTERESTS

The authors have not declared any conflict of interests.

ACKNOWLEDGEMENT

The authors wish to acknowledge the management of National Animal Production Research Institute (NAPRI) for the approval to use NAPRI animals and facilities according to NAPRI guidelines.

REFERENCES

Canadian Council on Animal Care Guide (CACC) (1993). Second edition Accessed 04.11.2015, 10pm. Available at: http://www.ccac.ca/Documents/Standards/Guidlines/Experimental_Animals_Voll.pdf

Fricke PM, Caraviello DZ, Weigel KA, Welle ML (2003). Fertility of dairy cows after resynchronization of ovulation at three intervals following first timed insemination. J. dairy sci. 86(12):3941-3950.

Fricke PM, Guesther JN, Wiltbank C (1998). Efficacy of decreasing the dose of GnRH used in a protocol for synchronization of ovulation andtimed AI in lactating dairy cows. Theriogenology 50(8):1275-1284.

HemoPharma (2014). Ovatide: A new highly potent hormonal formulation for induced breeding of fishes at low cost. Hemo pharmaceuticals PVT. Ltd.

Jeff S (2016). What is the best timed AI program? Reproduction. Hoard's Dairy man.

Martinez MF, Adams GP, Bergfelt DR, Kastelic JP, Mapletoft RJ (1999). Effect of LH or GnRH on the dominant follicle of the first follicular wave in beef heifers. Anim. Reprod. Sci. 57(1):23-33.

Martinez MF, Kastelic JP, Adams GP, Mapletoft RJ (2002b). The use of a progesterone-releasing device (CIDR-B) or melengestrol acetate with GnRH, LH, or estradiol benzoate for fixed-time AI in beef heifers. J. Anim. Sci. 80(7):1746-1751.

Naipagropediaraichur (2012). Induced breeding of Fishes with Ovatide. Available at: Agropedia.iitk.ac.in/content/induced-breeding-fishes-ovatide.

Navanukraw C, Reynolds LP, Grazul-Bilska AT, Redmer DA, Fricke PM. (2002). Effect of presynchronization on pregnancy rate to a timed artificial insemination protocol in lactating dairy cows. J. Dairy Sci. 85(Suppl 1):263.

Pullman NB (1978). Condition scoring of White Fulani cattle. Trop. Anim.Health Prod. 10:118-120.

Pursley JR, Mee MO, Wilkbank MC (1995). Synchronization of ovulation in dairy cows using $PGF2\alpha$ and GnRH. Theriogenology 44(7):915-923.

Rekwot PI, Oyedipe EO, Barje PP, Rwuaan JS (1998). Factors affecting the reproductive performance of cattle in Nigeria. Niger. Vet. J. 19:66-77. Sharma K, Yadava NK, Jindal M (2010). Effect of different doses of ovatide on the breeding performance of *Clarias batrachus* (Linn.). Livest. Res. rural Dev. 22(4).

RJ (2002a). The use of progestins in regimens for fixed-time artificial insemination in beef cattle. Theriogenology 57(3):1049-1059.

Voh AA Jr (1997). Fertility and embryonic mortality rates of Zebu cows following oestrus synchronization and artificial insemination. Ph.D. Thesis, Ahmadu Bello University, Zaria.

19

Newcastle disease virus antibody in serum and feather pulp of chickens vaccinated with thermostable vaccine coated on grains and brans in Zaria, Northern Nigeria

Helen Owoya Abah[1*], Paul Ayuba Abdu[2] and Jibril Adamu[3]

[1]Department of Veterinary Medicine, College of Veterinary Medicine, University of Agriculture Makurdi, Benue State, Nigeria.
[2]Department of Veterinary Medicine, Faculty of Veterinary Medicine, Ahmadu Bello University, Zaria, Nigeria.
[3]Department of Veterinary Microbiology, Faculty of Veterinary Medicine, Ahmadu Bello University Zaria, Nigeria.

Thermostable Newcastle disease vaccine virus strain I2 ($NDVI_2$) was investigated for its efficacy as foodborne vaccine using maize, sorghum and their brans as carriers. Immune response to vaccination and resistance to challenge were assessed by haemagglutination inhibition (HI) test. After primary and secondary vaccination at three and six weeks of age, sera and feather pulp samples were analyzed to determine the antibody titre in the different groups. The highest mean antibody titre of $7.39 \pm 0.42 \log_2$ was recorded for serum when the vaccine was administered through treated sorghum coated with gum Arabic (TSGG) and $7.28 \pm 0.37 \log_2$ for feather pulp in the group given maize bran (MZB) at eight weeks of age. There was no significant difference ($p > 0.05$) between the HI antibody titre in the feed groups from feather pulp samples at three weeks of age while a significant difference ($p < 0.05$) in the serum antibody titre was observed between all the feed groups at five weeks of age. There was correlation in antibody titre between serum and feather pulps only at two weeks after second vaccination. The protection rate after challenge in all the groups was low with the highest rate (14%) recorded when the vaccine was administered in treated maize (TMZ) and TSGG. The study concluded that the vaccine could be effective for the protection of village chickens as food-borne vaccine provided the carrier foods are adequately treated to remove antiviral agents. The use of feather samples as suitable alternative to serum for ND serology was discussed.

Key words: Chickens, maize, sorghum, Newcastle disease, thermostable vaccine.

INTRODUCTION

Newcastle disease (ND) is one of the major important viral disease of poultry which had caused huge economic loses to farmers in recent past (Aamir, 2014). Newcastle disease virus (NDV) has a wide range of hosts, as more than 250 bird species have been found to be susceptible by natural or experimental infections, although wild

*Corresponding author. E-mail: helenabah505@gmail.com.

waterfowl and shorebirds are regarded to be the reservoir of the virus in nature (Kaleta and Baldouf, 1988). Among avian species, the poultry flocks are commonly affected with this disease, chickens are most susceptible while ducks and geese are least susceptible to ND (Khan et al., 2000). ND is presently one of the most important endemic disease of poultry in Nigeria, causing high morbidity, mortality, decrease in eggs production and it constitutes a major constraint to the development of rural poultry production (Abdu et al., 1992).

In Nigeria, ND is controlled by vaccination of commercial birds with live thermolabile lentogenic or mesogenic NDV vaccines containing between 100 and 1000 bird dose per vial. The vaccines are administered intramuscularly, intraocularly or orally in water (Abdu et al., 2012). This is impracticable for a village farmer because the method of administration requires the catching and handling of birds and there is no guarantee that local birds will drink vaccine treated water (Abdu et al., 2012). The vaccine dose format is also not meant for village flocks containing between 7 and 29 birds (Otchere, 1990). Thermostable Newcastle disease virus (NDV) vaccines have been used widely to control ND for village poultry flocks, due to their independence of cold chains for delivery and storage (Guoyuan et al., 2015).

The NDV vaccine strain I_2 has undergone laboratory test in several countries and has proved to be protective against local virulent strains. In Vietnam, it has been officially recognized as the NDV vaccine for village chicken after extensive laboratory and village trials (Tu et al., 1998). In Tanzania, it has given protection for at least two months after vaccination (Wambura et al., 2000). Field records in Mozambique indicated that $NDVI_2$ vaccine provides approximately 80% protection in the field of an outbreak when given every month via eye drop (Pangani, 1999). The $NDVI_2$ vaccine is being tested in several African countries (Alders and Spradbrow, 2001).

The vaccine has been used successfully in village chickens populations in many countries in Asia and Africa including Nigeria (Jayawardane et al., 1990; Jagne et al., 1991; Ibrahim et al., 1992; Echeonwu et al., 2008a). Besides, the successes recorded by many researchers using the V4 and I_2 thermostable ND vaccine as feed based vaccine (Nasser et al., 1998; Wambura et al., 2000), there are some basic problems reported to be associated with feed-based vaccination (Cumming, 1992). Firstly, not all types of feed are suitable for the delivery of NDV vaccine in terms of suitability to the chicken and delivery of the virus for protection. Secondly, the type of food vehicle to be used is determined by the availability of that particular feed in a locality (Philemon et al., 2007).

The use of feather shafts of chickens for the diagnosis of viral infections and for monitoring vaccine viruses has been reported (Davidson, 2009). Other researchers (Dong-Hun et al., 2016) also detected viral antigens in feathers of chickens infected with viscerotropic velogenic NDV suggesting that feathers could act as source of viral

transmission. The threat of ND to the poultry industry requires routine seromonitoring of vaccinated chickens to show that they have been adequately immunized against the disease (Ameh et al., 2016). To do this effectively, serum samples need to be collected at regular intervals. However, farmers are generally reluctant to allow for collection of serum samples from their birds after vaccination. This study was therefore conducted to determine the suitability of maize and sorghum and their respective brans as delivery systems for $NDVI_2$ vaccines and also to study the suitability of using feather pulps as an alternative source of sample for seromonitoring of vaccinated chickens against ND in the study area.

MATERIALS AND METHODS

Study area

The study was conducted at the Nutrition Laboratory of the Veterinary Medicine Department of Ahmadu Bello University Zaria, Nigeria. Zaria is located in Kaduna State, Nigeria; it is a part of the central high plains of Northern Nigeria and about 670 m above sea level. Zaria is located at latitude 11.11°N and longitude 7.73°E. It has two distinct seasons: the dry or harmattan season (October to March) and wet season (April to September) with a population of 975,153 (Oladipo, 1985).

Experimental birds

Two hundred day-old unvaccinated cockerels were obtained from the Poultry Research Farm of the National Veterinary Research Institute Vom, Nigeria. The chicks were housed in a brooding room that was cleaned, washed, disinfected and fumigated. All chicks were placed under brooders with chicks mash and water provided *ad libitum*. At three weeks of age, 18 chicks each were randomly selected and placed in cages with wire mashed floors measuring 56.5 × 56.5 cm until the termination of the experiment.

Experimental design

The chicks were divided into 4 groups (A, B, C and D) at three weeks of age. Each group was subdivided into 2 subgroups each consisting of 18 birds. Groups: A1 (treated maize), A2 (treated sorghum), B1 (treated maize plus treated gum Arabic), B2 (treated sorghum plus treated gum Arabic), C1 (maize bran), and C2 (sorghum bran). All birds in subgroups A to C were vaccinated and challenged. Birds in subgroup D1 were not vaccinated but challenged and D2 were unvaccinated and unchallenged and served as positive and negative controls, respectively.

Source of NDVI2 vaccine and challenge virus

The $NDVI_2$ vaccine was obtained from the Viral Research Department, National Veterinary Research Institute (NVRI) Vom, Plateau State, Nigeria. The vials of the vaccines were 50 dose vials meant to be reconstituted in 50 ml of chlorine free water and to be giving orally at 1 ml/bird. The virus strain used for the challenge study was the NDV (Kudu 113 strain) isolated and characterized in a previous study (Echeonwu et al., 1993) with EID_{50} titre of $10^{7.5}$. The virus was obtained from the Virology Division of the NVRI, Vom.

Preparation and coating of food carrier with vaccine virus

Five kilograms each of maize, sorghum and their bran and 4 kg of gum Arabic were used. The maize and sorghum were milled once to remove the husk and then crushed into a gritty mash. These were soaked in chlorine free water for 72 h, while changing the water daily. The soaked grains were then washed with clean water, sieved and placed to dry in the sun. They were then weighed and packaged into polythene bags of 1 kg/package and stored at room temperature until used. The maize and sorghum brans were not subjected to any treatment; they were dried, packaged and kept at room temperature until used. About 2 kg of gum Arabic (used as additive) was soaked to dissolve overnight in 1,000 ml of distilled water. The gum Arabic was then boiled for an hour, allowed to cool and then autoclaved at 121°C for 15 min.

The method described by Alders and Spradbrow (2001) was used for coating the feed grain and brans with the vaccine virus. The quantity of grains or brans consumed by 18 birds (10 g per bird) was measured and the time taken to consume the vaccine feed was noted. Three vials of the 50 doses of $NDVI_2$ vaccines were reconstituted in 100 ml of PBS (pH 7.4). Then 50 ml of the treated diluted gum Arabic was thoroughly mixed with the reconstituted vaccine (total 150 ml) and then mixed with the feed in a bowl and then spread on trays and kept at room temperature for 30 min before administrating to the birds.

Vaccinations

First and second dose of $NDVI_2$ coated on the treated grains and bran were given to the birds at 3 and 6 weeks of age, respectively.

Serum samples

About 1 to 2 ml of blood was collected through the wing vein of each bird with a 2 ml syringe and 21 G needles on days 7, 14 and 21 before primary vaccination and at 2 and 3 weeks post vaccination. The blood samples were deposited into sterile test tubes and sera were separated by allowing the blood to clot in the test tubes slanted in racks at room temperature for 1 to 2 h. Sera collected were stored in a freezer at -20°C until tested.

Preparation of feather pulp for serology

The method described by Roy et al. (1998) with slight modification was used for preparing the feather pulp samples. Four down feathers, two from each wing were plucked from each bird, weighed and cut at the base to remove the pulp using a scissor. Laboratory pestle and mortar was used to grind the feather pulp which was then mixed with 2 ml of PBS, centrifuged at 2000 rpm for 5 min and the supernatant tested for NDV HI antibodies.

Haemagglutination (HA) and haemagglutination inhibition (HI) tests

Five millilitres of chicken blood was collected from newly hatched commercial chicks and transferred into 10 ml of Alsever's solution and gently mixed. The red blood cells (RBCs) were washed three times with PBS pH 7.2 by centrifugation at 2000 rpm for 5 min each. The concentration of the RBCs used was 1% in 99 ml of PBS. The titre of a live La Sota NDV strain antigen obtained from NVRI was determined by the HA test. Four HA units were used in the HI test. All sera collected were tested for NDV specific antibody by the haemagglutination inhibition (HI) test using methods described by OIE (2004). The antibody level for each serum and feather pulp sample was expressed as a log to the base two and recorded. The geometric mean titers (GM) were calculated. In this study, the published cut off value was used for the protective HI antibody titer (HI titer≥$\log_2$ 3, that is, GM≥3) for ND vaccination in chickens (Alexander et al., 2004; OIE, 2004).

Challenge studies

At nine weeks of age, three weeks after the second vaccination, all the birds except the negative controls were challenged with NDV Kudu 113 strain. Each bird received a dose of 0.2 ml through the oculonasal route. After challenge, the birds were observed for two weeks for clinical signs, gross lesions and death.

Data analysis

The mean HI antibody titre and percentage of birds with detectable ND antibody were calculated. Data collected were analyzed using Statistical Package for Social Sciences (SPSS) version 17 program. One way analysis of variance (ANOVA) was performed with Tukey post hoc multiple comparison, which determined statistical significant difference between subgroups at 95% confidence interval with $p<0.05$ considered as significant. The correlation coefficients were calculated to compare the mean HI ND antibody titres between serum and feather samples in the different groups. Mortality and protection rates were also calculated.

RESULTS

Antibody titre using serum

At three weeks of age the mean HI antibody titre was ≥ 3 $\log_2$ in all birds except those in group C2 (1.17 ± 0.38 $\log_2$) and D2 (1.67± 0.56 $\log_2$). Two weeks after primary vaccination (at five weeks of age), the HI ND antibody titre dropped in all groups with group A1 and C2 having the lowest mean HI ND antibody titre of 0.38 ± 0.23 $\log_2$. At six weeks of age, the lowest mean HI ND antibody titre was recorded in group A2 (0.33 ± 0.33 $\log_2$), while at eight weeks of age after secondary vaccination the highest mean HI ND antibody titre of 7.39± 0.42 $\log_2$ was recorded in groups B2 (Table 1).

Antibody titre using feather pulp

All the birds had low HI mean antibody titre before vaccination at three weeks of age with no detectable antibody titre in groups A1, A2 and C2 (Table 2). The response of birds to primary vaccination was high at five weeks of age with the highest mean HI antibody titre of 8.67 ± 0.58 $\log_2$ recorded in group A2; all other groups had mean HI antibody titre ≥ 3 $\log_2$. At six weeks of age the mean HI antibody titre in all the groups were ≥ 3 $\log_2$ except in group D2 which had the lowest HI antibody titre of 0.61 ± 0.39 $\log_2$. Antibody titre of birds in all the groups increased two weeks after booster vaccination (eight weeks of age) with the highest mean HI ND antibody titre recorded in group B2 (7.22 ± 0.58 $\log_2$) and 7.28 ± 0.37

Table 1. Mean haemagglutination inhibition antibody (log $_2$) titres from serum of birds vaccinated with Newcastle disease vaccine strain I$_2$.

Group	Vaccine carriers	No. of birds	Age (weeks) Mean±SD				
			3	5	6	8	9
A1	TMZ	18	4.27±0.51	0.38±0.23	5.27±0.82	2.28±0.58	2.39±0.38
A2	TSG	18	4.22±0.60	1.22±0.36	0.33±0.33	1.89±0.55	2.67±0.32
B1	TMZG	18	4.33±0.87	0.39±0.23	4.22±0.53	4.83±0.64	1.89±0.18
B2	TSGG	18	4.50±0.61	1.00±0.35	4.11±0.83	7.39±0.42	1.44±0.18
C1	MZB	18	3.89±0.72	0.72±0.30	4.78±0.64	6.89±0.58	1.44±0.17
C2	SGB	18	1.17±0.38	0.00±0.00	1.44±0.49	5.44±0.52	2.00±0.30
D1	Control 1	18	4.89±0.50	0.79±0.29	2.00±0.62	3.53±0.75	2.00±0.22
D2	Control 2	18	1.67±0.57	0.44±0.17	1.27±0.27	0.89±0.43	0.39±0.24

A1: Treated maize; A2: treated sorghum; B1: treated maize plus gum Arabic; B2: treated sorghum plus gum Arabic; C1: maize bran; C2: sorghum bran; D1 and D2: positive and negative controls not vaccinated.

Table 2. Mean haemagglutination inhibition antibody (log $_2$) titres from feather pulp samples of birds vaccinated with Newcastle disease vaccine strain I$_2$.

Group	Vaccine carriers	No. of birds	Age (weeks) Mean±SD				
			3	5	6	8	9
A1	TMZ	18	0.00±0.00	7.67±0.56	3.22±0.72	5.78±0.65	2.72±0.27
A2	TSG	18	0.00±0.00	8.67±0.58	3.27±0.73	5.22±0.67	2.22±0.17
B1	TMZG	18	0.17±0.12	4.28±1.11	3.28±0.65	5.17±0.72	1.72±0.25
B2	TSGG	18	0.17±0.17	6.61±0.18	5.22±0.68	7.22±0.58	3.72±0.32
C1	MZB	18	0.56±0.33	6.89±0.67	5.11±0.67	7.28±0.37	3.72±0.55
C2	SGB	18	0.00±0.00	7.11±0.87	4.50±0.72	3.11±0.83	4.06±0.47
D1	Control 1	18	0.26±0.17	3.26±0.91	3.63±0.83	0.26±0.15	3.32±0.28
D2	Control 2	18	0.06±0.06	3.89±1.05	0.61±0.40	0.33±0.14	2.56±0.64

A1: Treated maize; A2: treated sorghum; B1: treated maize plus gum Arabic; B2: treated sorghum plus gum Arabic; C1: maize bran; C2: sorghum bran; D1 and D2: positive and negative controls not vaccinated.

log$_2$ in group C, while the control groups had the lowest HI antibody titre of 0.26 ± 0.15 log$_2$ in group D1 and 0.33 ± 0.14 log$_2$ in group D2. At nine weeks of age, the mean HI antibody titre dropped again in all the groups except in groups B2, C1, C2 and D1 which had mean HI antibody titre ≥ 3 log$_2$ (Table 2).

Percentage of birds with ND antibody HI titres of ≥ 3 log$_2$ (serum)

At three weeks of age prior to primary vaccination, 88% of birds in group A1 and 94% of birds in group D1 had the highest HI antibody titre of ≥ 3log$_2$ (Table 3). At five weeks of age, 33% of birds in group A2 and 27% in group B2 had HI antibody titre of ≥ 3log$_2$. At six weeks of age, groups A1 and C1 had 77% of birds with HI antibody titre ≥ 3 log$_2$. At eight weeks of age, 100% of birds in group B1 had HI antibody titre ≥ 3 log$_2$. Prior to challenge at nine weeks of age, 44% of the birds in groups A1 and 50% in group A2 had HI antibody titres ≥ 3 log$_2$ (Table 3).

Percentage of birds with ND antibody HI titres of ≥ 3 log$_2$ (feather pulp)

At five weeks of age, 94% of the birds in groups A1, A2, and C1 had HI antibody titres of ≥ 3log$_2$, while group C2 had 83% of birds with ≥ 3 log$_2$ at five weeks of age. The highest percentage of birds (83%) with titres ≥ 3 log$_2$ at six weeks of age was recorded in group B2. All the birds (100%) in group C1 had HI antibody titres of ≥ 3 log$_2$ followed by 94% of the birds in group B2 and 83% of the birds in group A1 at eight weeks of age. At nine weeks of age, 77% of birds in group C2, 66% in group D1, and 11% in group B1 had HI antibody titres of ≥ 3 log$_2$ (Table 4).

Correlation analysis

The results of Pearson's and Spearman's rho correlation to compare the mean ND HI antibody titre between feather and serum are shown in Table 5. There was a

Table 3. Percentage of birds with $NDVI_2$ antibody titers of $\geq 3\ log_2$ in serum samples following vaccination at 3 and 6 weeks of age.

Group	Age in weeks				
	3	5	6	8	9
	Percent positive with titres of $\geq 3\ log_2$				
A1	88.9	11.1	77.8	38.9	44.4
A2	72.2	33.3	5.56	33.3	50.0
B1	61.1	11.1	72.2	83.3	22.2
B2	77.8	27.8	55.6	100	5.56
C1	66.7	11.1	77.8	94.4	5.56
C2	22.2	0.0	22.2	88.9	38.9
D1	94.4	22.2	38.9	61.1	5.56
D2	11.1	0.0	11.1	16.7	11.1

A1: Treated maize; A2: treated sorghum; B1: treated maize plus gum Arabic; B2: treated sorghum plus gum Arabic; C1: maize bran; C2: sorghum bran; D1 and D2: positive and negative controls not vaccinated.

Table 4. Percentage of birds with $NDVI_2$ antibody titres of $\geq 3\ log_2$ in feather pulp samples.

Group	Age in weeks				
	3	5	6	8	9
	Percent positive with titre of $\geq 3\ log_2$				
A1	0	94.4	55.6	83.3	50.0
A2	0	94.4	50.0	77.8	38.9
B1	0	44.4	55.6	77.8	11.1
B2	11.1	77.8	83.3	94.4	22.2
C1	11.1	94.4	77.8	100	72.2
C2	0	83.3	72.2	50.0	77.8
D1	11.1	44.4	50.0	0.0	66.7
D2	0.0	44.4	11.1	0.0	33.3

A1: Treated maize; A2: treated sorghum; B1: treated maize plus gum Arabic; B2: treated sorghum plus gum Arabic; C1: maize bran; C2: sorghum bran; D1 and D2: positive and negative controls not vaccinated.

Table 5. Results of correlation analysis for antibody titres in serum and feather pulp after vaccination of chickens with $NDVI_2$ at various ages.

Age (weeks)	Correlation coefficients	
	Pearson	Spearman's rho
3	0.041	0.080
5	0.098	0.076
6	0.193*	0.161
8	0.318**	0.301**
9	- 0.078	-0.032

*Correlation is significant at 0.05 level. **Correlation is significant at 0.01 level.

correlation only at eight weeks of age (two weeks after second vaccination).

Mortality rate and protection rate

The mortality and protection rates of birds challenged with NDV Kudu 113 are presented in Figure 1. The highest mortality rate (100%) was recorded in groups B1, C2 and the control group, while the lowest (78%) was recorded in groups A1 and B2. Groups A2 and C1 had 89% mortality rate. Protection rate after challenge was low for all the groups; A1 had (14%), A2 (1.2%), B2

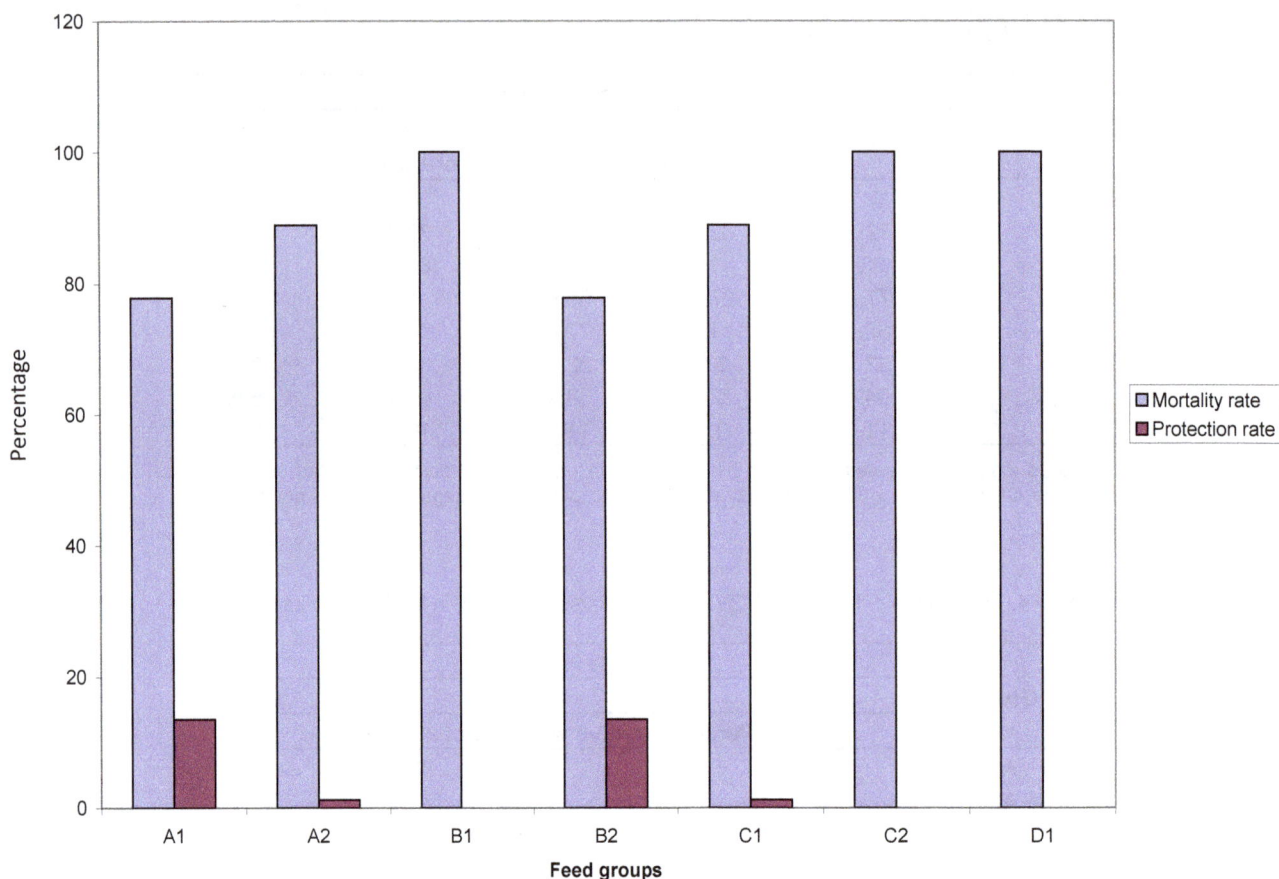

Figure 1. Mortality and protection rate in experimental birds after challenge with Newcastle disease virus Kudu 113 at three weeks after second vaccination. A1: Treated maize; A2: treated sorghum; B1: treated maize plus gum Arabic; B2: treated sorghum plus gum Arabic; C1: maize bran; C2: sorghum bran; D1 and D2: positive and negative controls not vaccinated.

(14%), C1 (1.2%), while B1, C2 and D1 were not protected (Figure 1).

DISCUSSION

The reported protective antibody titre for ND vaccines are HI $\geq$ 4 $\log_2$ (OIE, 2000) with reference to conventional ND vaccine designed for intensively reared commercial chickens. However, HI ND antibody titre of $\geq$ 3$\log_2$ was considered to be adequate for food-based vaccines orally administered to scavenging chickens (Echeonwu et al., 2007). The mean HI antibody titre at three weeks of age was low in all the groups with feather pulp samples in contrast to the high antibody titre recorded at same age in serum. The observed low antibody titre in the feather pulp might be due to movement of antibodies which was more in the central circulation than peripheral at three weeks of age and more in the peripheral circulation at five weeks of age. However, since the birds had no previous vaccination before the primary vaccination, the high antibody titre detected in serum at three weeks of

age could be due to the presence of maternal antibody which may also be responsible for the low antibody titre recorded in serum two weeks after primary vaccination at five weeks of age. It has been established that chicks from immunized parents possess high level of maternal antibody which protect the chicks against virulent virus and interferes with vaccine antigens (Saeed et al., 1988; Rahman et al., 2002). The percentage of vaccinated birds with HI antibody titres $\geq$ 3$\log_2$ showed a marked increase at six and eight weeks of age in both serum and feather pulp samples. Flock immunity reported by Boven et al. (2008) as the only means to prevent the transmission of NDV can only be achieved when $\geq$ 85% of vaccinated birds have antibody titres of $\geq$ 3$\log_2$. In the present study, this was achieved in groups B2, C1 and C2 for serum and groups B2 and C1 for feathers at eight weeks of age. However, prior to challenge at nine week of age, the percentage dropped in both serum and feather with none of the groups having percentage mean HI antibody titre sufficient to protect the birds from challenge. However, it was observed that some birds with low or undetectable ND HI antibody titres survived after challenge. This observation has been reported by Ibrahim et al. (1981) who concluded that low HI antibody titre following NDV4 vaccination were not indicative of susceptibility to challenge, an observation also confirmed by other researchers (Bell et al., 1995; Wambura et al., 2000; Tu et al., 1998). In addition to serum antibody, secretory antibody (IgA) at mucosal surfaces and cell mediated immunity are thought to play a role in resistance to challenge (Alexander, 2003).

There was a general increase in the HI ND antibody titre two weeks after secondary vaccination in serum and feather. Similar results were reported by other workers (Ideris et al., 1990; Spradbrow 1993) who stated that protective immunity is often not apparent until after the second oral vaccination. Similar findings were reported by Baba et al. (2006) and Nasser et al. (2000) that titres among vaccinated birds generally peaked by day 21 post vaccination and declined subsequently. The results of the current study show that administration of 2nd booster vaccination significantly and progressively increased HI antibody titer in all the treatment groups.

The duration of active protective immunity varies with the immune status of the bird and nature of the immune stimulus, which depends on the dose and strain of NDV vaccine and route of administration of the vaccine (Ibrahim et al., 1981; Westbury, 1984). Previous studies found that drinking water induced acceptable immune response and protection, but it is inappropriate particularly in cold weather because vaccination had to be conducted in the mornings, and not all chicken drink water in the mornings even after feeding (Mogoje, 2006). In another study, the administration of a partially thermostable ND vaccine via eye drop application gave the best response, while the vaccine administered via cooked maize meal gave the lowest response. Eye drop vaccination is impractical to implement in village environment (Mogoje, 2006).

There was positive correlation between the mean HI ND antibody titre of serum and feather pulp only at eight weeks of age. This is in contrast to the reports of Roy et al. (1998), who recorded consistent high ND HI antibody titre in serum than in feather three weeks after primary vaccination and three weeks after secondary vaccination in an experiment to compare ND vaccines by serology in tears and feather pulp samples. In the present study, fluctuations were observed in the level of ND HI antibody titre in both serum and feather after primary and secondary vaccination with a marked difference observed at three weeks of age in feather with very low antibody titre than serum and at five weeks of age, feather pulp samples had higher ND antibody titre than serum. These fluctuations could be due to the lack of uniformity of feather pulp samples, since the amount of pulp in each feather will produce some variation in results as reported by Garrido et al. (1992). Results from the present study showed high mortality and low protection rate in all the groups. The difference in the protection rate after

challenge with virulent NDV may be due to differences in the vehicles used in the administration of the vaccine. The highest mortality rate (100%) in vaccinated birds was recorded in birds vaccinated with TMZG and SGB. The lowest protection rate was also recorded in birds vaccinated via TMZG and SGB. However, birds vaccinated with TMZ and TSGG had the lowest mortality. These findings is similar to what was reported by Nasser et al. (2000) in vaccination trials in Ethiopia, where untreated and parboiled sorghum used as vaccine carriers for $NDVI_2$ gave low protection to vaccinated birds after challenge. Similarly, in Nigeria Musa et al. (2010) reported that untreated sorghum, parboiled sorghum, sorghum coated with gum Arabic and a commercial feed mash used as vaccine feed carriers for $NDVI_2$ gave low antibody titre and low protection following challenge with a velogenic NDV. The results of these investigations are in contrast to the findings of Echeonwu et al. (2007, 2008b) who tested $NDVI_2$ and V4 vaccines on millet, maize and guinea corn grains and bran in Nigeria and the vaccinated birds were protected after challenge.

Results from their study indicated that the vaccines could be effective for protection of village chickens as food-borne vaccines provided the carriers are adequately processed. Furthermore, different grains induced different level of HI antibody titer. This implies the presence of inherent variation in virus carrying capacity of different grains (Reta et al., 2016). This is an opportunity to screen grains of different species and varieties. Interestingly, treating grains (either cracking or parboiling) increased their efficacy as vaccine carrier. Similar results have been reported in Nigeria by Olabode (2010) as to the efficacy of treated grain particularly maize compared to untreated grain. Grains have been known to contain tannins, anthraquinone, cardiac glycosides and alkaloids. Some of these chemicals have been shown to have antiviral properties (Oakeley, 2000; Musa et al., 2010). The higher HI titer induced by treated grains than untreated ones could be due to the fact that cracking grains increase the surface area of the grains to adsorb the vaccine virus (Oakeley, 2000; Wambura et al., 2007; Olabode, 2010). Cracked maize and treated sorghum were found to be better vaccine carriers in this study, though the protection rate was low.

This is in contrast with the work of Lawal et al. (2016) in Nigeria using maize grit as vaccine carrier for $NDVI_2$. Their study showed that 94.3% of the vaccinated village chickens seroconverted with protective levels of antibodies against ND virus. However, it should be noted that the protection level of the grain based $NDVI_2$ vaccine varies under laboratory conditions, that is, >90% protection (Aini et al., 1990) and under real village conditions, that is, <60% (Aini et al., 1992) and with vaccine delivered by farmers (Aini et al., 1990). Hence, it is necessary to conduct pilot field trial at village level to evaluate the results of the current study under real village conditions.

Conclusion

The study concluded that treated maize, treated sorghum, untreated maize bran and untreated sorghum bran when used as feed carriers for NDVI$_2$ in this study gave low protection to vaccinated birds after challenge with velogenic NDV. The NDVI$_2$ vaccine could be useful for the protection of village chicken against ND provided the carrier feeds are adequately treated to remove antiviral substances. The use of different processing methods for maize and sorghum should be employed to treat these grains and other locally available feeds such as millet to reduce or eliminate possible antiviral substances in them and to test their suitability as ND vaccine carriers. Correlation was found between the NDV HI antibody titre in serum and feather pulp only at eight weeks of age and thus, feather pulp samples cannot be used as an alternative to serum for seromonitoring of vaccinated birds. However, feathers can be easily collected from live or dead birds, and thus can serve as suitable samples for diagnosis of NDV in chickens. The selection of feather for seromonitoring is important; however, since the amount of pulp in each feather will produce variation in results, further research is therefore necessary.

CONFLICTS OF INTERESTS

The authors have not declared any conflict of interests.

ACKNOWLEDGEMENTS

The authors appreciate the contributions of Prof. S. B. Oladele of the Department of Veterinary Microbiology, Ahmadu Bello University, Zaria, Dr. Musa U. of the Veterinary Research Institute, Vom and thank all staff of the Nutrition Laboratory, Faculty of Veterinary Medicine, Ahmadu Bello University, Zaria, for their technical assistance.

REFERENCES

Aamir S, Tanveer A, Mohammed U, Abdul R, Zahid H (2014). Prevention and control of Newcastle disease. Int. J. Agric. Innov Res. 3(2):454-460.

Abdu PA, Mera UM, Sa'iduL (1992). A study of chicken mortality in Zaria, Nigeria. Proceedings of the National Workshop on Livestock and Veterinary Services, Held at the National Veterinary Research Institute, Vom, pp. 51-55.

Abdu PA, Musa U, Joannis TM, Sa'idu L, Mera UM, Salami-Shinaba, JO, Haruna ES (2012). Vaccination of chickens against Newcastle disease with Lasota and V4 vaccines using brans, ground grains and water as vehicles. Vom. J. Vet. Sci. 9:1-10.

Aini I, Ibrahim AL, Spradbrow PB (1990). Field trials of a food-based vaccine to protect village chickens against Newcastle disease. Res. Vet. Sci. 49:216-219.

Aini I, Ibrahim AL, Spradbrow PB (1992). Efficacy of food pellet Newcastle disease vaccine: simulated village experiments. J. Vet.

Med. Malaysia 4:81-86.

Alders R, Spradbrow PB (2001).Controlling Newcastle Disease in Village Chicken. A field Manual. Australian centre for International Agricultural Research. Monograph 821:19.

Alexander DJ (2003). Newcastle disease and other Avian Paramixoviruses. In: Sairf YM, editor. Disease of poultry. 11th ed. Ames, Iowa: Iowa State press. pp. 63-87.

Alexander DJ, Bell JG, Alders RG (2004). Technology Review: Newcastle Disease. Rome: FAO Animal Production and Health Paper. pp. 1-26.

Ameh JA, Mailafia S, Olatunde H. Olabode BJA, God'spower RO, Martha EO, Dolapo IA (2016). Sero-prevalence of Newcastle disease virus antibodies in local and exotic chickens in Gwagwalada, Nigeria. J. Vet. Med. Anim. Health 8(11):193-198.

Baba SS, Heanacho CC, Ideris JM, El- Yugyda AD (2006). Food-based Newcastle disease vaccine in guinea fowl (*Numida Meleagris Galenta Pallas*) in Nigeria. Trop. Vet. 22(3):37-45.

Bell KG, Fotzo TM, Amara A, Agbebe G (1995). A field trial of the heat resistant V4 vaccine against Newcastle disease by eye drop inoculation in village poultry in Cameroon. Prev. Vet. Med. 25:19-25.

Boven Van M, Annemarie B, Teun HF, FabriElly K, Leo H, Guus K (2008). Herd immunity to Newcastle disease virus in poultry by vaccination. Avian Pathol. 37(1):1-5.

Cumming RB (1992). Newcastle disease research at the University of New England. In: P.B. Spradbrow (ed), Newcastle Disease in Village Chickens, Control with Thermostable Oral Vaccines. Proceedings no 39. Canberra: Australian Centre for International Agricultural Research. pp. 48-85.

Davidson I (2009). Diverse uses of feathers with emphasis on diagnosis of avian viral infections and vaccine virus monitoring. Br. J. Poult. Sci.11 (3):139-148.

Dong-Hun L, Jung-Hoon K, Jin-Yong N, Jae-Keun P, Seong-Su Y, Tseren-Ochir Erdene-Ochir, Sang-Soep N, Yong-Kuk K, Sang-Won L, Chang-Seon S (2016). Viscerotropic velogenic Newcastle disease virus replication in feathers of infected chickens. J. Vet. Sci. 17(1):115-117.

Echeonwu GON, Iroegbu CU, Ngene A, Junaid SA, Ndako J, Echeonwu IE, Okoye JOA (2008a). Survival of Newcastle disease virus (NDV) strain V4-UPM coated on three grains and exposed to room temperature. Afr. J. Biotechnol. 15:2688-2692.

Echeonwu BC, Ngele MB, Echeonwu GON, Joannis TM, Onovoh EM, Paul G (2008b). Response of chickens to oral vaccination with Newcastle disease virus vaccine strain I2 coated on maize. Afr. J. Biotechnol. 7(10):1594-1599.

Echeonwu GON, Iroegbu CU, Echeonwu BC, Ngene A, Olabode AO, Okeke OI, Ndako J, Paul G, Onovoh EM, Junaid SA, Nwankiti O (2007). Delivery of thermostable Newcastle disease (ND) vaccine to chickens with broken millet grains as the vehicle. Afr. J. Biotechnol. 6(23):2694-2699.

Echeonwu GON, Iroegbu CW, Emeruwa AC (1993). Recovery of velogenic Newcastle disease virus from dead and healthy free roaming birds in Nigeria. Avian Pathol. 22:383-387.

Garrido MF, Spencer JL, Chambers JR (1992). Feather pulp as a source of antibody to avain viruses. Avian Pathol. 21:333-337.

Guoyuan W, Chen C, Jing G, Zhenyu Z, Yu S, Huabin S, Qingping L, Jun Y, Hongling W, Hongcai W, Tengfei Z, Rongrong Z, GuofuC, Qingzhong Y (2015). Development of a novel thermostable Newcastle disease virus vaccine vector for expression of a heterologous gene. J. Gen. Virol. 96:1219-1228

Ibrahim AI, Ideris A, Babjee AM (1992). An overview of the use of food based Newcastle disease vaccine in Malaysia. In: Spradbrow PB (ed). Newcastle in Village Chickens Control with Thermostable Oral Vaccine. Australian Centre for International Agricultural Research Canberra, 1992.

Ibrahim AL, Chulan U, Babjee AM (1981). An assessment of the Australian V4 strains of Newcastle disease virus as a vaccine by spray, aerosol and drinking water administration. Austr. Vet. J. 57:227-280.

Ideris A, Ibrahim AL, Spradbrow PB (1990). Vaccination of chickens against Newcastle disease with a food pellet vaccine. Avian Pathol.19:371-384.

Jagne J, Aini I, Schat KA, Fennel A, Touray O (1991). Vaccination of village chickens in the Gambia against Newcastle Disease using heat-resistant, food pelleted V4 vaccine. Avian Pathol. 20:721-724.

Jayawardane GWL, de Alwis MCL, Dawwda B (1990). Oral vaccination of chickens against Newcastle disease with V4 vaccine delivered on processed rice grains. Austr. Vet. J. 67(10):364-366.

Kaleta EF, Baldouf C (1988). Newcastle Disease, Boston/Dordrect/London: Kluwer Academic Publishers. pp. 197-246.

Khan A, Ikhwan A, Muhammad A, Mushtaq A, Hamidullah A (2000). Prevalence of poultry diseases in Kohat. J. Sci. Tech. 24:25-28.

Lawal JR, El-Yuguda AD, Ibrahim UI (2016). Efficacy of feed coated Newcastle disease I2 vaccine in Village Chickens in Gombe State, Nigeria. J. Vet. Sci. Technol. 7:349.

Mogoje BL (2006). Evaluation of a thermostable Newcastle disease vaccine in free range chickens. Magister Technologiae Agriculture. Department of Animal Sciences, Tshwane University of Technology, South Africa. P 122.

Musa U, Abdu PA, Mera UM, Emmenna PE, Ahmed MS (2010). Vaccination with Newcastle disease vaccines strain I2 and LaSota in commercial and local chickens in Plateau state Nigeria. Nig. Vet. J. 31(1):46-55.

Nasser M, Lobr J, Mebratu Y, Zessein KH, Ademe Z (1998). Oral feed-based Newcastle disease vaccination trials in Ethiopia with the Australia V4 vaccine strain. Proceedings, Fourth Asian Pacific Poultry Health Conference, 22-26 November, 1998. Melbourne, Australia. P 129.

Nasser M, Lohr JE, Mebratu GY, Zessin KH, Baumann MPO, Ademe Z (2000). Oral Newcastle disease vaccination trials in Ethiopia. Avian Pathol. 29:27-34.

Oakeley RD (2000). The limitation of a feed/water based heat-stable vaccine delivery system for Newcastle disease control strategies for backyard poultry flocks in sub-Saharan Africa. Prev. Vet Med. 47:271-279.

Office International Des Epizootics (2000). Newcastle disease, Manual of Standards for Diagnostics Tests and Vaccines. pp. 104-124.

Office International Des Epizootics (OIE) (2004). Newcastle disease. In: OIE manual for diagnostic tests and vaccines for terrestrial animals. 5th ed. 1:270-283.

Olabode AO, James A, Ndako GON, Echeonwu GON, Anthony AC (2010). Use of cracked maize as a carrier for NDV4 vaccine in experimental vaccination of chickens. Virol. J. 7(67):1-5.

Oladipo EO (1985). Characteristics of thunderstorms in Zaria, Nigeria. Weather 40:316.

Otchere EO, Adeoye AT, Gefu JO, Adewuyi AA (1990). Preliminary observations on village poultry production in North-Central Nigeria. In: Proceedings of an International Workshop on Rural Poultry Development in Africa (Ed. EB Sonaiya), Ile-Ife, Nigeria, Thelia Publishers pp. 196-200

.Pangani P (1999). Stock breeding support programme in Gaza and Inhambane Provinces, Draft Activity Report by the Animal Health Advisor, October, 1999.

Philemon N, Wambura J, Meers P,Spradbrow PB (2007). Survival of avirulent thermostable Newcastle disease virus (strain I-2) in raw, baked, oiled and cooked white rice at ambient temperatures. J. Vet. Sci. 8:303-305.

Rahman MM, Bari ASM, Giasudin MJ, Islam RM, Sil AC (2002). Evaluation of maternal and humoral immunity against Newcastle disease virus in chicken. Int. J. Poult. Sci. 1:161-163.

Reta DA, Kasahun A, Olana M, Yilkal A, Eseyas G, Marta Y, Teshale Sori (2016). Serological response and protection level evaluation in chickens exposed to grains coated with I2 Newcastle disease virus for effective oral vaccination of village chickens. BMC Vet. Res. 8:12, 279.

Roy P, Koteeswaran A, Stridevi P, Venugopalan AT (1998). Comparison of Newcastle disease vaccines by serology using serum, tears and feather pulp samples. Trop. Anim. Health Prod. 30(1):31-35.

Saeed Z, Ahmad S, Rizvi AR, Ajmal M (1988). Role of maternal antibody in determination of an effective Newcastle disease vaccination programme. Pak. J. Vet. Res. 1:18-20.

Spradbrow PB (1993). Newcastle disease in village chickens. Poult. Sci. Rev. 5(2):57-96.

Tu TD, Phuc KV, Dinh NTK, Quoc DN, Spradbrow PB (1998). Vietnamese trial with a thermostable Newcastle disease (Strain I-2) in experimental and village chickens. Prev. Vet. Med. 34:205-214.

Wambura PN, Kapaga AM, Hyera JMK (2000). Experimental trials with a thermostable Newcastle disease virus (Strain I-2) in commercial and village chickens in Tanzania. Prev. Vet. Med. 43:75-83.

Wambura PN, Meers J, Spradbrow PB (2007). Survival of avirulent thermostable Newcastle disease virus (strain i-2) in raw, baked, oiled, and cooked white rice at ambient temperatures. J. Vet. Sci. 8:303-305.

Westbury HA (1984). Comparison of the immunogenicity of Newcastle disease virus strain V4, B1 and La Sota in chickens. Tests in susceptible chickens. Aust. Vet. J. 61:5-9.

20

Prevalence and risk factors associated to skin diseases in small ruminants in Gamo Gofa zone, south-Western Ethiopia

Bereket Molla[1]*, Haba Haile[2,3] and Sefinew Alemu[2]

[1]The Donkey Sanctuary Working Worldwide, Ethiopia Program, Ethiopia.
[2]University of Gondar, Gondar, Ethiopia.
[3]Gofa Universal College, Department of Animal Health, Sawla, Ethiopia.

A cross-sectional study was employed to estimate the prevalence of skin diseases in small ruminant and risk factors associated to its occurrence in Gamo Gofa zone from July, 2012 to April, 2014. The study areas were clustered into two agro-ecological zones; lowland and highland area. A total of nine hundred (450 sheep and 450 goats) were examined. Detailed physical examinations and systemic examinations, followed by skin scraping and laboratory tests were carried out to diagnose skin diseases. The Pearson's chi-square (χ^2) test was used to assess the degree of association between skin diseases and risk factors. The overall prevalence was found to be 42.33% (381/900). Significantly higher prevalence (p<0.05) of small ruminant skin disease was observed in goats (52.22%) than sheep (38.66%). Furthermore, the study also revealed significantly higher prevalence (p<0.05) in unvaccinated (42.92%) than vaccinated (29.52%) group of animals. The occurrence of skin diseases was statistically significantly associated with age and sex of animals. The prevalence was higher in males (30.38%) than females (22.49%), and in young age groups as compared to adults. The external parasites identified include manges (Sarcoptic, Chorioptic, Psoroptic and Demodectic), ticks (*Ambyloma varigatum, Rhipicephalus evertisi evertisi* and *Boophilus decloratus*), lice (*Bovicola* species and *Linognathus* species) and sheep ked (*Melophagus ovinus*). Viral infections, predominantly of pox virus infection were noted in sheep (10.44%) and goat (13.11%) and contagious ecthyma 2.44% on sheep and 2.00% on goats. The overall prevalence of viral disease showed significant association (p<0.05) with vaccination history and age of the study animals. The high prevalence of skin disease on small ruminant has shown there is urgent need for its strategic prevention and control, as skin and hides represent the second major export commodity of the country. It is recommended that external parasite control should be strategically designed and technologically verified in local context.

Key words: Ethiopia, external parasites, Gamo Gofa, goat, sheep, prevalence.

INTRODUCTION

Small ruminants contribute 35 and 14% of meat and milk consumption, respectively in Ethiopia (Kebede, 2013).

*Corresponding author. E-mail: mollabereket@gmail.com.

Hide and skin export has got the largest share of animal products next to live animal export and skin is the most important item in generating foreign currency, next to coffee (Kumsa et al., 2012). Ethiopia supplies a wide range of both processed and semi-processed sheep and goat skins to the world market (Kebede, 2013). Whereas hides and skins account for 12 to 16% of the total value exports in Ethiopia (Tefera, 2012). The current utilization of hides and skins is estimated to be 48% for cattle hide, 75% for goat skin and 97% for sheep skin with the expected off take rate of 33% and 75% for sheep, goat and cattle, respectively (Berhe, 2009; Yacob et al., 2008 and Tefera, 2012). In Ethiopia, hides, skins, leather and leather products are the most widely traded agro-based livestock commodities with an estimated value of over US$100 billion/year and continues to conspicuously exhibit a huge unexplored potential (Mekonnen et al., 2013). Even though small ruminants are important components of Ethiopian farming system, their contribution to food production, rural income and export income are far below the expected potential (Mekonnen et al., 2013). This is because small ruminant production not only in Ethiopia but in most of the developing countries is constrained by complemented effects of prevailing diseases, subclinical parasitism, poor feeding and managements (Abadi, 2000; Singla, 1995; Tefera, 2012; Yacob et al., 2008; Yacob, 2013). Over the last 10 years, there are indications that the quality of raw material has deteriorated with an increasing number of reject grades and the appearance of skin diseases like "*Ekek or cockle*" that is mainly due to sheep ked and lice infestation (Assefa et al., 2011). The low quality of skins undermines the competitiveness of the industry, as it leads to low factor inputs productivity especially in the tanning process (Mekonnen et al., 2013).

Among the diseases of small ruminant skins, infestations by mange mites, ticks and infections by pox disease and dermatophilosis possess considerable economic losses, particularly to the skin export due to various defects (Dessie et al., 2010). Losses from these diseases and other skin abnormalities are leading to downgrading and rejections of skins; unfitness to the leather industries (Kebede, 2013; Kumsa et al., 2012). Skin diseases in small ruminants were reported from different parts in Ethiopia. Kumsa et al. (2012) reported the prevalence of 48.1% in central Ethiopia, Dessie et al. (2010) reported a mange mites prevalence in Wolaita area of southern Ethiopia 1.98 and 3.85% in sheep and goats, respectively. A study of tick infestation in small ruminants in Bedelle district, Western Ethiopia, revealed prevalence of 66.12 and 80.7% in goats and sheep, respectively reported by Fufa et al. (2012). Many other studies and reviews conducted at different regions of the country reported the importance of small ruminant's skin diseases (Kebede, 2013; Yacob, 2013; Assefa et al., 2012; Tewodros et al., 2012; Dessie et al., 2010; Yacob et al., 2008; Tefera, 2012; Haffiz, 2001; Abadi, 2000). Despite various study on the prevalence and associated

risk factors in different parts of the country, it is not known in Gamo Gofa zone of Southern Ethiopia. Furthermore, this area is known to border with the major pastoral livestock production area of South Omo zone, and serving as a route of market from the lowland pastoral production areas to the highland meat value chain areas of highland markets. In due concern to the above facts, and to seek as whether there is need and/or serve as baseline information, this study was initiated. The objectives were to estimate the prevalence and assess associated risk factors of skin diseases, and to determine the etiological agents of skin diseases in small ruminants.

MATERIALS AND METHODS

Study area

The study was conducted on three districts, categorized into two agro-ecological zones, namely Demba Gofa and Zala district, representing lowland, and Geze Gofa district for highland. Lowland categories were areas ranging from 800 to 1500 meter above sea level (masl) but those ranging from 1500 to 2800 masl were considered as highland. The average annual rainfall of the study areas were varying from 950 to 1150 mm, characterized by a bi-modal type of distribution. The mean annual minimum and maximum temperature were 15.4°C and 37.2°C in the highland and lowland, respectively.

Study animals

The study population animals were extensively managed, almost all are reared in mixed species herd type as an individually owned herd or a group based. A total of 900 small ruminants (450 goats and 450 sheep) were sampled with systematic random sampling. Ages of animals were addressed in two category, young (below 2 years) and adult (above 2 years) of age according to (Bersisa et al., 2013; Gatenby, 1999). The body condition score (BCS) was considered in three categories, poor (BCS of 1 and 2), medium (BCS of 3) and good (BCS of 4 and 5) according to Desta et al. (2001) and Tefera (2012).

Sampling method and sample size

Study districts were selected purposively to represent different agro-ecology and accessibility whereas study Peasant Associations (PA) was randomly selected. 10% of shoat herds were selected from each PA's and individual animals were selected from the population by systematic random sampling approach. The sample size was determined according to Thrusfield, 1995, with expected prevalence of 50%, as there were no such study in the area and 95% confidence interval was considered. Despite this, the calculated sample size was 380, it was increased to 450 from each species and a total of 900 animals were included in the study.

Study designs

A cross-sectional study design was employed to estimate the prevalence of skin diseases and identify the causal factors for different skin diseases of small ruminants. The age, sex, species, body condition scoring, geographical location, season of the year and vaccination were considered as test variables to see if these were risk factors associated with disease occurrence or not. Animals with visible skin problems suspected for bacterial and fungal infections were subjected to skin scrapings. Both skin scrapings and visible external parasites such as ticks, sheep ked and lice were shifted to universal sampling bottle, labelled, preserved and transported to Gofa Universal college department of animal health for species identifications and subsequent laboratory confirmation. 70% ethyl alcohol or 10% formalin were used to preserve adult external parasites recovered and 10% potassium hydroxide (KOH) was used as a cleaning agent for skin scrapings. Species identification and laboratory test on skin scraping was conducted according to Soulsby (1982) and Urquhart et al. (1996).

Sample collection and identification of etiological agents

Physical inspection was conducted to assess the presence of external parasites and gross skin lesions, followed by palpation of all parts of the body. External parasites, sheep keds, ticks and lice were manually collected using tissue forceps and identified under stereomicroscope according to the morphological keys described by (Soulsby, 1982; Urquhart et al., 1996; Taylor et al., 2007). Skin scrapings were collected when suspected for mange mites, fungal and bacteriological lesions. This was done by clipping the hair around the lesion, scrapping the edges of lesions with scalpel blade until capillary oozing was evident (Bersisa et al., 2013; Urquhart et al., 1996). The scrapped materials were either directly shifted to clean microscopic slide or container for laboratory examination. A few drops of 10% potassium hydroxide (KOH) was added to skin scrapings and allowed to stand to 24 h until the time of examination under 4x, 10x, and 40x magnifications of light microscope (Bersisa et al., 2013). Laboratory tests were limited only to bacteriological, fungal and parasitological examinations (arachino-entomology). Skin scrapings suspected for bacterial infections were handled aseptically in clean and disinfected sampling bottles and test tubes. Gram staining was the principal bacteriological test conducted for samples suspected for Dermatophilosis and Giemsa staining was used to test fungal pathogens suspected. Viral diseases like sheep and goat pox (SGP) and contagious ecthyma were tentatively diagnosed on the bases of field level physical clinical examinations.

Data management and statistical analysis

The data entered into Microsoft excel spreadsheet, imported to statistical software for social science (SPSS) version 20.0 for windows. Descriptive statics such as tables, graphics, averages and percentages were used to summarize and present the results of the collected data. The Pearson's chi-square (χ^2) test was used to assess the degree of association between skin diseases with the various risk factors. In all cases, 95% confidence interval (CI) and 5% absolute precision was used for statistical analysis.For all conditions, a p-value of less than 0.05 (p < 0.05) was taken as significant association.

RESULTS

Prevalence of skin diseases

Animal was classified as positive to skin disease if it has at least one of the clinical abnormalities associated to skin disease or is infested with an external parasite. The overall prevalence of skin diseases in small ruminants was found to be 42.33% (381/900). On species bases,

the prevalence was 52.22 and 38.66% in goats and sheep, respectively. Small ruminants from lowland agro-ecology revealed higher prevalence (43.43%) of skin diseases than the highland (37.85%) (Tables 1 and 2).

On species bases, statistically significant (p=0.026) variation in prevalence of skin disease was observed on goats 235 (52.22%) than sheep population 174 (38.66%). Except at Geze Gofa district, in which comparatively larger sheep populations manifested skin disease 52 (48.6%). In the rest two districts, higher prevalence was seen on goat population than sheep populations (Table 2).

On age bases, there is statistically significant (p=0.003) difference on prevalence of skin diseases in young and adult small ruminants. Greater prevalence was recorded in young age groups as compared to adults (Table 3). Whereas, there were no statistically significant difference in the occurrence of skin diseases in small ruminants on sex bases (Table 4), body condition scores and season of the year (Table 6). On the bases of vaccination history, there was statistically significant difference (p=0.000) on occurrence of skin diseases in the study area. The study revealed higher prevalence of skin diseases, 61.45% in unvaccinated small ruminants as compared to vaccinated ones, 23.96 % (Table 5).

Prevalence of external parasites

The study revealed significantly higher prevalence of external parasites (p<0.05) in goat population than sheep population. Furthermore, the study also revealed significantly higher prevalence (p<0.05) of external parasite infestation in males (30.38%) than in females (22.49%). When external parasite infestation was calculated, in goats: 78 (43.33%), 57 (28.50%) and 9 (12.85%) were infested at Demba Gofa, Zala and Geze Gofa Woredas, respectively. However, the prevalence of external parasites in goats was not showing statistically significant difference (P>0.05) among the three Woredas (Table 7). The current study also revealed the external parasite prevalence of 34 (17.62%), 27 (18.00%) and 32 (29.90%), respectively on sheep population from Demba Gofa, Zala and Geze Gofa Woredas. However, there was no statistically significant difference (P>0.05) in prevalence of external parasites of sheep among the three Woredas of Gamo Gofa zone (Table 8). In infested goats, the predominant external parasite identified was tick species (Ambyloma varigatum, Boophilus decoloratus and Rhipicephalus evertisi evertisi) accounted to be 23 (12.77%), 22 (11.00%) and 2 (2.85%), respectively at Demba Gofa, Zala and Geze Gofa Woredas. However the variation in prevalence of ticks was not statistically significant (P>0.05) with respect to agro-ecological zones, age, sex and body condition scoring. In goats, the other external parasite identified next to ticks was pediculosis (lice infestation) occurring with the prevalence of 13.33, 7.5 and 2.85% at Demba Gofa, Zala and Geze

Table 1. Prevalence of small ruminant skin diseases on agro-ecology bases in Gamo Gofa zone.

Agro-ecology	Total examined	Total infected	Prevalence (%)
Lowland Woredas	723	314	43.43
Highland Woredas	177	67	37.85
Total	900	381	42.33

P-value = 0.121, Chi-square (χ^2_{cal}) = 2.399.

Table 2. Prevalence of small ruminant skin diseases on to species bases in Gamo Gofa zone.

Agro-ecology	Total examined		Total infected		Prevalence (%)	
	Goats	Sheep	Goats	Sheep	Goats	Sheep
Lowland Woredas	380	343	220	122	57.95	35.57
Highland	70	107	15	52	21.42	48.60
Total	450	450	235	174	52.22	38.66

P-value=0.026, Chi-square (χ^2_{cal}) = 4.929.

Table 3. Prevalence of small ruminant's skin diseases on age bases in GamoGofa zone.

Agro-ecology	Total examined		Total infected		Prevalence (%)	
	Adults	Youngs	Adults	Youngs	Adults	Youngs
Demba Gofa	258	115	125	63	48.44	54.78
Zala Woreda	295	55	118	28	40.00	50.90
Geze Gofa	140	37	50	17	35.71	45.94
Total	693	207	293	108	42.27	52.17

DF: 1, p-value = 0.003, and Chi-square (χ^2_{cal}) = 8.651.

Table 4. Prevalence of skin diseases on sex and body condition bases in Gamo Gofa zone.

Woreda	Sex		Body condition scoring		
	Male (%)	Female (%)	Poor (%)	Medium (%)	Good (%)
Demba Gofa	87 (48.87)	101 (51.59)	19 (42.22)	51 (39.84)	118 (59.00)
Zala Woreda	49 (49.00)	77 (30.80)	26 (44.10)	66 (36.67)	34 (30.63)
Geze Gofa	30 (33.33)	37 (42.53)	9 (45.00)	26 (32.91)	32 (41.02)
Total	166 (45.10)	215 (40.41)	54 (43.54)	143 (36.95)	184 (47.30)

DF: 1, χ^2_{cal} = 1.709, p-value = 0.191 for sex. DF: 2, χ^2_{cal} = 2.519 and p-value: 0.284 for body condition score.

Table 5. Prevalence of skin diseases on the bases vaccination history in Gamo Gofa zone.

Agro-ecology	Total examined		Total infected		Prevalence (%)	
	Vaccinated	Unvaccinated	Vaccinated	Unvaccinated	Vaccinated	Unvaccinated
Demba Gofa	194	179	70	118	36.08	65.92
Zala Woreda	195	155	28	98	14.35	63.22
Geze GofaWoreda	70	107	12	55	17.14	51.40
Overall	459	441	110	271	23.96	61.45

DF: 1, χ^2_{cal} = 17.302 and p-value: 0.000.

Table 6. Prevalence of skin diseases on the bases of season of the year in Gamo Gofa zone.

Agro-ecology	Total examined		Total infected		Prevalence (%)	
	Dry	Wet	Dry	Wet	Dry	Wet
Demba Gofa	200	173	116	72	58.00	41.61
Zala Woreda	221	129	100	26	45.21	20.15
Geze Gofa Woreda	101	76	48	19	47.52	25.00
Overall	522	378	264	117	50.57	30.95

DF: 1, χ^2_{cal} = 0.015, and p-value: 0.903.

Table 7. Prevalence of external parasites and skin disorders in goats in three Woredas of Gamo Gofa zone.

Skin diseases	Demba Gofa n (%)	Zala Woreda n (%)	Geze Gofa n (%)
External parasites	*78 (43.33)*	*57 (28.5)*	*9 (12.85)*
Sarcoptes scabies	10 (5.55)	9 (4.50)	2 (2.85)
Chorioptes spp	3 (2.77)	5 (2.50)	0 (0.00)
Demodex caprae	18 (10.00)	6 (3.00)	3 (4.28)
Ticks	23 (12.77)	22 (11.00)	2 (2.85)
Pediculosis	24 (13.33)	15 (7.50)	2 (2.85)
Skin disorders	*46 (25.55)*	*42 (21.00)*	*6 (8.57)*
Goat pox	26 (14.14)	28 (14.00)	5 (7.14)
Contagious ecthyma	6 (3.33)	3 (1.50)	0 (0.00)
Dermatophilosis	3 (2.77)	1 (0.50)	0 (0.00)
Dermatophytosis	7 (3.88)	4 (2.00)	0 (0.00)
Wounds and scratches	4 (2.22)	5 (2.50)	1 (1.14)
Photosensitization	2 (1.11)	1 (0.50)	0 (0.00)
Overall	124 (68.89%)	99 (49.50)	15 (21.42)

Table 8. Prevalence of external parasites and skin disorders in sheep in three Woredas of GamoGofa zone.

Skin diseases	Demba Gofa (n = 193)	Zala Woreda (n = 150)	Geze Gofa (n = 107)
External parasites	**34 (17.62)**	**27 (18.00)**	**32 (29.90)**
Sarcoptes scabies	7 (3.62)	4 (2.66)	5 (4.67)
Chorioptes ovis	2 (1.04)	0 (0)	3 (2.80)
Psorptes ovis	0 (0)	3 (2.00)	1 (0.93)
Demodex ovis	3 (1.55)	9 (6.00)	3 (2.80)
Ticks	13 (6.74)	4 (2.66)	9 (8.41)
Pediculosis	9 (4.66)	7 (4.66)	14 (13.08)
Skin disorders	**41 (21.24)**	**20 (13.33)**	**20 (18.69)**
Sheep pox	21 (10.88)	12(8.00)	14 (13.08)
Contagious ecthyma	7 (3.63)	3(2.00)	1 (0.93)
Dermatophilosis	4 (2.07)	1 (0.50)	3 (2.80)
Dermatophytosis	7 (3.63)	2 (1.33)	2 (1.87)
Wounds and scratches	2 (1.04)	2 (1.33)	0 (0.00)
Overall	75 (38.86%)	47 (31.33)	52 (48.60)

Gofa Woredas, respectively. The prevailing lice species identified were Linognathus species and Bovicola species from sucking and biting groups of lice (Table 7 and 8). As far as mange mite infestation in goat population was concerned, Sarcoptic mite was occurring at the prevalence of 5.55, 4.5 and 2.85% in Demba Gofa, Zala and Geze Gofa Woredas, respectively. Chorioptic mite (2.77, 2.50, and 0%), and *Demodex caprae* (10.00, 3.00, and 4.28%) were also recorded in the three respective Woredas above (Table 7 and 8). External parasites identified on the sheep was lice infestation, accounted to be 13.08, 4.66, and 4.66%, respectively at Geze Gofa, Zala and Demba Gofa Woredas. Similar species of lice as recovered in goats. Prevalence of pediculosis was not statistically significantly different (P > 0.05) among sheep of the three Woredas of Gamo Gofa Zone (Table 8). Ticks were the other dominant external parasites observed even though the prevalence was not showing statistically significant difference (P > 0.05) among small ruminants of the 3 Woredas of Gamo Gofa zone, Southern Ethiopia. Sarcoptic mite, Chorioptic mite, Psoroptic mite and *Demodex ovis* were also identified in sheep population, but their prevalence was at very low rate.

Prevalence of bacterial, fungal and viral infections

The predominant viral infection on small ruminants was caused by pox disease, prevalence of 14.44, 11.00, and 7.14% in goats and, 10.88, 10.66 and 9.35% in sheep at Demba Gofa, Zala and Geze Gofa Woredas, respectively. Occurrence of pox disease was not statistically significantly associated (P>0.05) with agro-ecology, species, sex and body condition scores, whereas, there was statistically significant variation (p<0.05) on age group base; higher in young as compared to adult (Table 8). The occurrence of pox disease in both sheep and goat was limited only to unvaccinated small ruminants.

DISCUSSION

The current study revealed the overall prevalence of 42.33% for small ruminant skin diseases. The record of significantly higher skin disease prevalence from goat species than sheep was suggested as due to variation in animal husbandry system. Traditionally, sheep and sheep products like skin are relatively expensive than goat and goat products in all three Woredas of the study areas and this finding is in agreement with the explanation underlined by Tekle et al. (2009) and Yacob (2013). So, the underlying reason for increased exposure of goats to skin disease was lack of care in terms of veterinary service, feeding, vaccination and housing. The finding of current study is in agreement with Rahmeto et al., (2011) who had reported an overall skin disease prevalence of 51.7% on sheep and 59.60% on goats at Tigri Regional State of Ethiopia and, a 48.1% overall skin disease prevalence reported by Yalew (2014) at Wolita-Sodo, Southern Ethiopia.

However, the current result is higher than that of previous works conducted by Dessie et al. (2010), on small ruminant mange mite; 1.98% on sheep and 5.85% on goats at three ecological zones of Wolita-Sodo, Southern Ethiopia. The variations could be attributed due to seasonal variation, variation in animal husbandry system and/or geographical location of the study areas. Relatively higher overall prevalence in current study (42.33%) could be due to very limited intervention for external parasite prevention and control in the area and overall poor veterinary facility in the area. The sharing of different flocks of animals to communal watering and grazing sites could have facilitated the establishment and spread of external parasite infestation and contagious skin infections in the area. This finding is also in agreement to Yacob et al. (2013). Statistically significant difference in prevalence (p<0.05) was observed from unvaccinated small ruminants than vaccinated groups. The finding suggests that immunizing the animals is an important strategy to prevent skin diseases especially those originated from bacterial and viral groups. Furthermore, the study revealed significantly higher overall small ruminant skin disease prevalence in young animals than adults, which could be because of their low acquired resistance compared to adults. Many previous works agrees with the finding of this research (Yacob et al., 2013; Fufa et al., 2012). The finding of higher prevalence of external parasite in goats than sheep in current report is in agreement with previous reports by Dessie et al. (2010), Kebede (2013), Yacob (2013) and Zenaw and Mekonnen (2012). The higher prevalence of external parasite in male small ruminants of both species could be due to the fact that anatomically the skins of male goats and sheep have heavy course grain nature that lacks tensile strength, while female skins have better strength in nature (Tekle, 2009), not favourable for external parasite infestation. The tick species identified by this study were *Ambyloma varigatum*, *Rhipcephalus evertisi evertisi* and *Boophilus decoloratus* in agreement to Yacob et al. (2008); reported the presence of these three tick genera in Ethiopia. The occurrence of small ruminants infested by ticks by current study is comparatively lower than the previous reports; 66.12% in goats and 80.7% in sheep by Fufa et al. (2012) around Bedelle district of Oromia regional state, Ethiopia. The current study revealed both burrowing (Sarcoptic mange, Demodectic mange) and non-burrowing mites (Chorioptic and Psoroptic mange) in both species of the study animals. These findings are in agreement to the reports of Dessie et al. (2010), Yacob et al. (2008) and Haffiz (2001), whereas, relatively larger prevalence of mange mites in sheep (69.3%) and goat (57.3%) was reported Kassa et al. (2013).

CONCLUSION AND RECOMMENDATIONS

Ethiopia has a huge small ruminant population, endowed

with great potential of attractive global market for skin. However, the contribution of skin in the national export income and enhancing the earnings from the skin to its producers are disproportionately small as a result of various skin diseases. The causes of deteriorated quality of skin were external parasites infestation, bacterial, viral and fungal diseases, and the poor animal husbandry practices such as poor nutrition and improper slaughter and flying operations. Moreover, poor veterinary infrastructure, lack of awareness and absence of a designed strategy in prevention and control of skin diseases continued to be a problem of deterioration of skin quality.

1. Therefore, awareness creation among farmers about the impacts of skin diseases and improving livestock extension system was recommended.
2. Control of external parasites through combination rotational grazing, sound husbandry practices and application of acaricides should also be encouraged.
3. More importantly, vaccinating both sheep and goat population against pox diseases and bacterial pathogens across the study Woredas was also suggested.
4. Further study should be conducted in designing integrated skin diseases prevention and control regimen on the bases of species dynamicity and seasonal occurrence.

ACKNOWLEDGEMENTS

The authors would like to express heartfelt thanks and appreciation to Dr Gizat Almaw from Sebeta National Veterinary Research Institute and Yetinayet Aragaw from Addis Ababa University for their technical support. Deep appreciation also goes to staffs of Gofa Universal College, Department of Animal Health and the management of the college for allowing the use of their laboratory.

CONFLICT OF INTERESTS

The authors have not declared any conflict of interests.

REFERENCES

Abadi Y (2000). Current problems of leather industry: The opportunities and challenges of enhancing goat production in East Africa: Proceedings of Conference held at Debub University, Hawassa, Ethiopia. *E(kika) de la Garza* institute for Goat research. OK: Langston pp. 139-143.
Assefa M, Tesfaye D, Taye M (2011). A study on the prevalence of sheep and goat skin defects in Bahir Dar tannery, Ethiopia. Onl. J. Anim. Feed Res. 2(4):384-387.
Berhe A (2009). Assessment of hides and skin marketing in Tigri region. The case of Atsbi Wemberta Woreda, Eastern Tigri: *Msc thesis*: Addis Ababa University School of Graduate Studies College of Development Studies, pp. 1-37.

Bersisa M, Jemberu A, Tamirat M (2013). Skin defects of small ruminants in Africa. Ethiop. Vet. J. 321-322.
Dessie S, Hailu D, Dereje B (2010). Epidemiological study of small ruminant mange mites in three agro-ecological zones of Wolita, Southern Ethiopia. Ethiop. Vet. J. 14(1)31-38.
Desta H, Girma A, Alemu Y (2001). Body condition scoring of sheep and goat. Technical Bulletin Number 8. Ethiopian Sheep and Goat Productivity Improvement Program (ESGPIP), Addis Ababa, Ethiopia, 2:109-134.
Fufa A, Josen T, Alemayehu R (2012). Status of tick infestation in small ruminants of Bedelle district: Oromia region, Ethiopia. Glob. Vet. 8(5):459-462.
Gatenby R (1999). Sheep major health in tropical production system. In: The Tropical Agriculturalist, Macmillan Education. London: UK pp. 7-8.
Haffiz M (2001). Study on skin disease of small ruminants in central Ethiopia. *DVM thesis:* Faculty of Veterinary Medicine, Addis Ababa University, DebreZeit, Ethiopia, pp. 12-32.
Kassa B, Asegid S (2013). Enhancing economic growth through control of livestock skin diseases in Ethiopia. 27th EVA Annual Conference Proceedings, Addis Ababa, Ethiopia. Ethiop. Vet. J. pp. 85-93.
Kebede M (2013). Effects of small ruminant ecto-parasites in tanning industry in Ethiopia: O Revion. J. Anim. Sci. Adv. 3(9)424-430.
Kumsa B, Beyecha K, Goleye M (2012). Ectoparasites of sheep in three -agro-ecological zones in central Oromia region, Ethiopia. J. Vet. Res. pp. 1-8.
Mekonnen H, Nicholas M, Mwinyikione M (2013). Unlocking the potential of Ethiopian leather value chain: Livestock based extension role. COMESA Leather and Leather Products Proceedings (LLPI): 27th Ethiopian Veterinary Association Proceedings, Addis Ababa, Ethiopia. Ethiop. Vet. J. pp. 51-66.
Rahmeto A, Dessie S, Mekalash T, Bekele M, (2011). Prevalence of small ruminant external parasites and associated risk factors in selected districts of Tigri region, Ethiopia. Glob. Vet. 7(5)433-437.
Singla D (1995). A note on sub-clinical gastro-intestinal parasitism in sheep and goats in Ludhiana and Faridkot districts of Punjab. Indian Vet. Med. J. 19:61-62.
Soulsby E (1982). Helminthes, arthropods and protozoa of Domesticated animals London: Bailliere Tindal. pp. 92-106, 136-166.
Taylor M, Coop R, Wall R (2007). Veterinary Parasitology. 3rd ed . Oxford, UK: Blackwell Publishing, pp. 459-475.
Tefera S (2012). Investigations on external parasites of small ruminants in selected sites of Amhara regional state and their impact on tanning industry. MSC thesis, Faculty of Veterinary Medicine, Addis Ababa University, Ethiopia, pp. 1-37.
Tekle Z, Alemu Y, Merkel R (2009). Common defects of sheep and goat skins in Ethiopia and their causes: *Technical Bulletin* at Addis Ababa, Ethiopia, pp. 1-59.
Tewodros F, Tsegedingle Y, Mersha C (2012). Bovine demodicosis: Threat to leather industry in Ethiopia. Asian J. Agric. Sci. 4(5)314-318.
Thrusfield M (1995). Veterinary Epidemiology. 2 nd ed, Blackwell Science.
Urquhart M, Armor J, Duncan L, Dunn A, Jennings F (1996). Veterinary Parasitology. 2nd ed. London: Blackwell Science, pp. 123-192.
Yacob H (2013). Skin defects in small ruminants and their nature and economic importance: The case of Ethiopia. Glob. Vet. 11(5):552-559.
Yacob H, Nesanet B, Dinka A (2008). Prevalence of major skin diseases in cattle, sheep and goats at Adama Veterinary Clinic, Oromia Regional State, Ethiopia. Rev. Med. Vet. 159:8-9.
Yalew T (2014). Study on the prevalence of ecto-parasites in small ruminants in and around Wolita Sodo, Southern Ethiopia. Trop. Anim. Health Prod. 47:27-35.
Zenaw Z, Mekonnen A (2012). Assessment of major factors that cause skin defects at Bahir Dar Tannery, Ethiopia. Adv. Biol. Res. 6(5)177-181.

21

Study on calf coccidiosis in dairy farms in and around Holeta Town, Finfine Zuria Liyu Zone, Oromia, Ethiopia

Zerihun Adugna Regasa[1], Belay Mulatea[1] and Temesgen Kassa Getahun[2]*

[1]Faculty of Veterinary Medicine and Animal Health, Wollo University, Ethiopia.
[2]Animal Health Research, Holeta Agricultural Research Center, Ethiopian Institute of Agricultural Research, P. O. Box 31, Holeta, Ethiopia.

Bovine coccidiosis is a protozoan infection caused by different species of *Eimeria* which has a worldwide distribution. The disease which mainly affects calves belongs to large herd size where hygiene is not well managed and is associated with poor body condition. A cross-sectional study was conducted from November 2016 to April 2017 to determine the prevalence of bovine coccidiosis and identify the associated risk factors in semi intensive and extensive dairy farms in and around Holeta town, Finfine Zuria Liyu Zone, Oromia Regional State, Ethiopia. Fecal samples were randomly collected from three hundred and eighty four calves belonging to dairy farms and examined for the presence of the oocyts of *Eimeria* by floatation technique using saline solution. The study revealed that the overall prevalence of coccidiosis was 26.04%. The risk factors considered were age, sex, breed, production system, herd size, fecal consistency, body condition and hygienic status of the house. The prevalence of coccidiosis was higher within calves in poor hygienic (58.6%) dairy farms than calves from better hygienic farms (14.6%). There was also significant difference (P<0.05) in the prevalence of coccidiosis between different herd sizes with higher prevalence in herd size >10 animals (39.3%). The highest prevalence of coccidiosis was recorded in calves with diarrheic faeces (91.7%) than calves with soft, constipated and normal fecal consistency (P<0.05). Appropriate monitoring and control of the disease is advisable in the study farms.

Key words: Calf, coccidiosis, dairy farms, *Eimeria*, Holeta, prevalence.

INTRODUCTION

Ethiopia is endowed with abundant livestock resources of varied and diversified genetic roles with specific adaption to its wide range of agro ecologies (CSA, 2015). This great livestock potential is not properly exploited due to many prevailing socio economic values and attitudes, traditional management methods, limited genetic potential and rampant disease.

Gastrointestinal parasite infections are a problem for both small and large scale farms; however, their impact is greater in sub-Saharan Africa. The prevalence of

*Corresponding author. E-mail: Temesgen.kassa@yahoo.com.

gastrointestinal parasites and the severity of infection vary considerably depending on the genera of helminth and protozoan parasites involved, animal species, local environmental conditions such as humidity, temperature, rainfall, vegetation and management practices (Debela, 2002; Sandhu and Singla, 2005; Wadhawa et al., 2011).

The most important disease problems in the young calf are pneumonia and diarrhea. The pathogens associated with calf diarrhea are rotavirus, corona virus, *Salmonella* species, protozoan parasites, *Eimeria* and *Cryptosporidium* species (Bhat et al., 2012; Brar et al., 2017). Bovine coccidiosis is a protozoan disease of the intestinal tract caused by microscopic organisms called coccidia; and is one of the most common and important disease of cattle worldwide(The Merck Veterinary Manual, 2005). This disease is usually the most known and devastating protozoan disease in calves under age of one year (Ernst et al., 1987).

Previous works which were conducted in different parts of Ethiopia showed that coccidiosis is a paramount important protozoan disease in younger calves (<12 months) which were kept in poor hygienic status as well as improperly nourished with colostrum (Abebe et al., 2008; Mehreteab et al., 2012; Alemayehu et al., 2013; Temesgen, 2016). Although, coccidiosis is an important cause of calf morbidity and mortality in Ethiopia in general, and in the study area in particular, there is no previous detail information on its prevalence coccidiosis in the study area.

Therefore, this study was conducted to determine the prevalence and associated risk factors of calf coccidiosis in farms in and around Holeta, Finfine Zuria Liyu zone, Ethiopia.

MATERIALS AND METHODS

Study area

The present study was conducted in extensive and semi intensive farms found in and around Holeta town located in Finfine Zuria Liyu Zone, Oromia Regional State, Ethiopia during the period between November 2016 and April 2017 to determine calf coccidiosis and its putative risk factors. Holeta is located 45 km west of Addis Ababa at altitude 2400 m above sea level. It is geographically located between 9° 3′N latitude and 38° 30′ E longitudes. The area experienced bimodal rainfall pattern with a short rainy season from February to April and the long rainy season from the middle of June to end of September. The remaining months are dry periods. The area gets an annual rain fall of 1000 to 1100 mm and the annual temperature ranges between 18 and 24°C. The total cattle population of the study area is estimated to be 175,741, out of which 172,769 (98.3%) heads of cattle are local breeds and 2972 (1.7%) are crosses kept under extensive and semi intensive management systems (WoWAHA, 2015).

Study animals

The study was carried out on 384 calves within the age of 1 month to 1 year old. The samples were randomly collected from calves reared under semi intensive and extensive management systems. Examined calves were categorized based on their age and grouped into three as: group I (1 to 4 months age), group II (5 to 8 months) and group III (9 to 12 months of age), based on house hygiene grouped into three (good, moderate and poor) and also based on size of herd grouped into three (<10, 11-20 and >20 head of calves).

Study design and sample size determination

The type of study was cross sectional with simple random sampling technique conducted between November 2016 and April 2017 to determine the prevalence and associated risk factors of calf coccidiosis in and around Holeta town. The desired sample size for this study was determined by using the single population proportion formula according to Thrusfield (2005). Since there is no previous report on calf coccidiosis in the study area, the sample size was established based on the 50% expected prevalence, 5% desire absolute precision and 95% confidence level (CI).

$$n = \frac{z * Pex(1 - Pex)}{d^2}$$

Where, n = required sample size; z=1.96²; p_{ex} = expected prevalence; d = desired absolute precision.

Thus, the desire sample size for P_{ex} = 0.5 is n= 384 calves included in this study. While collecting faecal samples, data related to age, sex, bred, herd size management system, body condition, fecal consistency and hygienic status of barn were properly recorded.

Faecal sample collection and examination

A total of 384 faecal samples were collected directly from the rectum of each sampled animal with strict sanitation, and placed in air and water tight sample vials. After collection, the samples were transported in ice box to Holeta Agricultural Research Center (HARC) Parasitological Laboratory for fecal examination using simple floatation technique with saline solution (Yu et al., 2011; Gupta and Singla 2012).

Data management and analysis

All data collected were entered and managed in MS-Excel software program and analyzed using SPSS 20.0 statistical software version. Descriptive statistics such as percentage was used to approximate the prevalence of calf coccidiosis in the study area. Prevalence was calculated as number of positive calves harboring *Eimeria* oocytes divided by the total calves examined. Chi-square (x^2) statistics were used to test the association between variables. At p <0.05 was taken as statistically significant.

RESULTS

Overall prevalence

In the present study, out of total 384 samples tested, 100 (26.04%) were positive for the presence of *Eimeria* oocyts.

The prevalence was higher in Barfata (37.5%) as compared to other study localities (p <0.05) as shown in Table 1.

Table 1. Prevalence of caves Coccidiosis in the study localities.

Study locality	No. of animals examined	No. of positive	Prevalence (%)	x^2	p-Value
Holeta	206	37	18		
Barfata	98	37	37.5	15.698	0.000
WajituHarbu	80	26	32.5		
Total	384	100	26.04		

Potential risk factors

The analysis of putative risk factors was made by Chi-square analysis. The result showed strong significant associations between coccidian infection and herd size (x^2 =16.387, P = 0.000), different body condition scores (x^2 = 51.447, P = 0.000), faecal consistency (x^2 = 44.668, P = 0.000) and hygienic status of the house (x^2 = 29.393, P= 0.000). However, no significant difference was observed between the prevalence of coccidiosis and different age groups (x^2=3.363, P =0.186), sexes (x^2 = 0.437, p = 0.508), breeds (0.103, P =0.748) and different management systems (x^2 = 0.281, P =0.596) as shown in Table 2.

DISCUSSION

Calf coccidiosis causes a significant economic loss through morbidity and mortality worldwide. The result of the present study conducted in three localities of Holota town and its environs showed an overall prevalence of 26.04% coccidian infection in calves. The 26.04% prevalence of coccidiosis in this study is in line with previous studies of Bekele et al. (2012) [22.7%] in Dire Dawa, Temesgen (2016) [24.3%] in South Wollo Zone Amhara region, Ethiopia, Toaleb et al. (2011) [24.2%] in Egypt. However, the prevalence result of the present study is much lower than many of the previous reports in Ethiopia, namely, 68.1% in Addis Ababa and Debre Zeit Dairy Farms (Abebe et al., 2008), 31.9% in Kombolcha, south Wollo (Alemayehu et al., 2013), 62.5% in Asella town (Ibrahim, 2016) and 38.9% in and around Asella town dairy farms (Tsegaye, 2016). The findings of this study are also much lower than that of other countries of the world. For instance, a prevalence of 47.1% was reported in China (Dong et al., 2012). The results of the present study, however, is higher than previous reports by Gillhuber et al. (2014) (13.3%) in Southern Germany, Hussin (2016) (9.5%) in Iraq and Das et al. (2015) (11.9%) in India. Such inconsistency in the prevalence rate of coccidiosis may be due to the variation in diagnostic tests, age of the animals, susceptibility of different breeds to the disease, stress level, handling, climatic and other factors of agro-ecology, variation in the study season, number and target group of the study animals and husbandry practices(Radostitis et al., 2007a; Abebe et al., 2008; Heidari et al., 2014).

This study showed variation in the prevalence of calf coccidiosis between different study localities (18% to 37.5%). Similar results were obtained in different parts of Zimbabwe (17.4 to 32.6%) (Pfukenyi et al., 2007), Al-Baha, Saudi Arabia (29.84 to 32.51%) (Ibrahim et al., 2015) and in Addis Aababa and DebreZeit, Ethiopia (57.2 to 76.4%) (Abebe et al., 2008). This geographical difference in distribution of positive cases could be explained by the management practices and the bio-security followed by the farm owners.

Analysis of risk factor with regard to the age of the calves revealed that there is no statistically significant association ($\chi2$= 3.363, P= 0.186) between the age of the calves and coccidian infection. This result agrees with the reports of Abebe et al. (2008), Tsegaye (2016), Alemayehu et al. (2013), Bekele et al. (2012) and Gillhuber et al. (2014). This similarity could be due to the fact that animal husbandry practices in the study areas are identical, and also, different age groups were kept and housed together without separation.

There was no statistically significant difference in prevalence of coccidian infection between male and female animals ($\chi2$ = 0.437, p =0.508), which is in agreement with the reports of Abebe et al. (2008), Heidari and Gharekhani (2014), Alemayehu et al. (2013) and Ibrahim (2016). This might be associated with the fact that different sex groups kept in similar husbandry system might have equal chance of accessing the oocyts. Despite this, previous studies done on adult cattle showed higher prevalence of *Eimeria* in female animals than in males (Manya et al., 2008; Rehman et al., 2011). Nevertheless, this could be attributed to the physiological stress loaded on female animals in relation to pregnancies and giving birth as compared to males (Radostits et al., 2007a).

The breed related prevalence of coccidian infection in the present study showed no statistical significant difference between breeds ($\chi2$ = 0.103, p =0.748), which is in agreement with the findings of Abebe et al. (2008) and Alemayehu et al. (2013).

The possible explanation for this similarity could be the fact that calf rearing condition in the study areas was identical and different breeds were housed together without separation. In contrast to the current findings, susceptibility differences were reported between local and cross breeds (Ibrahim, 2016). This breed susceptibility difference could be related to the dose of oocytes ingested and the species of *Eimeria* involved in

Table 2. Prevalence of calf coccidiosis in relation to various risk factors.

Risk factor		No. of sampled calves	No. of positive	Prevalence (%)	χ^2	p-Value
Age (Months)	1-4	204	58	28.4		
	5-8	102	28	27.5	3.363	0.186
	9-12	78	14	17.9		
Sex	Female	208	57	27.4	0.437	0.508
	Male	176	43	24.4		
Breed	Local	124	31	25	0.103	0.748
	Cross	240	69	26.5		
Herd size	≤10 Animals	92	22	23.9		
	11-20 Animals	117	46	39.3	16.387	0.000
	>20 Animals	175	32	18.3		
Management	Semi intensive	296	79	26.7	0.281	0.596
	Extensive	88	21	23.9		
Body condition score	Good	171	20	11.7		
	Moderate	164	50	30.5	51.447	0.000
	Poor	49	30	61.2		
Fecal consistency	Normal	302	59	19.5		
	Soft	67	28	41.8		
	Constipated	3	2	66.7	44.668	0.000
	Diarrheic	12	11	91.7		
Barn hygiene	Good	164	24	14.6		
	Moderate	191	59	30.9	29.393	0.000
	Poor	29	17	58.6		

the infection (Taylor et al., 2007).

In the current study, coccidian infection was significantly higher in calves reared in large herd size than in small size ($\chi2$ = 16.387, P = 0.000). This finding is in line with the report of Nasir et al. (2009). This similarity might be due to rapid spread of infection from calf to calf as well as greater contamination of feeding and watering troughs when animals are communally feed and overcrowded (Radostitis et al., 2007a). However, the current finding disagrees with that of Abebe et al. (2008). This variation might be due to the differences in the study seasons, husbandry practices and the treatment regime given to the calves.

There was no significant difference ($\chi2$ = 0.281, p = 0.596) in the prevalence of coccidiosis and management systems. This result agrees with the report of Abebe et al. (2008), Alemayehu et al. (2013) and Temesgen (2016). This similarity might be due to equal chance of accessing the oocysts when grazing from contaminated field.

However, the current finding is in contrast with the previous report of Abisola (2004). This variation might be due to hygienic condition of the barn, nutritional status of the calves, contamination level of the feed, water, floor and treatment given to the animals.

There was statistically significant ($\chi2$=44.668, P=0.000) difference in prevalence rate between fecal consistency and coccidian infection which agrees with the findings of Pundit (2009) and Alemayehu et al. (2013). However, this finding disagrees with the report of Abebe et al. (2008). In the present study, 91.7% diarrheic calves were found tobe positive to *Eimeria*. However, there were no apparent clinical signs in most of the animals sampled for the study.

A strong significant association ($\chi2$= 51.447, P= 0.000) was recorded between body condition score and coccidian infection in the current study. Similarly, Mehreteab et al. (2012) reported a higher infection rate in calves with poor body condition score than in calves with good and moderate body condition score. This might be due to the weak immune status of the calves with poor body condition score. As a result, malnutrition and other parasitic infections result in immune compromised calves. This condition produces a higher infection rate in poor state animals than in good-state animals (Radostits et al., 2007b).

In the current study, association of *Eimeria* infection in relation to the hygienic status of calf house was verified ($p < 0.05$). This result agrees with the report of Bekele et al. (2012) Mundt et al. (2005a, b) and Dawid et al. (2012). The similarity implies that poor sanitation in the calving and calf housing areas as well as poor management of housing favors infection of coccidiosis. Obviously, poor ventilation, droughts, poor calf nutrition, group pens, heavy stocking, cows present with calves, soiled bedding are regarded as risk factors for coccidiosis (Radostits et al., 2007b).

CONCLUSION AND RECOMMENDATION

In conclusion, this study provides proof of a coccidian infection in dairy farms in Holeta and its environs. Hygiene of calf's house can be considered as a risk factor for the occurrence of coccidia. Large herd size, diarrheic faeces and poor body condition of the calves also increased the risk of infection with coccidia. However, sex, age, breed and management system of calves did not show any difference with the occurrence of protozoan parasite infection. In general, different risk factors were considered to affect the rate of infection of calves with this protozoan parasite.

Based on these findings, it was recommended that calves with severe diarrhea be isolated and treated with appropriate drugs; any possibility of fecal contamination of the farm and the calves be minimized. Further epidemiological investigations are required to determine the protozoan parasite species composition and their economic impact.

CONFLICT OF INTERESTS

The authors declare that there is no conflict of interest.

REFERENCES

Abebe R, Wossene A, Kumssa B (2008). Epidemiology of Eimeri infections in calves in Addis Ababa and DebreZeit Dairy Farms, Ethiopia. Int. J. Appl. Res. Vet. Med. 6(1):24-30.

Abisola TO (2004). Studies on Bovine coccidian. [Apicomplexia: eimeriidae] In: Parts of Plateau State, Nigeria. Available at: http://dspace.unijos.edu.ng/jspui/handle/123456789/129

Alemayehu A, Nuru M, Belina T (2013). Prevalence of bovine coccidia in Kombolcha district of South Wollo, Ethiopia. J. Vet. Med. Anim. Health 5(2):41-45.

Bekele M, Ferid D, Yeshitila A (2012). Calf coccidiosis in selected dairy farms of Dire Dawa, Eastern Ethiopia. Glob. Vet. 9(4):460-464.

Bhat SA, Juyal PD, Singla LD (2012). Prevalence of cryptosporidiosis in neonatal buffalo calves in Ludhiana district of Punjab, India. Asian J. Anim. Vet. Adv. 7(6):512-520.

Brar APS, Sood NK, Kaur P, Singla LD, Sandhu BS, Gupta K, Narang D, Singh CK and Chandra M (2017). Periurban outbreaks of bovine calf scour in Northern India caused by Cryptosporidium in association with other enteropathogens. Epidemiol. Infect. 145(13):2717-2726.

Central Statistical Agency (CSA) (2015). Federal Democratic Republic of Ethiopia: Central Statical Agency Agricultural sample survey, Volume II, report on Livestock and Livestock chracterstics, Bulletin No.578. Addis Ababa. pp. 12-15.

Das M, Deka DK, Sarmah PC, Islam S, Sarma S (2015). Diversity of Eimeria spp. in dairy cattle of Guwahati, Assam, India. Vet. World 8(8):941-945.

Dawid F, Amede Y, Bekele M (2012). Calf coccidiosis in selected dairy farms of Dire Dawa, Eastern Ethiopia. Glob. Vet. 9 (4):460-464.

Debela E (2002). Epidemiology of gastro-intestinal helminthiasis of Rift Valley goats under traditional husbandry system in Adami Tulu district, Ethiopia. Ethiop. J. Sci. 25: 35-44.

Dong H, Zhao Q, Han H, Jiang L, Zhu S, Li T, Kong C, Huang B (2012). Prevalence of coccidian infection in dairy cattle in shanghais, China. J. Parasitol. 98(5):963-966.

Ernst JV, Stewart TB, Witlock DR (1987). Quantitative determination of coccidian oocysts in beef calves from the coastal plain area of Georgia (USA). Vet. Parasitol. 23(1-2):1-10.

Gillhuber J, Rügamer D, Pfister K, Scheuerle MC (2014). Giardiosis and other enteropathogenic infections: A study on diarrhoeic calves in Southern Germany. BMC Res. Notes 7:112-120.

Gupta SK, Singla LD (2012). Diagnostic trends in parasitic diseases of animals. In: Veterinary Diagnostics: Current Trends. Gupta RP, Garg SR, Nehra V and Lather D (Eds), Satish Serial Publishing House, Delhi. pp. 81-112.

Heidari H, Gharekhani J (2014). Detection of Eimeria species in Iranian native cattle. Int. J. Adv. Res. 2(7):731-734.

Heidari H, Sadeghi-Dehkordi Z, Moayedi R, Gharekhani J (2014). Occurrence and diversity of Eimeria species in cattle in Hamedan province, Iran. Vet. Med. 59(6):271-275.

Hussin AG (2016). Prevalence and Associated Risk Factors of Eimeria spp. in cattle of Baghdad, Iraq. J. Appl. Anim. Sci. 9(1):37-44.

Ibrahim DAYDN (2016). Prevalence and associated risk factors of calf coccidiosis in and around Asela Town, Southeast Ethiopia. Prevalence 6(3).

Ibrahim MM, Soliman MF, Alghamdi AO (2015). Subclinical bovine coccidiosis in Al-Baha Area, Saudi Arabia. Int. J. Vet. Sci. Res. 1(1):023-028.

Manya P, Sinha SR, Sinha S, Verma SB, Sharma SK, Mandal KG (2008). Prevalence of bovine coccidiosis at patna. J. Vet. Parasitol. 22:5-12.

Mehreteab B, Ferid D, Yeshitila A (2012). Calf coccidiosis in selected dairy farms of Diredawa, eastern Ethiopia. Glob. Vet. 9:460-464.

Mundt HC, Bangoura B, Rinke M, Rosenbruch M, Daugschies A (2005a). Pathology and treatment of Eimeria zuernii coccidiosis in calves: investigations in an infection model. Parasitol. Int. 54(4):223-230.

Mundt HC, Bangaura B, Mengel H, Keidel J, Daugschies A (2005b). Control of clinical coccidiosis of caslves due to E. bovis and E.zuerni with toltrazuril under field conditions. Parasitol. Res. 97:134-142.

Nasir A, Avais M, Khan MS, Ahmad N (2009). Prevalence of Cryptosporidium parvum infection in Lahore (Pakistan) and its association with diarrhea in dairy calves. Int. J. Agric. Biol. 11(2):221-224.

Pfukenyi DM, Willingham AL, Mukaratirwa S, Monrad J (2007). Epidemiological studies of parasitic gastrointestinal nematodes, cestodes and coccidia infections in cattle in the highveld and lowveld communal grazing areas of Zimbabwe. Onderstepoort J. Vet. Res. 74(2):129-142.

Radostits OM, Gay CC, Blood DC, Hinchcliff KW (2007a). Veterinary Medicine - A Textbook of the Diseases of Cattle, Horses, Sheep, Pigs and Goats, 10th edition reviewed by Sameeh M. Abutarbush, BVSc, MVetSc, Diplomate ABVP, Diplomate ACVIM Saunders, USA Available at: https://www.ncbi.nlm.nih.gov/pmc/articles/PMC2857440/

Radostits OM, Gay CC, Hinchcliff KW, Constable PD (2007b). Diseases associated with protozoa. Veterinary Medicine: A Textbook of the Diseases of Cattle, Sheep, Goats, Pigs and Horses. 10th ed. Philadelphia, Pennsylvania: Saunders Elsevier. pp. 1498-1515.

Rehman TU, Khan MN, Sajid MS, Abbas RZ, Arshad M, Iqbal Z, Iqbal A (2011). Epidemiology of Eimeria and associated risk factors in cattle of district Toba Tek Singh, Pakistan. Parasitol. Res. 108(5):1171-1177.

Sandhu BS, Singla LD (2005) Coccidiosis in bovines: an increasing problem. In: Compendium of Winter School on Novel Approaches for Diagnosis and Control of Parasitic Diseases of Domestic and Wild Animals held from 07-27 October, 2005 at PAU, Ludhiana. pp. 190-194.

Taylor MA, Coop RL, Wall RL (2007). Veterinary Parasitology. 3rd ed. Oxford, UK: Blackwell Publishing. Available at: http://trove.nla.gov.au/work/26713022

Temesgen GK (2016). Epidemiological studies on calf coccidiosis in dairy farms in South Wollo Zone Amhara Region, Ethiopia. J. Vet. Sci. Technol. 7(392):2.

The Merck Veterinary Manual (2005). Merck & Co. Inc. and Merial Limited introduce the Ninth Edition of the Merck Veterinary Manual. Available at: http://veterinarynews.dvm360.com/merck-merial-publish-2005-merck-veterinary-manual-0

Toaleb NI, El-Moghazy FM, Hassan SE (2011). Diagnosis of eimeriosis in cattle by ELISA using partially purified antigen. World Appl. Sci. J. 12:33-38.

Thrusfield M (2005).Veterinary Epidemiology. 3rd Ed., Blackwell Science Ltd., Oxford, UK. pp.233-261.

Tsegaye E (2016). Occurrence of coccidiosis in diarrheic calves in and around Asella town dairy farms. World J. Biol. Med. Sci. 3(3):48-54.

Wadhawa A, Tanwar RK, Singla LD, Eda S, Kumar N and Kumar Y (2011). Prevalence of gastrointestinal helminths in cattle and buffaloes in Bikaner, Rajasthan, India. Vet. World 4(9):417-419.

WoWAHA(2015).WolmeraWereda Animal Health Agency. Statistical Abstract. Wolmera, FinfineLiyuZuria Zone, Oromia, Ethiopia.

Yu SK, Gao M, Huang N, Jia YQ, Lin Q (2011). Prevalence of coccidian infection in cattle in Shaanxi province, Northwestern China. J. Anim. Vet. Adv. 10:2716-2719.

22

A study on gross and histopathological pulmonary lesions of cattle slaughtered at Abergelle Abattoir, Mekelle, Tigray, Ethiopia

Kidane Workelul Yalew[1*], Nesibu Awol[2], Yishak Tsegay[1], Haftay Abraha[1] and Hailesilassie W/mariam[1]

[1]Department of Veterinary Medicine, College of Veterinary, Mekelle University, Kelamino, Mekelle, Ethiopia.
[2]Department of Veterinary Medicine, School of Veterinary, Wollo University, Dessie, Ethiopia.

Animals in sub-Saharan African countries are used as source of milk, meat, hides and skin where animal diseases are one of the primary constraints in increasing the productivity of food animals. Studies were conducted to examine various respiratory problems of cattle with purpose of identifying the gross and histopathological lesions in lungs of slaughtered cattle at Abergelle Export Abattoir from April 2015 to June 2015 Mekelle, Tigray, Ethiopia. A total of 240 lungs of cattle originating from different parts of Tigray regions were examined and as many as 208 lung samples with gross pulmonary lesions were collected for further confirmatory histopathological study. The prevalence of pulmonary lesions of cattle in this study was 86.6% (n=208). The case of pneumonia was found to be highest followed by lung emphysema and congestion besides cases of oedema, hydatidosis, abscess and atelectasis. These results indicated that respiratory problem is still a major health problem in cattle production.

Key words: Lung, pneumonia, pulmonary lesion, Ethiopia.

INTRODUCTION

Domestic animals in Ethiopia are mainly used as drought animals, source of milk, meat, hide and skin and as pack animals. Animal diseases are one of the primary constraints in increasing the productivity of food animals in sub-Saharan Africa (Lemma et al., 2001).

Lopez (2012) stated diseases affecting the respiratory system are generally the leading causes of morbidity and mortality in large domestic animals. The management and environmental stress are often the decisive factors for the development of clinical diseases (Howard, 1993).

Environmental and management stresses like over work, undue exposure to cold winds and rain, sudden change of climate, insufficient food and chronic diseases particularly trypanosomosis are responsible for respiratory diseases (Andrews and Kennedy, 1997; Dungworth, 1993). Pulmonary tissues are damaged by potential bacterial pathogens especially *Pastuerella* infection that normally reside in the upper respiratory tract (Carter, 1984). Even the lung tissues can be found infected with food borne parasitic zoonotic infections

*Corresponding author. E-mail: kiduney06@gmail.com.

(Sandhu et al., 1995; Chhabra and Singla 2009).

The reaction of the lung tissue may be in the form of an acute fibrinous process as in pasteurellosis, a necrotizing lesion as infection with *Fusobacterium necrophonrum* or as a more chronic caseous or granulomatous lesion in *Mycobacterial* or *Mycotic* infections (Radostits et al., 2007).

The gross and histopathological characterization of the pulmonary disease has not yet been studied in Mekelle and around slaughter at Abergelle Export Abattoir; for this reason this study is designed with the objective to assess the major pulmonary lesion of the slaughter cattle based on lobular distribution of the infected lung and to identify as well as characterize the types of gross and histopathological lesions in lungs of cattle slaughtered at Abergelle Export Abattoir.

MATERIALS AND METHODS

Study area

The study was conducted in Abergelle Export Abattoir, Mekelle. Mekelle is the capital city of Tigray Region. It is located around 780 km north of the Ethiopian capital City Addis Ababa, at a latitude and longitude of 13°29′N 39°28′E, with an elevation of 2084 m above sea level. The mean annual rainfall of the area is 628.8 mm. The annual minimum and maximum temperature is 11.8 and 29.94°C, respectively (RSTBARD, 2009).

Study type and study animals

A cross-sectional study was undertaken to establish the prevalence of gross and histopathological pulmonary lesions of cattle slaughtered at Abergelle Export Abattoir, Mekelle. The study was conducted purposively on 240 cattle subjected to slaughter from different parts of Tigray region. All cattle examined in this study were male greater than six years of age and have good body condition were apparently healthy during ante-mortem inspection.

Sample collection and processing

Immediately after slaughter, post-mortem examination was made by visual examination, palpation and incision for the presence of any lung lesion. The gross appearance, location as well as size of the lesions and observations made on incision were also recorded .Out of 240 cattle lungs examined, a total of 208 lung tissue samples with gross pulmonary lesions were collected for histopathological study. Tissue samples having a thickness of up to 2 to 3 cm were collected from every pulmonary lesion. They were taken from the margin of healthy and affected tissue parts and fixed in 10% buffered neutral formalin (BNF) immediately. Each sample was fixed separately and transported to pathology laboratory for processing. After fixing tissue samples for 24 h, all samples collected for histopathological study were dehydrated in alcohol, embedded in paraffin, sectioned at 4 to 6 µm thickness and stained with Haematoxyline - Eosin stain. The stained samples were examined using light microscope. Sample collection and processing was done as per the method described by Assegedech (2005) and Bancroft et al. (1996).

Data analysis

The data was entered into Microsoft excel spread sheet and coded appropriately. For data analysis, SPSS version 15 was used. In this data analysis, descriptive statistic was used to determine the proportion of the different respiratory lesions and their lobular distributions. Chi-square was used to test the lobular distributions of pulmonary lesions.

RESULTS

Pulmonary lesions

Out of the total 240 slaughtered cattle examined during the study, 208 cattle (86.6%) were found to have pulmonary lesions. On the basis of gross and microscopic examination pneumonia, pulmonary emphysema, pulmonary congestion and oedema, hydatidosis, pulmonary abscesses and atlectiasis were identified with prevalence of 33.33% (n=80), 31.25% (n=75), 12.08% (n=29), 6.67% (n=16), 2.08% (n=5) and 1.25% (n=3), respectively. The frequency and prevalence of pulmonary lesions identified in this study was summarized in Table 1. The lobular distribution of pneumonia, pulmonary emphysema, and pulmonary congestion and edema were significantly (*p-value* = 0.000) higher in the right cranial lobe than the other lobes of lungs. However, pulmonary abscess was significantly (*p-value* = 0.000) higher in the right middle and caudal lobes of the lungs compared to the other lung lobes. Hydatidosis, was also most frequently encountered in the right caudal lobe (*p-value* = 0.000). In addition, atelectasis was most commonly encountered in the caudal lobes of both right and left lungs with *p-value* < 0.321. The lobular distributions of pulmonary lesions were summarized in Table 2. Representative images of some pulmonary lesions are indicated in Figure 1.

DISCUSSION

Out of 240 cattle lungs examined, 86.6 % had pulmonary lesions. This result was in agreement with the report of Gebrehiwot et al. (2015) and Abayneh (1999) who reported pulmonary lesions of cattle with prevalence of 86.2 and 83.87%, respectively. However, the result of this study was higher than the findings of Amene et al. (2012) and Ahmed et al. (2013) who reported pulmonary lesions with prevalence of 46.22 and 44.6%, respectively. These all results showed that respiratory diseases are highly prevalent in cattle production area. This high prevalence of pulmonary lesions could be due to the older age of the animals at slaughter with possibility of exposure to one of the agents which causes respiratory disease through time at least once.

The overall prevalence of pneumonia in this study was 33.33%. This agree with the report of Ahmed et al. (2013) who reported pneumonia in cattle at a prevalence of 28.7% but higher than the results of Yifat (2011) and Amene et al. (2012) who reported 1.8 and 1.11%

Table 1. Prevalence of pulmonary lesions in lungs of cattle slaughtered at Abergelle Export Abattoir, Mekelle.

Pulmonary lesion	Frequency	Prevalence (%)
Pneumonia	80	33.33
Emphysema	75	31.25
Pulmonary congestion and edema	29	12.08
Hydatidosis	16	6.67
Pulmonary abscesses	5	2.08
Atlectiasis	3	1.25

Table 2. Lobular distributions of pulmonary lesions.

Lesion	Percentage of distribution of pulmonary lesions (%) in different lobes of the lungs							Chi-square	
	RCC	RCD	RM	RD	LCC	LCD	LD	x^2	P-value
Pneumonia	86.25	32.5	36.25	18.75	20	15	2.5	168	0.000
Emphysema	62.67	18.67	25.33	12	13.33	6.67	2.67	299	0.000
Pulmonary congestion and Oedema	72.41	17.24	27.59	31.03	20.69	17.24	3.45	104	0.000
Hydatidosis	6.25	18.75	31.25	62.5	0	6.25	25	61.1	0.000
Pulmonary abscess	0	20	40	40	0	20	20	17.4	0.008
Atelectasis	33.33	33.33	0	66.67	33.33	33.33	66.67	7	0.321

RCC, Right Cranial Cranial; RCD, Right Cranial Caudal; RM, Right Middle; RD, Right Caudal; LCC, Left Cranial Cranial; LCD, Left Cranial Caudal; LD, Left Caudal.

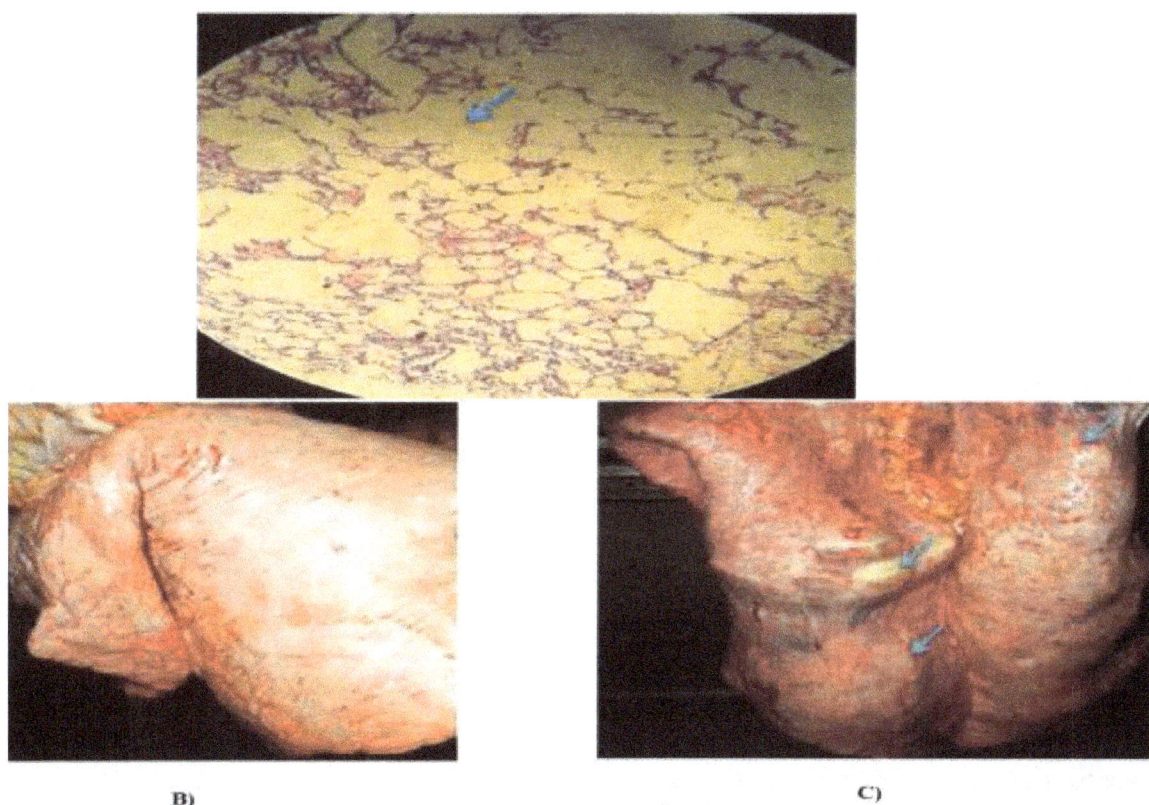

B)   C)

Figure 1. Microscopic and gross representative images of typical pulmonary lesions. (A) Emphysema with ruptured alveolar wall and coalescence of alveolar space (arrow); (B) Gross lesion of emphysematous lungs; (C) Multiple hydatid cysts in lungs (arrows).

prevalence of pneumonia in cattle, respectively. The factors affecting are different in management systems, breed of animals, nutrition, climatic factors, and animal health extension services etc.

Emphysema was found to be the second most prevalent lesion with a prevalence of 31.25%. This result coincides with the report of Gebrehiwot et al. (2015) where emphysema was observed on 36.3% of cattle and higher than the studies of Abayneh (1999) and Amene et al. (2012) who reported emphysema at prevalence of 16.53 and 6.77%, respectively. The emphysema could be due to excessive destruction of alveolar walls as a result of an imbalance between proteases produced by phagocytes and antiproteases produced in the lungs as a defense mechanism, secondary to obstruction of outflow of air or agonal at slaughter as indicated by Lopez (2012) and Dungworth (1993). Emphysema was encountered more frequently on the right cranial lobes of the lung.

Pulmonary oedema and congestion occurred at a prevalence of 12.08% and this was higher than the results of Amene et al. (2012) and Ahmed et al. (2013) who reported a prevalence of 2.33 and 6.5%, respectively. However, the result of this study was lower than the results of Rahman et al. (2003) and Gebrehiwot et al. (2015), who reported pulmonary oedema and congestion in cattle at a prevalence of 61.53 and 38.5%, respectively. Pulmonary oedema and congestion provides an ideal environment for the growth of pathogens of relatively low virulence.

Hydatidosis was encountered in 6.67% of the examined cattle lungs and lower than the findings of Rahman et al. (2003), Gebrehiwot et al. (2015) and Amene et al. (2012) who reported prevalence of 25, 18.3 and 35.88%, respectively. This difference in the prevalence of hydatidosis may be due to variation of dogs and wild carnivore population. Hydatid cycts were distributed most frequently on the right caudal lobes of the lungs. This could be due to the larger size of the caudal lobes, which in effect get a greater volume of blood supply (Lopez, 2012).

Pulmonary abscesses were encountered in 2.08% of the cases. This result was higher than the result of Amene et al. (2012) (0.11%) and lower than that of Gebrehiwot et al. (2015) (7.1%) and Ahmed et al. (2013) (9.4%). Pulmonary abscess arise from either focal residues of severe, supportive lobar or bronchopneumonia or from septic emboli lodging in the pulmonary vascular bed. The most common sources of septic emboli include ruptured hepatic abscess in cattle, suppurative metritis, mastitis, septic arthritis, omphalophebitis in farm animal and bacterial endocarditis (right side) in all species (Lopez, 2012; Dungworth, 1993). Additionally the two less common causes of pulmonary abscess are aspiration of foreign bodies and direct traumatic penetration of the lungs (Lopez, 2012; Dungworth, 1993).

The prevalence of atelectasis in this study was 1.25%.

Atelectasis is common when collateral ventilation is less (Lopez, 2012). The cause of usual atelectasis is occlusion of the bronchus or bronchiole, which supplies it. This results most often from a plug of mucus or purulent exudates. The air contained at the time the bronchus is closed is absorbed in a short time as is regularly the case with entrapped gases. The airless alveoli then collapse under surrounding pressures (Lopez, 2012; Jone and Hunt, 1983). It also accompanies space occupying lesions in the thoracic cavity or on the lung parenchyma like neoplasia, granuloma, hydatid cyst etc and the accumulation of transudate and exudates when their volume is large (Lopez, 2012; Jone and Hunt, 1983; Dungworth, 1993). In all types of atelectasis the collapsed lung is prone to secondary infections (Lopez, 2012).

CONCLUSION AND RECOMMENDATIONS

Out of the total 240 lungs of cattle examined, 86.6% were found with one or more pulmonary lesions, indicating pulmonary diseases as an important constraint of cattle production. The lesions encountered in this study will also play a role as a predisposing factors for respiratory disease outbreak under the influence of stress factors such as environmental change, extremes of climatic conditions, transportation and shortage of feeds and water or alone. Therefore, the prevailing environmental condition undue exposure to cold winds and rain, sudden change of climate coupled with the management stresses like over work might reverse these hidden inactive lesions and thereby contribute for the higher occurrence of respiratory diseases in cattle's.

Taking these facts into consideration the following recommendations are forwarded:

1. Further and subsequent study is recommended on a larger scale with specific data about the origin of animals slaughtered.
2. Awareness of the public about hydatidosis should be increased through public education and infected organs should be properly disposed.
3.Strong collaboration among governmental organization, nongovernmental organization, veterinarian (researchers) and livestock owners should be made in order to determine the impact of respiratory disease on cattle production and to design control and prevention strategies.

CONFLICT OF INTERESTS

The authors have not declared any conflict of interests.

ACKNOWLEDGMENT

The author sincerely would like to appreciate Mekelle

University College of Veterinary Medicine for provision of the laboratory and other facilities. They also extend their thanks to the Abergelle Export Abattoir for providing their facility to conduct the study.

REFERENCES

Abayneh L (1999). Pulmonary lesions of cattle slaughtered at Assela abattoir, Ethiopia. DVM Thesis, AAU, FVM, Debre Zeit, Ethiopia, pp. 1-21.

Ahmed AM, Ismail SAS, Dessouki AA (2013). Pathological lesions survey and economic loss for male cattle slaughtered at Ismailia abattoir. Inter. Food Res. J. 20(2):857-863.

Amene F, Eskindir L, Dawit T (2012). The cause, rate and economic implication of organ condemnation of cattle slaughtered at Jimma municipal abattoir, Southwestern Ethiopia. Glo. Vet. 9(4):396-400.

Andrews GA, Kennedy GA (1997). Respiratory diseases in diagnostic pathology Veterinary Clinical. North America: Food Animimal. Practies. 13(3):515-547.

Assegedech S (2005). Histopathology. In: Standard Veterinary Laboratory Diagnostic Manual, (Vol. V). Ministry of Agriculture and Rural Development, Animal Health Department. Addis Ababa, Ethiopia. pp. 1-60.

Bancroft JD, Stevans A, Turner DR (1996). Theory and practice of histological techniques. 4th Ed. Churchill Livinigstone, Edinburgh, London, Melbourne, New York.

Carter GR (1984). Diagnostic Procedures in Veterinary Bacteriology and Mycology, 4th ed. Charles C. Thomas, Springfield, Illinois, U.S.A. pp. 3-166.

Chhabra MB, Singla LD (2009). Food-borne parasitic zoonoses in India: Review of recent reports of human infections. J. Vet. Parasitol. 23(2):103-110.

Dungworth DL (1993). The respiratory system. In: K.V.F. Jubb, P.C. Kennedy and Palmer (eds), Pathology of Domestic Animals 2. Academic Press, INC. Harcourt Brace Jovanovich, Publishers, San Diego, U.S.A. pp. 539-699.

Gebrehiwot T, Verma PC, Berhanu H (2015). Study on gross pulmonary lesions in lungs of slaughtered animals and their economic importance in Tigray, Ethiopia. Momona Ethiop. J. Sci. 7(1):46-54.

Howard JL (1993). Current Veterinary therapy 3rd ed: Food Animal practice. Saunders company, Philadelphia, U.S.A. pp. 633-642.

Jone TC, Hunt RD (1983). The respiratory system. In : Veterinary pathology, 5th (ed). Lea and Febiger, Philadephia, U.S.A. pp. 1208-1249.

Lemma M, Kassa T, Tegen A (2001). Clinically manifested major health problems of cross breed dairy herds on urban and peri-urban production system on the central high lands of Ethiopia. Trop. Anim. Health and Prod. 6:34-43.

Lopez A (2012). Respiratory system. In Cariton, W.W., Mc Gavin, M.D. (eds), Thomson's Special Veterinary pathology. 5th ed, Chicago pp. 116-174.

Radostits OM, Gay CC, Blood DC, Kenneth H (2007). Veterinary Medicine- Text Book of the Diseases of cattle, sheep, pig, goats and horses. 9th edition, W.B. Saunders, Tottenham Court Road, London, pp. 431-441.

Rahman A, Nooruddin M, Begum N, Lee J (2003). Epidemiological study of pulmonary lesions and diseases in slaughtered cattle. Korean J. Vet. 26(1):81-88.

Regional State of Tigray Bureau of Agriculture and Rural Development (RSTBARD) (2009). Estimated animal population of Tigray region.

Sandhu BS, Brar RS, Singla LD, Singh H, Brar APS (1995). Sarcocystis in alveolar tissue of buffalo lungs. Ind. J. Vet. Pathol. 19(1):53.

Yifat D (2011). Major causes of organ condemnation and financial significance of cattle slaughtered at Gondar Elfora Abattoir, Northern Ethiop. Glob. Vet. 7(5):487-490.

23

Sero-prevalence and associated risk factors for *Brucella* sero-positivity among small ruminants in Tselemti districts, Northern Ethiopia

Mulalem Zenebe Kelkay[1*], Getachew Gugsa[2], Yohannes Hagos[3] and Habtamu Taddelle[3]

[1]Tigray Agricultural Research Institute, Mekelle, Ethiopia.
[2]School of Veterinary Medicine, Wollo University, Dessie, Ethiopia.
[3]College of Veterinary Medicine, Mekelle University, Mekelle, Ethiopia.

A cross sectional study design was employed with the aim to determine sero-prevalence of brucellosis among sheep and goats and identify factors associated with sero-positivity to *Brucella*. A total of 558 sera were collected randomly and aseptically from small ruminants from November, 2015 till October, 2016 in Tselemti district, Northern Ethiopia, following proper restraining. All the sera were primarily screened for the presence of *Brucella* antibodies using Rose Bengal Plate test (RBPT) and then confirmed by Complement Fixation Test (CFT). The overall sero-prevalence of disease in the study area was 1.79% (n=10). Most of the risk factors including peasant association, species, sex, age, parity, herd size, lactation, and pregnancy status had no significant effect on the sero-positivity to *Brucella* (P>0.05), whereas animals with previous history of abortion and retained fetal membrane had significant effect (P<0.05). Hence, the odds of being sero-positive to *Brucella* was found to be 5.68 (COR=5.68; 95% CI: 1.13, 28.53) and 4.05 (AOR=4.05; 95% CI: 1.01, 16.22) times higher in animals with previous history of retained fetal membrane and abortion when compared with animal with no history of retained fetal membrane and abortion, respectively (P<0.05). The results of the current study demonstrated that brucellosis is endemic and the cause for reproductive loss and failure. Hence, the finding suggests that there is a need for implementation of better management practice such as culling of positive animals from the flock, burning/burial of aborted or retained fetal membrane, and also community awareness about zoonotic importance of the disease should be raised.

Key words: Risk factors, small ruminants, sero-prevalence, Tselemti districts.

INTRODUCTION

Ethiopia owns a huge resource of small ruminant population with an estimated number of 27.34 and 28.16 million heads of sheep and goats, respectively (CSA, 2014). Small ruminants provide various benefits particularly to smallholder farmers. They may be used as a source of immediate cash income, meat, milk, skin,

*Corresponding author. E-mail: m.zenebe2007@gmail.com.

manure, risk spreading, and various social functions (Berhanu et al., 2006). Besides this, small ruminants are also considered as means of investments and insurance for the small holder farmers in order to provide income for the purchase of food during the seasons of crop failure because sheep and goats have high fertility rates, short generation interval, and small feed requirement and adaptability to harsh environmental conditions as compared to large ruminants which make them best suited for smallholder farming practice in the country (Berhanu et al., 2006; Tsedeke, 2007).

The current levels of contributions of the livestock sector in Ethiopia, at either the macro or micro level are below the country's potential. The levels of foreign exchange earnings from livestock and livestock products are also much lower than would be expected, given the size of the livestock population (Berhanu et al., 2007). This is due to the prevailing animal disease, feed shortage both in quality and quantity, low genetic potential and management problems. Of these, infectious diseases are the major constraints for enhancing small ruminant production all around the globe including Ethiopia (Singla, 1995; Getahun, 2008; Gizaw, 2010; Kaur et al., 2013).

Brucellosis is a zoonotic infectious disease affecting a wide range of species of animals and humans with an estimated half a million human cases reported annually. It is caused by different Brucella species of the genus Brucella. It is facultative intracellular Gram negative bacteria. The disease is one of the most widespread zoonoses and is endemic in many developing countries (Corbel, 2006; Pal et al., 2013).

Brucella melitensis is the most important cause of brucellosis which primarily affects sheep and goats and also very pathogenic for human beings. The disease is also caused by Brucella ovis which severely affects sheep. Although the disease has preferred hosts, the bacteria have an ability to cross infect other domestic animals. Hence, sporadic infections in small ruminants could also be caused by Brucella abortus or Brucella suis, but such cases are rare (Corbel, 2006; OIE, 2015).

Small ruminant brucellosis mainly affects the reproductive tract of animals which is manifested by late term abortions, retention of placenta in the case of female animals, epididymitis and orchitis in males. Additionally, the disease also poses major constraint to international trading of animal and animal products (Benkirane, 2006; Radostits et al., 2007; Seleem et al., 2010).

As the disease often goes undetected, identification of infected herd and animals is of prime importance for control of the disease. Having huge livestock resource at hand coupled with intermingling of livestock species may cause uninfected animals to easily get exposed to the disease from multiple sources such as abortion discharges and direct contact with infected animals. Mixed farming especially raising goats and sheep along with cattle was also reported by many researchers to be

a risk factor for Brucella transmission between different animal species (Godfroid et al., 2013; Padilla et al., 2010).

In Ethiopia, the existence of small ruminant brucellosis has been reported from different parts of the country. Most of the authors used serological surveys to determine the prevalence and associated risk factors. Such kind of information on the status of small ruminant brucellosis in Tselemti district, Northwestern Zone of Tigray Regional State is absent, although there are cases of abortion and retained placenta among small ruminants according to oral information given by farmers, local authorities, and experts. This problem is probably because of brucellosis. So far, the existence of the disease in small ruminants is little known in the study area and so is the circulating Brucella spp. in sheep and goats. As there are major risk factors for the occurrence of the disease, a detailed study on small ruminant brucellosis is necessary to establish disease effective control program.

Therefore, the aims of this study were to estimate the sero-prevalence of brucellosis in small ruminants in Tselemti district and to determine risk factors associated with Brucella sero positivity.

MATERIALS AND METHODS

Study area

The study was conducted from November, 2015 till October, 2016 in Tselemti district of Northwestern Zone of Tigray Regional State, Northern part of Ethiopia. The study area is situated at 38°15' E and 13°48' N and 1178 km away from the capital city of Addis Ababa. The study area is among the six districts of the Northwestern zone of Tigray and border with districts of Asgede Tsimbla on the North, Welkayit on the West, Tanqua Abergelle on the East and Amhara region on the South.

In Tselemti districts, six Peasant Associations (PA) were used for the current study. Geographically, the Medinealem which is located at longitude 13°35'21" N and 38°8'48" E with an altitude of 1361 m, Wihdet at 13°33'0" N and 38°5'48" with 1156 m, Mayteklit at 13°37'42" N and 38°3'4"E with 1227 m, Mayayni at 13°40'38"N and 38°9'51" E with 1413 m, Maytsebri at 13°58'04" N and 38°14'17"E with 1370, Mayambesa at 13°37'29"N and 38°13'2"E with 1405 m and Mayayni located at 13°40'38"N and 38°9'51"E with altitude of 1413 m. The area coverage of the district is approximately 2702.5 km^2 with an altitude ranging from 800 to 2870 m above sea level. The mean annual temperature of the area ranges from 16 to 38°C. The annual rainfall also ranged from 758 to 1100 mm and has a mono-modal pattern.

In addition to this, the livestock production system is predominated by extensive production system. The dominant ruminant species in the study area are cattle and goats and followed by sheep with an estimated number of 268, 647, 264, 429, and 13,276 thousands of cattle, goats, and sheep, respectively (OoARDT, 2014).

Study design and study animals

A cross-sectional study design was employed to estimate the sero-prevalence of brucellosis in small ruminants in Tselemti districts.

The current study was conducted on small ruminants kept under extensive production system. Sheep and goats within the age of 6 months and above and both sexes in the selected flock with no previous history of vaccination against brucellosis were included in the study. Individual animals belonging to the study household flock were selected randomly for blood sampling to examine for brucellosis using serological tests. All data related to potential risk factors were also collected.

Sampling techniques

A combination of purposive and two stage random sampling were used to select district, PA, and individual animals. A two stage cluster sampling was employed to determine the sero-prevalence of brucellosis considering districts as primary clustering units and PA as the secondary clustering units. There are six districts, namely, Medebay Zana, Tahtay Koraro, Asgede Tsimbela, Tselemti, Lalay, and Tahtay Adiyabo in the Northwestern zone of Tigray. From the six districts, Tselemti was selected purposively based on high livestock population and ease of transportation service in order to synchronize the present study with research activities of the Shire-Maitsebri Agricultural Research Center. In Tselemti districts, there were 25 PA, of which 6 were selected purposively for the study based on proximity to the main roads and ease of transportation. Finally, individual households having sheep or goats or both species were selected randomly for blood sampling from the selected PA.

Sample size determination

The sample size for the study was determined according to the formula given by Thrusfield (2005) for random sampling method. A 5% absolute precision and 95% confidence interval was used to determine the sample size. An expected prevalence of 50% was taken to determine the maximum sample size. Accordingly, 384 animals were used during the study period. In order to increase the accuracy, the sample size was increased to 558 animals.

$$n = 1.96^2 \times P_{exp} (1 - P_{exp}) / d^2$$

Where, n=total sample size; d=absolute precision; and Pexp=expected prevalence.
   Accordingly,

$$n = 1.96^2 \times 0.5 (1 - 0.5) / (0.05)^2$$

Sample collection

About 10 ml of blood sample was collected aseptically from the external jugular vein of each animal using plain vacutainer tubes after the animal was restrained properly. All samples were serially identified and labeled properly using permanent marker. The blood sample was allowed to clot in slant position at room temperature and transported using an ice box to the Maitsebri Veterinary Clinic. After 24 h of collection, serum was then separated gently by decanting into 2 ml cryo vials tubes following centrifugation at 3000 rpm for 3 min and stored at -20°C in Maitsebri Veterinary Clinic until tested. The sera were then transported to Mekelle University College of Veterinary Medicine and National Animal Health Diagnostic and Investigation Center (NAHDIC) for serological diagnosis.

Serological diagnosis

The Rose Bengal Plate Test (RBPT) and Complement Fixation Test

(CFT) were used as screening and confirmatory tests for brucellosis (OIE, 2009).

Rose Bengal Plate Test (RBPT)

Initially, the entire serum sample was tested using Rose Bengal Plate Test (RBPT) by adding an equal volume of antigen (30 µl) and serum onto glass slides. The antigen and test serum were then mixed thoroughly by plastic applicator, shaken for 4 min and the degree of agglutination was observed visually and recorded immediately as positive for the presence of agglutination and negative for its absence of agglutination (OIE, 2009).
   Agglutination was then recorded as 0, +, ++, +++ according to the degree of agglutination where 0 indicates absence of agglutination, + indicates barely visible agglutination, ++ indicates fine agglutination, and +++ indicates coarse clumping. The samples identified with no agglutination (0) were recorded as negative, while those with +, ++, and +++ were regarded and recorded as positive.

Complement fixation test (CFT)

All the sera tested positive to RBPT were confirmed using Complement Fixation Test (CFT). A known antigen was incubated at 37°C with test and control sera to form immune complexes. A defined amount of complement was added to reaction mixtures. An immune complex was then produced in positive antigen and antibody reaction which was suggestive of the complement was fixed or consumed. In negative sera, an immune complex was not produced.
   An animal is considered positive if tested for sero-positive on both RBPT and CFT in serial interpretation. The use of RBPT/CFT combinations, the most widely used serial scheme, is generally recommended (Dohoo et al., 2003).

Data collection and statistical analysis

Data obtained on serological test was entered and stored on Microsoft excel sheet. Statistical analysis was performed using STATA version 11.1 statistical software. Chi-square and univariate logistic regression analysis were used to check the association between the outcome and explanatory variables and the degree of association was then expressed as odds ration and 95% confidence interval. Those independent variables that were statistically significant were again subjected to multivariate logistic regression. For all analysis, a cut-off point of $P<0.05$ was used for significance difference. The final model was developed using a step wise reaction. In the final model, all variables with a P value < 0.05 were considered statistically significant and retained in the model.

RESULTS

A total of 558 animals sera comprising 145 sheep and 413 goats were examined for the presence of *Brucella* antibodies. A total of 13 and 10 sera were found positive for RBPT and CFT tests, respectively. Accordingly, the overall sero-prevalence of brucellosis in the study area was 1.79% (10/558). The higher prevalence was recorded in goats (2.18%, 9/413) as compared to sheep (0.69%, 1/145). This observed difference was found to be statistically insignificant ($P>0.05$) (Table 1).
   In the present study, explanatory variables such as PA,

Table 1. Sero-prevalence of small ruminant brucellosis in Tselemti district.

Test variable	Total sera examined	Serological tests	
		RBPT positive N (%)	CFT positive N (%)
Sheep	145	2 (1.38)	1 (0.69)
Goats	413	11 (2.66)	9 (2.18)
Total	558	13 (2.33)	10 (1.79)
P-value	-	0.37	0.24

sex, age, species, pregnancy status, lactation status, parity and herd size had no effect on being sero-positive to Brucella (P>0.05). However, animals with previous history of abortion and retained fetal membrane were found to be statistically associated with small ruminant brucellosis (P<0.05) (Table 2).

More importantly, the sero-positivity to brucellosis was higher in small ruminants with previous history of abortion (5.17%) as compared to animals with no previous history of abortion (1.08%). The odds ratio indicates that animals with previous history of abortion were found to be 4.05 (AOR=4.05; 95% CI: 1.01, 16.22) times more likely prone to the infection when compared with animals with no previous history of abortion. The difference observed was found to be statistically significant (P<0.05).

The prevalence of the disease was also found to be higher in those animals with previous history of retained fetal membrane (9.09%) as compared to animals with no previous history of retained fetal membrane (1.73%). Accordingly, the odds of being sero-positive to Brucella were found to be 5.68 (COR=5.68; 95% CI: 1.13, 28.53) times higher in sheep and goats with previous history of retained fetal membrane as compared to animal with no history of retained fetal membrane (P<0.05).

DISCUSSION

The present study indicates that the overall prevalence of small ruminant brucellosis was 1.79%. Several authors in Ethiopia have reported different sero-prevalence values of the infection in different parts of the country. Prevalence of 1.76% in Debrezeit and Modjo export abattoirs (Tsegay et al., 2015) and 1.9% in Somali (Teshale et al., 2006) was reported which is comparable to the current finding. However, higher prevalence of the disease was also recorded with 16% in Afar (Teshale et al., 2006), 13.6% in Afar (Adugna et al., 2013), and 3.5% in Southern part of Tigray (Teklue et al., 2013). Conversely, relatively low prevalence of 0.7% was also recorded in Kombolcha (Tewodros and Dawit, 2015). The difference in the prevalence rates in the current study and other studies might be due to differences in management practice and agro ecology.

Statistically, species of the animals had no significant effect on the sero-positivity in the current study. Sheep and goats were found equally susceptible to the infection but the magnitude of the disease was higher in goats (2.18%) as compared to sheep (0.69%). This finding is in agreement with those of Teklue et al. (2013) and Bekele et al. (2011). As opposed to the current study, there are significant differences in species susceptibility to the infection in which goats were found at higher risk of getting the infection than sheep as reported by Teshale et al. (2006), Ashenafi et al. (2007), Adugna et al. (2013), and Tegegn et al. (2016). This observed difference could be due to the fact that cattle and goats are the principal livestock species in the study area, while sheep is domesticated and raised in small pocket areas of the district which might not be the same in other study areas.

Additionally, statistically insignificant difference was also noted between sex of the animals and sero-positivity to Brucella in which higher prevalence was recorded in females as compared to males. Similar findings were also reported by Teshale et al. (2006), Ashenafi et al. (2007), Bekele et al. (2011), Debassa et al. (2013), Teklue et al. (2013), and Tsehay et al. (2014). Conversely, sex had an effect on the prevalence of the disease as reported by Tegegn et al. (2016). Lack of difference between the female and male animals on the prevalence of the disease observed in the current study and other study might be due to smaller samples of male animals used. Small ruminants especially male goats are considered as first candidates for marketing and serve as immediate source of income to satisfy house hold demands and purchase of agricultural inputs. Another reason for such variation in the present study and others might be small number of male animals kept as sires for the purpose of breeding in the study area.

Similarly, higher sero-positivity to Brucella was detected in adult animals as compared to young animals. The difference observed was found to be statistically insignificant (P>0.05). The present study was consistent with the work of Teklue et al. (2013), Tewodros and Dawit, (2015), and Tsehay et al. (2014). Contrary to the present study, there was significant association between age of the animal and sero-positivity to Brucella spp. as reported by Adugna et al. (2013), Ashenafi et al. (2007), and Bekele et al. (2011). The variation observed might be related to small sample size used in the present study. Additionally, there is high market and consumer preference for small ruminants especially when the age

Table 2. Logistic regression analysis of the effect of risk factors on prevalence of small ruminant brucellosis.

Variable	Total examined	Positive [N (%)]	COR (95% CI)	P-value	AOR (95% CI)
Peasant Association					
Maytsebri	98	1 (1.02)	-	0.53	-
Medhinealem	188	4 (2.13)	-	-	-
Wihdet	160	5 (3.13)	-	-	-
Mayteklit	59	0	-	-	-
May Ambesa	17	0	-	-	-
May Ayni	36	0	-	-	-
Sex					
Male	73	0	-	0.21	-
Female	485	10 (2.06)	-	-	-
Age					
Young	73	0	-	-	-
Adult	485	10 (2.06)	-	-	-
Species					
Sheep	145	1 (0.69)	-	0.24	-
Goats	413	9 (2.18)	-	-	
Lactation status					
Lactating	259	4 (1.54)	-	0.39	-
Non lactating	226	6 (2.65)	-	-	-
Pregnancy status					
Non pregnant	329	8 (2.43)	-	0.40	-
Pregnant	156	2 (1.28)	-	-	-
History of abortion					
No	369	4 (1.08)	1	-	1
Yes	116	6 (5.17)	4.97 (1.37, 17.95)	0.01	4.05 (1.01, 16.22)
History of retained fetal membrane					
No	463	8 (1.73)	1	-	1
Yes	22	2 (9.09)	5.68 (1.13, 28.53)	0.03	2.44 (0.42, 14.03)
Herd size					
1-20	111	1 (0.90)	-	0.42	-
>20	447	4 (2.01)	-	-	-
Parity					
No	56	0	-	0.29	-
1-3	269	7 (2.60)	-	-	-
>3	160	3 (1.88)	-	-	-

of the animals reaches 6 to 12 months in the districts.

Higher sero-positivity to brucellosis was found in animals with previous history of abortion (5.17%) than animals with no history of abortion (1.08%). Accordingly, the odds ratio (OR) indicates that sheep and goats with previous history of abortion were found to be 4.05

(AOR=4.05; 95% CI: 1.01, 16.22) times more likely prone to brucellosis as compared to animals with no previous history of abortion (P<0.05). The present finding was in agreement with reports of Teklu et al. (2013) and Tadeg et al. (2015). This is due to the fact that there exist tropism/preference of *Brucella* spp. to the key target cells called trophoblasts. Growth of *Brucella* inside trophoblasts is apparently enhanced synergistically in the presence of high concentration of steroid hormones and erythritol during the final gestation of ruminants. The capacity to replicate rapidly and extensively in trophoblasts can compromise the integrity of the placenta and infection of the fetus, resulting in abortion or birth of weak offspring (OIE, 2012; Xavier et al., 2009).

Likewise, the odds of being sero-positive to *Brucella* were 5.68 times higher in (COR=5.68; 95% CI: 1.13, 28.53) sheep and goats with previous history of retained fetal membrane as compared to goats and sheep with no history of retained fetal membrane. The observed difference was statistically found to be significant (P<0.05). The current study was found to be consistent with the work of Tadeg et al. (2015).

Conclusions

The current study revealed that the prevalence of small ruminant brucellosis is low in the study area as compared to previous works. Risk factor analysis also revealed that factors such as species, age, lactation and pregnancy status, parity, and herd size had no significant effect on the sero-positivity of *Brucella* spp. However, small ruminants with previous history of abortion and retained placenta had significant effect on sero-positivity to *Brucella* spp. More importantly, animals with history of abortion were identified as a risk factor in the final model. The existence of positive animals in the flock can serve as foci of infection to in contact animals and humans and responsible for the spread of the infection. Hence, implementation of better management practices like introducing brucellosis free animals, the use of maternity pen of separation for animals during parturition, use of personal protective equipments, proper disposal of fetal membranes and/or aborted fetus, culling of positive animals, and proper cleaning and disinfection activity. Moreover, extensive extension service including health education must be launched to make animal owners, animal attendants and the consumers aware of the public health significance of the disease.

CONFLICT OF INTERESTS

The authors have not declared any conflict of interests.

ACKNOWLEDGEMENTS

The authors are very much indebted to many individuals and organizations for their support and encouragement. Their utmost gratitude goes to farmers, Bureau of Agricultural and Rural Development of Tselemti District, Tigray Bureau of Agricultural and Rural Development, Tigray Agricultural Research Institute, Mekelle University and National Animal Health Diagnostic and Investigation Center for their invaluable, persistent and unlimited encouragement and support given.

REFERENCES

Adugna W, Tesfaye ST, Simenew K (2013).Sero-prevalence of small ruminants brucellosis in four districts of Afar National Regional State, Northeast Ethiopia. J. Vet. Med. Anim. Health 5(12):358-364.

Ashenafi F, Teshale S, Ejeta G, Fikru R, Laikemariam Y (2007). Distribution of brucellosis among small ruminants in the pastoral region of Afar, Eastern Ethiopia. Rev. Sci. tech. Off. Int. Epiz. 26:731-739.

Bekele M, Mohammed H, Tefera M, Tolosa T (2011). Small ruminant brucellosis and community perception in Jijiga District, Somali Regional State, Eastern Ethiopia. Trop. Anim. Health Prod.43:893-898.

Benkirane A (2006). Ovine and caprine brucellosis: World distribution and control/ eradication strategies in West Asia/ North Africa region. Small Ruminant Res. 62(1):19-25.

Berhanu G, Hoekstra D, Azege T (2006). Improving the Competitiveness of Agricultural Input Markets in Ethiopia: Experiences since 1991, Paper presented at the Symposium on Seed-fertilizer Technology, Cereal productivity and Pro-Poor Growth in Africa: time for New Thinking 26th Triennial Conference of the International Association of Agricultural Economics (IAAE), August 12 – 18, 2006, Gold Coast, Australia.

Berhanu G, Hoekstra D, Samson J (2007). Heading towards commercialization: The case of live animal marketing in Ethiopia, Improving Productivity and Market Success (IPMS) of Ethiopian Farmers, Project Working Paper 5. ILRI (International Livestock Research Institute), Nairobi, Kenya. P 73.

Central Statistical Agency (CSA) (2014).Federal Democratic Republic of Ethiopia, Central Statistical Agency, Agricultural sample survey 2013/14 (2006 E.C). Vol II. Report on livestock and livestock characteristics (Private Peasant Holdings). Statistical Bull. P 573.

Corbel MJ (2006). Brucellosis in humans and animals. Produced by WHO in collaboration with the FAO of the United Nations and OIE, Geneva. WHO/CDS/EPR/2006.7

Debassa G, Tefera M, Addis M (2013). Small ruminant brucellosis: serological survey in Yabello District, Ethiopia. Asian J. Anim. Sci. 7(1):14-21.

Dohoo I, Martin W, Stryhn H (2003). Veterinary Epidemiologic Research, AVC Inc., Prince Edward Island, Canada. ISBN 0-919013-41-44.

Getahun L (2008). Productive and economic performance of small ruminant production in production system of the highlands of Ethiopia. PhD Dissertation, University of Hohenheim, Stuttgart, Hoheinheim, Germany.

Gizaw S (2010 Sheep and goat production and marketing systems in Ethiopia: Characteristics and strategies for improvement (No. 23). ILRI (aka ILCA and ILRAD).

Godfroid J, Al Dahouk S, Pappas G, Roth F, Matope G, Muma J, Marcotty T, Pfeiffer D, Skjerve E (2013). A`` One Health`` surveillance and control of brucellosis in developing countries: Moving away from improvisation. Comp. Immunol. Microbial. Infect. Dis. 36(3):241-248.

Kaur S, Singla LD, Hassan SS, Juyal PD (2013). Application of indirect plate ELISA in early diagnosis of paramphistomosis using purified polypeptides of somatic antigen of *Paramphistomumepiclatum*. Trends Parasitol. Res. 2(1):9-15.

Office International *des* Epizooties Terrestrial Manual (OIE) (2012).Bovine brucellosis (Chapter 2.4.3). In: OIE Manual of diagnostic tests and vaccines for terrestrial animals. Paris: Off. Int. Epizoot. 616-650.

Office of Agricultural Rural Development of Tselemti district (OoARDT) (2014). Description of Agro climatology and Livestock population Tselemti District, Livestock development and Animal Health Core process, Office of Agricultural Rural development of District Tselemti, Maytsebri.

Office of International *des* Epizooties (OIE) (2009).Chapter 2.7.2.Caprine and ovine brucellosis (excluding *Brucellaovis*), OIE Terrestrial Manual.1-10.

Pal M, Tesfaye S, Dave P (2013). Zoonoses occupationally acquired by abattoir workers. J. Environ. Occup. Sci. 2(3):155-162.

Padilla Poiester F, Nielsen K, Ernesto Samartino L, Ling Yu W (2010).Diagnosis of Brucellosis. Open Vet. Sci. J. 4:46.

Radostits OM, Gay CC, Hinchcliff KW, Constable PD (2007). Diseases of the cardiovascular system. Veterinary medicine: a text book of the diseases of cattle, horses, sheep, pigs and goats.10:399-438.

Seleem MN, Boyle SM, Sriranganathan N (2010). Brucellosis: A re-emerging zoonosis. Vet. Microbiol.140:392-398.

Singla LD (1995). A note on sub-clinical gastro-intestinal parasitism in sheep and goats in Ludhiana and Faridkot districts of Punjab.Indian Vet. Med. J. 19:61-62.

Tadeg WM, Gudeta FR, Mekonen TY, Asfaw YT, Birru AL, Reda AA (2015). Seroprevalence of small ruminant brucellosis and its effect on reproduction at Tallalak district of Afar region, Ethiopia. J. Vet. Med. Anim. Health 7(4):111-116.

Tegegn AH, Feleke A, Adugna W,Melaku SK (2016).Small Ruminant Brucellosis and Public Health Awareness in Two Districts of Afar Region, Ethiopia. J. Vet. Sci. Technol. 7(335):2.

Teklue T, Tolosa T, Tuli G, Beyene B, Hailu B (2013). Sero-prevalence and risk factors study of brucellosis in small ruminants in Southern Zone of Tigray Region, Northern Ethiopia. Trop. Anim. Health Prod. 45:1809-1815.

Teshale S, Muhie Y, Dagne A, Kidanemariam A (2006). Sero prevalence of small ruminant brucellosis in selected districts of Afar and Somali pastoral areas of Eastern Ethiopia: the impact of husbandry practice. Revue. Med. Vet.157 (11):557-563.

Tewodros AE, Dawit AA (2015). Sero-Prevalence of Small Ruminant Brucellosis in and around Kombolcha, Amhara Regional State, North-Eastern Ethiopia. J. Vet. Sci. Med. Diagn. 4(5).

Thrusfield M (2005). Veterinary Epidemiology, 3rd edition, Blackwell Science limited, Oxford,UK. pp. 233-234.

Tsedeke K (2007). Production and marketing of sheep and goats in Alaba, Southern Nations Nationalities and Peoples Region, MSc thesis, Hawassa University, Awassa, Ethiopia.

Tsegay A, Tuli G, Kassa T, Kebede N (2015). Sero prevalence and risk factors of Brucellosis in small ruminants slaughtered at DebreZiet and Modjo export abattoirs, Ethiopia. J. Infect. Dev. Ctries. 9(4):373-380.

Tsehay H, Getachew G, Morka A, Tadesse B, Eyob H (2014). Sero prevalence of brucellosis in small ruminants in pastoral areas of Oromia and Somali regional states, Ethiopia. J. Vet. Med. Anim. Health 6(11):289-294.

Xavier MN, Paixão TA, Poester FP, Lage AP, Santos R (2009). Pathological, immuno-histochemistry, and bacteriology of tissues and milk of cows and fetuses experimentally infected with *Brucella abortus*. J. Comp. Pathol.140:149-157.

24

Nigerian Veterinarians' attitude and response to small animal pain management

Cecilia Omowumi Oguntoye* and Oghenemega David Eyarefe

Department of Veterinary Surgery and Radiology, University of Ibadan, Ibadan, Oyo state, Nigeria.

Received 12 June, 2017: Accepted 10 October, 2017

Nigerian veterinarians' attitude and responses to pain management predominantly in small animals were evaluated using a structured questionnaire. The questionnaires were administered to representatives of seventy small/large animal clinics and hospitals distributed across ten states of the country. The respondents possess the Doctor of Veterinary Medicine (DVM) (58.6%), Master of Veterinary Science MVSc (32.9%) degrees, fellowship diplomas (5.7%) and PhD (2.9%) degree. Majority of the respondents (92.9%) had less than 20 years of post DVM clinical experience. Seventy-nine percent (79%) had good understanding of animal pain perception while 43% still hold the misconception that some degree of pain is beneficial to an animal after surgery. Pain rating excellently assigned to fracture reduction by 83% of practitioners, but inappropriately assigned by 66% of practitioners to caesarean section, 66% to laparotomy, 63% to ovariohysterectomy, 60% to mastectomy and 60% to dental procedures. Xylazine, lignocaine and ketamine were anaesthetic/analgesics commonly used. Respondents (98%) recognized pain based on animal's response to painful body part palpation, attitude of animal (97%), history by care giver (80%) and inappetence (73%). Determinants of analgesic drug choice for dogs/cats were: analgesic efficacy (99/29%); potential for toxicity (95/38%); availability (93/43%), side effect (86/42%), cost (82/37%), availability of information on the drug (76/36%), and ability of analgesic drug to cause sedation in the animal (65/33%). Respondents sourced information for analgesic therapeutics from: literature (73%), internet (80%), and drug leaflet (98%). In conclusion, most veterinarians surveyed had understanding of animal pain perception and use anaesthetic protocols that provide analgesia. Nonetheless, some of them still hold on to the misconception that minimal pain perception is beneficial to the patient at the post-operative period which may have influenced their non-provision of additional analgesia post-operatively.

Key words: Pain, management, small animals, Nigerian veterinarians.

INTRODUCTION

Global response to pain concerns of veterinary patients' is on the increase (Joubert, 2001; Brearley, 2003; Flecknell, 2008; Lorena et al., 2014). Animals experience significant pain perception contrary to previous assumptions (Flecknell, 2008). Recent advances in research have shown that animal species; reptiles, birds,

*Corresponding author. E-mail: wumcel06@yahoo.com.

and mammals, possess the neuro-anatomic and neuro-pharmacologic components necessary for the transduction, transmission and perception of noxious stimuli (Flecknell, 2008; Lorena et al., 2014).

Pain types, be it nociceptive; inflammatory or pathologic, induce complex systemic derangements with severe physiologic and emotional consequences (Flecknell, 2008; Zaki, 2013, Epstein et al., 2015). This makes animal pain alleviation not just a professional obligation by veterinarians, but a key element of compassionate, humane patient care necessary to successful management outcomes. Professional approach to pain management demands pre-empting and recognising pain perception, understanding relief modalities and instituting the best pain therapy. Despite the large empirical data on animals' pain perception studies (Capner et al., 1999; William et al., 2005; Hewson et al., 2006; Joubert, 2006; Weber et al., 2012), there is still an overall general low usage of analgesics in veterinary medicine (Flecknell, 2008; Bell et al., 2014).

Following Hansen and Hardie`s (1993) report on the attitude of veterinarians to pain recognition and management in companion animals, several articles have been published on the subject (Capner et al., 1999; William et al., 2005; Hewson et al., 2006; Joubert, 2006; Weber et al., 2012). A position paper by the American Animal Hospital Association (AAHA) and the American Association of Feline Practitioners (AAFP) has also helped to standardize approach to pain management in dogs and cats (Epstein et al., 2015). Similar articles have evaluated veterinarians attitude on analgesic usage in dogs and cats among Brazilian (Lorena et al., 2014), New Zealand (Williams et al., 2005), French (Hugonnard et al., 2004), Finnish (Raekallio et al., 2003), Canadian (Hewson et al., 2006), South African (Joubert, 2001) and the British (Capner et al., 1999) practitioners.

There is however a dearth of information on veterinarians attitude and perception of analgesic usage in clinical practice in Nigeria. If humane animal patient care through proper usage of analgesic modalities will be achieved globally, assessment of a country's veterinarians' perception, attitude and use of analgesics for animal pain management cannot be over-emphasized. This paper therefore reports veterinary practitioners' perception and attitude to analgesic usage especially in small animal patient management in Nigeria.

MATERIALS AND METHODS

Survey instrument design, pre-test and reliability

A structured questionnaire was developed to evaluate and access veterinarians' perception of analgesia need and its provision to small animals in Nigeria. The questionnaire consisted of seven parts with questions pertaining to: Clinician's demography, practice type and case load, assessment of veterinarians' understanding of/ attitude to pain and pain control in animals, assessment of pain rating for various surgical procedures,

assessment of criteria for pain recognition/ evaluation, assessment of determinants of analgesic drug choice, assessment of analgesic type for selected surgical procedures in dogs and cats, and assessment of source of knowledge for pain recognition and treatment. The Likert's scale was adopted as respondent indicator for the study. A draft version of the questionnaire was validated through experienced veterinarians, and their comments used to modify the final version of the instrument. Additional validity and reliability (internal consistency) of instrument sample data was high with the Cronbach Alpha reliability coefficient of 0.76.

Instrument administration

The questionnaires were administered between December 2016 and March 2017. Some of the questionnaires were administered at state's veterinary medical association meetings while others were delivered to clinicians at their practice locations.

Enrolment criteria

Veterinary practitioners in small and mixed practice were enrolled. One questionnaire was served to each practice even when more than one clinician works in the same clinic or hospital. Incompletely filled questionnaires were not used in the analysis.

Data analysis

The responses (Practitioners' bio-data and questions) were coded and entered into Microsoft windows excel spread sheet (Version 2010). Data generated within each section were presented in percentages with standard deviations.

RESULTS

Demography, location and practice type of respondents

Representatives, (males, 51 and females -19) of 70 veterinary clinics distributed across 10 states of Nigeria (Figure 1) participated in the survey. Majority of the respondent veterinarians have less than twenty years post DVM clinical experience (92.9%) with very few (7.2%) having over 20 years' experience. The highest academic qualification of many of the respondents is DVM (58.6%) while the lowest qualification is PhD (2.9%). A total of 32.9% respondents have a second degree (MVSc) and 5.7% have fellowship diplomas. The largest percentage of the clinics (58.6%) operated mixed practice (small and large animals), while 40% handle small animal patients alone with 1.4% handling only large animal patients.

Assessment of veterinarians' attitudes to pain relief

Most of the respondents (79%) agreed that animals feel pain. Some respondents (56%) believe that pain control is necessary following animal surgeries, while others (43%) feel some degree of pain is beneficial to the animal after surgery (Table 1).

Assessment of practitioner's pain rating of surgical procedures

If analgesic was not administered within 24 h following surgical procedures, 83% of practitioners rated fracture reduction to elicit the most severe pain, followed by caesarean section (66%), laparotomy (66%), ovariohysterectomy (63%), mastectomy (60%), and dental procedures (60%). Procedures rated as producing mild to moderate pain by a large number of respondents included surgical repair of aural haematoma (83%), burn wound debridement (78%), wound stitching (74%) and orchiectomy (72%). Cherry eye and skin tumour excision were rated to produce moderate to severe pain by 72 and 70% respondents respectively. One or two respondents indicated that the animal feels no pain without analgesic provision in the first 24 h of surgery following aural haematoma, skin tumour excision, caesarean section, laparotomy, dental procedures, orchiectomy, wound stitching and cherry eye repair (Table 2).

Assessment of criteria for pain recognition/evaluation

Most respondents (98%) recognize pain based on the animal's response to palpation of painful body part, followed by the animal's attitude (97%), information by care-giver (80%) and inappetence (73%) (Table 3).

Assessment of factors influencing analgesic choice

Analgesic efficacy, potential for toxicity and drug availability were the major factors that influence choice of analgesics among other factors by practitioners (Table 4).

Assessment of analgesic drugs used for surgical procedures in respondents' practices

Lignocaine by site infiltration was mostly used for aural haematoma (surgical repair) (46%); wound repair, (51%); orchiectomy (46%); wound debridement (44%) and dental procedures (29%). Xylazine was mostly used for skin tumour excision (33%); cherry eye repair (31%); fractures (31%); laparotomy (30%) and ovariohysterectomy (30%). Ketamine, lignocaine and bupivacaine were mostly used for caesarean section (Table 5).

Assessment of source of knowledge about recognition and treatment of pain

All the respondents had knowledge about pain recognition and treatment through practice experience,

and additional knowledge through literature (87%), internet (79%) and drug leaflet (77%) (Table 6).

DISCUSSION

The results of this study showed that Nigerian veterinary practitioners have understanding of animals' pain indicators and the need for pain amelioration. It is noteworthy that the survey of veterinary clinics and hospitals representatives rather than individual practitioner may have been responsible for the smaller sample size in comparison with previous studies (Dohoo and Dohoo, 1996a,b; Watson et al., 1996; Capner et al., 1999; Lascelles et al., 1994; Williams et al., 2005; Hewson et al., 2006; Joubert, 2006; Weber et al., 2012).

Survey of clinic and hospital representatives was necessary to prevent repetition of information that may defeat the objective of the survey. Most of the veterinarians surveyed manage small animals predominantly, although a good number do see few large animal patients. Most of the respondents had their practice in the Southern part of Nigeria. Previous studies have established the predominance of small and mixed practice in the southern part of the country due to predominance of dogs for companionship and security concerns (Eyarefe and Oyetayo, 2016). The greater percentage of male than female respondents may not reflect the actual picture of male to female veterinary practitioner's ratio in the country, since the statistics captured practice representatives although a previous study had also given a capture with similar ratio (Eyarefe and Oguntoye, 2016).

Pain relief is very important in animal patient management, irrespective of pain type (nociceptive; inflammatory or pathologic). Some Nigerian practitioners however still uphold the misconception that some amount of inflammatory pain is beneficial to animal patient following surgery (Table 1). This shows that many veterinary practitioners may require more awareness on current information about animal pain perception and management in line with global best practice (Mathews et al., 2014).

Majority of the practitioners assigned pain rating for fractures correctly but pain rating for other procedures incorrectly (Table 2). A clinician's pain rating skill could influence his sense of judgment of analgesia requirement for a patient, and this could be a disadvantage to the patient if his pain assessment skill is imperfect (Mathews, 2000; Epstein et al., 2015). Virtually, all the respondents recognized pain based on patients' attitude (Table 3). Behavioral change often accompanies pain, and therefore, a key point in pain recognition, and management (Fox, 2014).

Practitioners' choice of analgesic drug for dogs and cats were influenced by drug efficacy, availability and cost among others (Table 4). Noticeably, more than half

Table 1. Assessment of veterinarians attitudes to pain relief in animals.

S/N	Statements	No response (%)	Strongly agree (%)	Agree (%)	Disagree (%)	Strongly disagree (%)	$\bar{x}$	SD
1	Animals do not feel pain	4 (5.7)	6 (8.6)	5 (7.1)	6 (8.6)	49 (70)	1.43	1.02
2	Pain threshold in animals is higher than in man (humans feel more pain than animals for the same type of surgery)	6 (8.6)	8 (11.4)	29(41.4)	16(22.9)	11 (15.7)	2.31	1.14
3	Some degree of pain following surgery is beneficial in animals	4 (5.7)	5 (7.1)	25(35.7)	21 (30)	15(21.4)	2.17	1.04
4	Pain control is unnecessary following animal surgeries	2 (2.6)	2 (2.6)	4 (5.7)	23 (32.9)	39 (55.7)	1.50	0.78

SD, Standard deviation.

Table 2. Assessment of pain rating for various procedures.

S/N	Procedure	No response (%)	No pain (%)	Mild pain (%)	Moderate pain (%)	Severe pain (%)	$\bar{x}$	SD
1	Aural haematoma (surgical repair)	1(1)	1(1)	18 (26)	40 (57)	10 (14)	1.90	0.76
2	Wound repair (stitching)	1(1)	2(3)	19 (27)	33 (47)	15 (21)	1.91	0.81
3	Wound debridement (burn wounds)	1(1)	0(0)	27 (38.6)	27 (38.6)	15 (21.4)	1.86	0.80
4	Cherry eye repair	5(7.1)	2(2.8)	13 (18.6)	30 (42.9)	20 (28.6)	2.24	1.06
5	Skin tumour excision	2(2.9)	1(1)	11 (16)	29 (41)	27 (39)	2.27	0.85
6	CS	2(3)	1(1)	5 (7)	16 (23)	46 (66)	2.63	0.77
7	Laparatomy	1(1)	1(1)	6 (9)	16 (23)	46 (66)	2.59	0.77
8	Fractures	3(4)	0(0)	2 (3)	7 (10)	58 (83)	2.90	0.54
9	Mastectomy	0(0)	0(0)	8 (11)	20 (29)	42 (60)	2.49	0.70
10	Ovariohysterectomy	1(1)	0(0)	8 (11)	17 (24)	44 (63)	2.54	0.72
11	Dental procedures	1(1)	1(1)	10 (14)	16 (23)	42 (60)	2.46	0.81
12	Orchiectomy	1(1)	1(1)	18 (26)	32 (46)	18 (26)	2.00	0.80

SD, Standard deviation.

of the respondents did not give any response concerning cats (Table 4). This may be because they either rarely see cats or have never seen cats before in their practice. The low case load of cats in the survey is due to the general negative myths associated with cat keeping (Eyarefe and Oyetayo, 2016). Drug availability for pain management is an important factor influencing drug choice in poor resource settings. Apart from tramadol and pentazocine which are available as human preparations, no other commonly used opioid analgesics in veterinary medicine is readily available in the market for veterinary use except the practitioner places a special order for them from outside the country (personal observation). The study result also showed that lignocaine (site infiltration), xylazine and ketamine were drugs used for various procedures for provision of

Table 3. Assessment of criteria for pain recognition/evaluation.

S/N	Statements	No response (%)	Strongly agree (%)	Agree (%)	Disagree (%)	Strongly disagree (%)	$\bar{x}$	SD
1	Animals' attitude	2 (3)	56 (80)	12 (17)	0 (0)	0 (0)	3.71	0.75
2	Information by care giver	6 (9)	16 (23)	40 (57)	6 (9)	2 (3)	3.26	3.77
3	Animals' response to palpation of painful part	1 (1)	59 (84)	10 (14)	0 (0)	0 (0)	3.80	0.58
4	Inappetence	3 (4)	20 (29)	31 (44)	14 (20)	2 (3)	2.90	0.96

SD, Standard deviation.

Table 4. Determinants of choice of analgesic.

S/N	Factor	Dogs					Cats				
		No Response (%)	SA (%)	A (%)	D (%)	SD (%)	No Response (%)	SA (%)	A (%)	D (%)	SD (%)
1	Availability	0 (0)	35 (50)	30 (43)	1 (1)	4 (6)	39 (56)	14 (20)	16 (23)	1 (1)	0 (0)
2	Cost	1 (1)	18 (26)	39 (56)	5 (7)	7 (10)	39 (56)	9 (13)	17 (24)	4 (6)	1 (1)
3	Side effect	4 (6)	27 (39)	33 (47)	2 (3)	4 (6)	38 (54)	13 (19)	16 (23)	1 (1)	2 (3)
4	Potential for toxicity	3 (4)	32 (46)	34 (49)	0 (0)	1 (1)	41 (59)	15 (21)	12 (17)	0 (0)	2 (3)
5	Difficulty in getting exact dose	4 (6)	4 (6)	22 (31)	16 (23)	24 (34)	38 (54)	5 (7)	9 (13)	11 (16)	7 (10)
6	Record keeping requirements	10 (14)	5 (7)	19 (27)	15 (21)	21 (30)	40 (57)	4 (6)	11 (16)	7 (10)	8 (11)
7	Causation of sedation	8 (11)	15 (21)	31 (44)	7 (10)	9 (13)	40 (57)	4 (6)	19 (27)	2 (3)	5 (7)
8	Analgesic efficacy	1 (1)	38 (54)	31 (45)	0 (0)	0 (0)	40 (57)	15 (21)	14 (20)	1 (1)	0 (0)
9	Availability of information on the drug	9 (13)	27 (39)	26 (37)	1 (1)	7 (10)	42 (60)	14 (20)	11 (16)	2 (3)	1 (1)

SA, Strongly agree; A, agree; D, disagree; SD, strongly disagree.

analgesia by the respondents. The frequent usage of lignocaine and xylazine reported here is contrary to results from a survey in Canada where a low usage of local anaesthetics and alpha-2 agonists was observed (Hewson et al., 2006). However, both local anaesthetics and alpha-2 agonists are powerful adjuncts in perioperative pain management (Pascoe, 2000; Lemke and Dawson, 2000; Lemke, 2004), and the low prevalence of their usage in the Canada survey was one of the reasons given for inadequate analgesia provision by veterinarians in that survey (Hewson et al., 2006).

Only very few respondents filled the option of additional analgesia with any other agent which may be due to unavailability of analgesics packaged for veterinary use (personal observation). With the exception of tramadol and pentazocine no other commonly used opioids or nonsteroidal anti-inflammatory drugs (NSAIDs) for veterinary medicine is readily available in the country (personal observation) as earlier

mentioned. It may also be that practitioners feel that there is adequate analgesia provision since the xylazine, ketamine and lignocaine all possess analgesic properties. This situation is similar to what was reported in a survey in South Africa (Joubert, 2001) where a high number of the respondents did not include any drugs specifically for their analgesic properties in the premedication and induction of cats (83.6%) and dogs (80.75%) undergoing routine sterilization. However, when the author included premedication and induction

Table 5. Analgesic type enquiry.

S/N	Procedure	Ketamine (%)	Xylazine (%)	Site infiltration with lignocaine (%)	Epidural block with lignocaine (%)	Epidural with bupivacaine (%)	Diclofenac (%)	None (%)	Others (specify) (%)
1	Aural haematoma (surgical repair)	16 (23)	14 (20)	32 (46)	0 (0)	0 (0)	3 (4)	4(6)	1 (1)
2	Wound repair (stitching)	12 (17)	14 (20)	36 (51)	0 (0)	0 (0)	3 (4)	4(6)	1 (1)
3	Wound debridement (burn wounds)	7 (10)	10 (14)	31 (44)	1 (1)	0 (0)	7 (10)	13 (19)	1 (1)
4	Cherry eye repair	21 (30)	22 (31)	6 (9)	1 (1)	1 (1)	5 (7)	12 (17)	2 (3)
5	Skin tumour excision	13 (19)	23 (33)	21 (30)	1 (1)	0 (0)	3 (4)	8 (11)	1 (1)
6	CS	21 (30)	15 (21)	5 (7)	15 (21)	3 (4)	3 (4)	7 (10)	1 (1)
7	Laparatomy	19 (27)	21 (30)	7 (10)	11 (16)	2 (3)	3 (4)	6 (9)	1 (1)
8	Fractures	20 (29)	22 (31)	7 (10)	4 (6)	1 (1)	5 (7)	9 (13)	2 (3)
9	Mastectomy	18 (26)	14 (20)	14 (20)	9 (13)	0 (0)	2 (3)	12 (17)	1 (1)
10	Ovariohysterectomy	19 (27)	21 (30)	5 (7)	11 (16)	2 (3)	4 (6)	7(10)	1 (1)
11	Dental procedures	11 (16)	18 (26)	20 (29)	4 (6)	0 (0)	8 (11)	8 (11)	1 (1)
12	Orchiectomy	12 (17)	14 (20)	32 (46)	3 (4)	0 (0)	3 (4)	5(7)	1 (1)

Table 6. Assessment of Source of knowledge about recognition and treatment of pain.

S/N	Knowledge source	No response (%)	Strongly agree (%)	Agree (%)	Disagree (%)	Strongly disagree (%)	$\bar{x}$	SD
1	Experience from practice	2 (3)	56 (80)	12 (17)	0 (0)	0 (0)	3.81	0.39
2	Internet	6 (9)	16 (23)	40 (57)	6 (9)	2 (3)	2.76	1.00
3	Drug leaflet	1 (1)	59 (84)	10 (14)	0 (0)	0 (0)	2.84	1.03
4	Literature	3 (4)	20 (29)	31 (44)	14 (20)	2 (3)	3.06	1.01

SD, Standard deviation.

agents with analgesic properties, this percentage was reduced to 34.2%. The author concluded that a large number of practitioners were unaware of the pharmacology of many of the drugs. Nevertheless, in order to provide optimal analgesia making the animal feel more comfortable a multimodal approach of analgesia should be employed (Lascelles et al., 1994; Lundeberg, 1995; Mathews et al., 2014).

A few practitioners in this study use diclofenac for analgesia provision (Table 5). Multimodal analgesia involves the combining of different classes of analgesic drugs that allows the veterinarian to optimize the management of pain, while limiting the occurrence of side effects. Drugs most commonly used in multimodal analgesia include opioids, NSAIDs, local anaesthetics, NMDA antagonists and alpha 2 adrenoceptor agonists. Furthermore, the lack of indication of any other analgesic agent by most of the respondents suggests that they do not consider post-operative analgesia provision highly necessary otherwise it may be that they think the analgesia provided by the most frequently used drugs after the lignocaine, that is, ketamine and xylazine are adequate. Indeed, alpha 2-adrenergic agonists are known to have potent analgesic

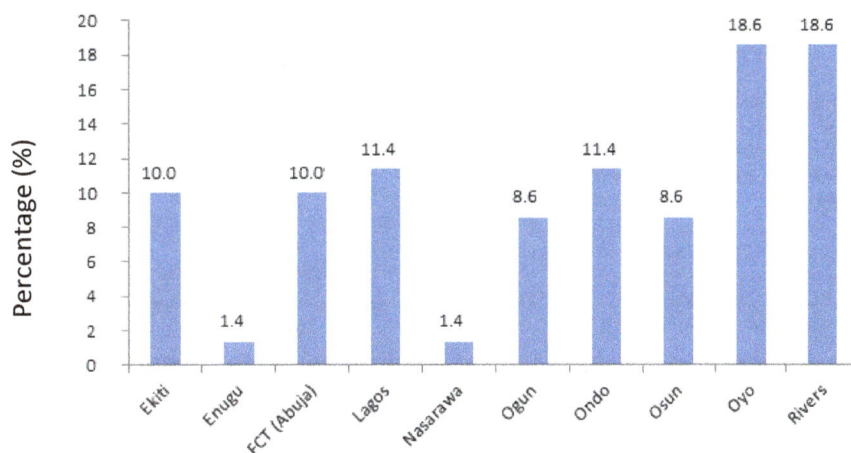

Figure 1. Percentage distribution of surveyed respondents per state.

properties (Paddleford and Harvey, 1999; Clarke et al., 2001) and sub anaesthetic doses of ketamine given pre-operatively have been shown to be effective in reducing post-operative pain (Slingsby and Waterman-Pearson, 2000).

Nevertheless, the analgesic effect of alpha 2 adrenergic agonists does not last as long as the sedative effect (Paddleford and Harvey, 1999), therefore xylazine does not contribute much to post-operative analgesia (Lascelles et al., 1994).

Conclusion

A substantial number of the veterinarians surveyed are well informed about animal pain perception, and use anaesthetic protocols that provide analgesia. Nonetheless, some of them still hold on to the misconception that minimal pain perception is beneficial to the patient at the post-operative period which may have influenced their non-provision of additional analgesia post-operatively.

CONFLICT OF INTERESTS

The authors have not declared any conflict of interests.

REFERENCES

Bell A, Helm J, Reid J (2014). Veterinarians' attitudes to chronic pain in dogs. Vet. Rec. 175(17):428.
Brearley JC (2003). Veterinary Analgesia: State of the art. Domenica Giugno 1(1):22. Available at: http://www.isvra.org/PDF/VRA/Brearley%20JC%20-%20Veterinary%20analgesia%20state%20of%20the%20art.pdf
Capner CA, Lascelles BD, Waterman-Pearson AE (1999). Current British veterinary attitudes to perioperative analgesia for dogs. Vet. Rec. 145(4):95-99.
Dohoo SE, Dohoo IR (1996a). Postoperative use of analgesics in dogs

and cats by Canadian veterinarians. Can. Vet. J. 37: 546-551.
Dohoo SE, Dohoo IR (1996b). Factors influencing the postoperative use of analgesics in dogs and cats by Canadian veterinarians. Can. J. 37(9):552.
Epstein M, Rodan I, Griffenhagen G, Kadrlik J, Petty M, Robertson S (2015). 2015 AAHA/AAFP pain management guidelines for dogs and cats. J. Feline Med. Surg. 17(3):251-272.
Eyarefe OD, Oguntoye CO (2016). Honey, an unexplored topical wound dressing agent in Nigerian veterinary practice. Sokoto J. Vet. Sci. 14(3):8-17.
Eyarefe OD, Oyetayo NS (2016). Prevalence and pattern of small animal orthopaedic conditions at the Veterinary Teaching Hospital, University of Ibadan. Sokoto J. Vet. Sci. 14(2):8-15.
Flecknell P (2008). Analgesia from a veterinary perspective. Brit. J. Anaesth. 101(1):121-124.
Fox SM (2014). Pain Assessment in Small Animal Medicine in Textbook of Pain Management in Small Animal Medicine, CRC Press, USA. pp 32-33.
Clarke KW, Trim CM, Hall LW (2014). Principles of sedation, anticholinergic agents, and principles of premedication. Vet. Anaesth. 79-100.
Hansen B, Hardie E (1993). Prescription and use of analgesics in dogs and cats in a veterinary teaching hospital: 258 cases (1983-1989). J. Am. Vet. Med. Assoc. 202(9):1485-1494.
Hewson CJ, Dohoo IR, Lemke KA (2006). Perioperative use of analgesics in dogs and cats by Canadian veterinarians in 2001. Can. Vet. J. 47(4):352.
Hugonnard M, Leblond A, Keroack A, Cadore JL, Troncy E(2004). Attitudes and concerns of French veterinarians towards pain and analgesia in dogs and cats. Vet. Anaesth. Analg. 31:154-163.
Joubert KE (2001). The use of analgesic drugs by South African veterinarians: continuing education. J. South Afr. Vet. Assoc. 72(1):57-60.
Joubert KE (2006). Anaesthesia and analgesia for dogs and cats in South Africa undergoing sterilisation and with osteoarthritis-an update from 2000: report. J. South Afr. Vet. Assoc. 77(4):224-228.
Lascelles BDX, Butterworth SJ, Waterman AE (1994). Postoperative analgesic and sedative effects of carprofen and pethidine in dogs. Vet. Rec. 134(8):187-191.
Lemke KA (2004). Perioperative use of selective alpha-2 agonists and antagonists in small animals. Can. Vet. J. 45(6):475.
Lemke KA, Dawson SD (2000). Local and regional anesthesia. Veterinary Clinics: Small Anim. Pract. 30(4):839-857.
Lorena ERS, Luna PL, Lascelles XD, Corrente JE (2014). Current attitudes regarding the use of perioperative analgesics in dogs and cats by Brazilian veterinarians. Vet. Anaesth. Analg. 41:82-89.
Lundeberg T (1995). Pain physiology and principles of treatment. Scandinavian J. Rehabilitation Med. Suppl. 32:13-41.

Mathews KA (2000). Pain assessment and general approach to management. Veterinary Clinics of North America: Small Anim. Pract. 30(4):729-755..

Mathews K, Kronen PW, Lascelles D, Nolan A, Robertson S, Steagall PV, Wright B, Yamashita K (2014). Guidelines for recognition, assessment and treatment of pain. J. Small Anim. Pract. 55(6).

Paddleford RR, Harvey RC (1999). Alpha2 agonists and antagonists. Veterinary Clinics of North America: Small Anim. Pract. 29(3):737-745.

Pascoe PJ (2000). Perioperative pain management. Veterinary Clinics: Small Anim. Pract. 30(4):917-932

Raekallio M, Heinonen KM, Kuussaari J, Vainio O (2003). Pain alleviation in animals: attitudes and practices of Finnish veterinarians. Vet. J. 165(2): 131-135.

Slingsby LS, Waterman-Pearson AE (2000). The post-operative analgesic effects of ketamine after canine ovariohysterectomy-a comparison between pre-or post-operative administration. Res. Vet. Sci. 69(2):147-152.

Watson AD, Nicholson A, Church DB, Pearson MR (1996). Use of anti-inflammatory and analgesic drugs in dogs and cats. Australian Vet. J. 74(3):203-210.

Weber GH, Morton JM, Keates H (2012). Postoperative pain and perioperative analgesic administration in dogs: practices, attitudes and beliefs of Queensland veterinarians. Australian Vet. J. 90(5):186-193.

Williams VM, Lascelles BD, Robson MC (2005). Current attitudes to, and use of, peri-operative analgesia in dogs and cats by veterinarians in New Zealand. New Zealand Vet. J. 53(3):193-202.

Zaki S (2013). Pain Assessment and Management in Companion Animals Veterinary Update. Boardtalk Insert 1:1-8.

Prevalence and economic significance of bovine hydatidosis at Adama Municipal Abattoir, Adama, Ethiopia

Muhammadhussien Aman[1], Diriba Lemma[2]*, Birhanu Abera[2] and Eyob Eticha[2]

[1]Gindhir District Livestock and Fishery Resource Development Office, Bale Zone, Gindhir, Ethiopia.
[2]Asella Regional Veterinary Laboratory, Asella, Ethiopia.

A cross sectional study was conducted to assess the prevalence and economic significance of bovine hydatidosis at Adama municipal abattoir. A total of 500 cattle were examined and 191 (38.2%) of them were found infected. Also, 253 visceral organs were found harboring one or more hydatid cyst. Prevalence of lung and liver cyst accounted for 94.5% and the involvement of other organs as many as 20 cysts were recovered from a single lung. Proportionally 35.7, 34.6, 20.8 and 8.82% of the cysts were calcified, small, medium and large sized, respectively. In addition, sterile and fertile cysts represent 46.2 and 18.1%, respectively. The rate of calcification is higher in liver than lungs, while that of most fertile cysts were recovered from lungs. The annual economic loss due to bovine hydatidosis at Adama abattoir is estimated to be about 171,436.36 Eth Birr (ETB). This information shows the risk of hydatid cyst distribution and economic significance in the study area. Therefore, appropriate control measures should be undertaken which include public awareness education program and a more aggressive effort that should include a reduction of stray dog population.

Key words: Adama abattoir, economic significance, hydatid cyst, fertility, prevalence.

INTRODUCTION

Hydatidosis (cystic echinococcosis) is a cosmopolitan food borne parasitic zoonoses caused by the larval stages of cestodes belonging to the genus *Echinococcus* (Family Taeniidae) (Chhabra and Singla, 2009). Larval infection (hydatidosis) is characterized by long term growth of metacestode (hydatid cysts) in the intermediate host. The two major species of veterinary importance are *Echinococcus granulosus* and *Echinococcus multilocularis* which cause cystic Echinococcosis (CE) and alveolar Echinococcosis (AE), respectively. Both CE and AE are serious diseases, the latter especially so, with a high fatality rate and poor prognosis if not managed properly. Hydatid cysts of *E. granulosus* develop in internal organs (mainly the liver and lungs) of humans and other herbivores intermediate hosts (sheep, horses, cattle, pigs, goats and camels) as unilocular fluid filled

*Corresponding author. E-mail: diribalema@gmail.com.

bladders. These consists of two parasites derived layers, inner nucleated germinal layer and an outer acellular laminated layer surrounded by a host-produced fibrous capsule and protoscoleces bud off from the germinal membrane (Thompson and McManus, 2001).

E. granulosus is the smallest of all tape worms with only three proglottids (Eckert and Deplazes, 2004; OIE, 2004). The body or strobila has a number of reproductive units (proglottids), the mature penultimate proglottid and the terminal proglottid (Soulsby, 1982; Adem, 2006). The latter is gravid and is usually more than half the length of the worm. This gravid uterus/proglottid has 12-15 short lateral diverticuli and is usually filled with 100-1500 thick shelled eggs. The gravid proglottids and or eggs are shed in the feaces (McManus et al., 2003). The eggs are brown in color and morphologically indistinguishable from those of other tape worms of the genus *Taenia*. The egg has a single hexacanth embryo, the oncosphere, which has three pairs of hooks (Thompson and McManus, 2001).

Hydatidosis caused by *E. granulosus* is a serious concern in public health which is much more common on the rural areas of Ethiopia where dogs and domestic animals live in a very close association usually sharing the same accommodation with human. Man becomes infected by an accidental injection of onchospheres from contaminated food, water and environments, where as the dog is the commonest final host (FH), which becomes infected by ingestion of infected offals (Urquahart et al., 1996).

The disease has also an advert effect on the productivity of animal with huge economic losses. The level of which has not until now been precisely determined (Polydorous, 1992). In addition to its direct effect on livelihood of domestic animals and man, *Echinococcus* causes great economic losses. The losses due to this parasite is considerable when one considers its effect on the productivity of animals, the condemnation of infected viscera or even the whole carcass and costs incurred for its control (Hubbert et al., 1975).

Several researchers from different parts of the country (Abebe and Yilma, 2011; Kebede et al., 2010, 2011; Jobre et al., 1996) have reported a prevalence range of 13.7 to 72.4% in cattle slaughtered at Dire Dawa, Gonder, Adama and Asella, respectively by indicating its highly importance and existence of the disease. To establish the prevalence and estimated economic loss of hydatid disease in animals depend on mainly collection of data in slaughter houses. Prevalence of the disease in domestic food animals' show that sheep are the most commonly infected domestic intermediated host (IH), though cattle and various other types of live stock are also affected. Infection does not usually result in any sign in livestock (Soulsby, 1986).

Echinococcus parasites are difficult to detect in faeces of definitive host, due to their small size. Diagnosis has been performed by examination of purge contents for the presence of *E. granulosus* even though the techniques have some disadvantage such as poor sensitivity, incomplete purgation, adverse reactions to the drugs in some dogs and infectivity of the purge material for the personal involved. The more recently developed serological tests, for the diagnosis of hydatid disease are enzyme linked Immuno sorbent assay (ELISA), radio immuno assay (RIA), immune electro phoresis (IEP) and indirect haem agglutination (IHA) (Sewell and Brockles, 2002).

In general, different organs lung, liver, spleen, heart and kidney (rarely) involved in hydatidosis of which lung and livers are the primary (most commonly) condemned organs due to hydatidosis, among cattle slaughtered. Nevertheless, study on prevalence and proper evaluations of economic losses due to this disease in different species of animals in the nation is lacking to which other wise is of great relevance where economic realities often determine the type and scope of the control measures to be envisaged. The principal objectives of this study were therefore to determine the prevalence of hydatidosis in cattle at Adama municipal abattoir and to estimate the magnitude of economic losses incurred due to hydatidosis.

MATERIALS AND METHODS

Study area

The study was conducted from November, 2008-May 2009, in Adama town, East Shoa zone of Oromo Regional State, Central Ethiopia. The town is located at 99 km South East of Addis Ababa at 39.1 N and 8.31 E, at an elevation of 1770 m above sea level and receives the annual rainfall raining from 400 to 800 mm; the temperature range is 13.9 to 27.7°C (NMSA, 2016).

Adama town is one of the most populous town ships in the country with important multi directional trade route. The town ship has one municipality Abattoir that supplies the inspected meat to more than 150,000 inhabitants and 61 legally registered butcheries. Backyard slaughter is also significant in spite of some pressure from the government authorities to ban this activity.

Study animal and design

The study was conducted on local breed cattle that originated from neighboring provinces such as Bale, Arsi, Harar, areas around Adama and Borena zone of Ethiopia. Almost all cattle presented for slaughter were male and adult.

A cross-sectional study type was carried out from November, 2008 to May 2009 by collecting data on events associated with hydatidosis in cattle slaughtered at Adama Municipality Abattoir.

Sample size determination

The sample size determined according to Thrustfield (2007) by using expected prevalence of hydatidosis 50% then the sample size required was 384 cattle at 95% confidence level and 5% expected error. But, in order to increase accuracy of the study, the sample sizes were increased to 500 cattle.

Study methodology

Post-mortem examination

During post mortem examination organs of the abdominal and thoracic cavities namely liver, lungs, heart, spleen and kidneys were systematically inspected for presence of hydatid cyst by applying the routine meat inspection procedures. The inspection procedure used during the post mortem examination consisted primary examination followed by a secondary examination if evidence of hydatid cyst were found. The primary examination involved, visualization and palpations of organs and muscles, whereas secondary examination involves further incision into each organ in case where a single or more hydatid cysts were found. Whenever and wherever hydatid cysts were apparent the number and the size of the cysts as well as calcified cysts per organ and per animal were recorded. The size of the cyst was categorized into three groups small (1-5<5 cm) in diameter, medium 5-8 cm in diameter and large (>8 cm in the diameter).

In organs with hydatid cysts, the cysts were carefully removed using a knife, collected in a clean container (ice box) and brought to Asella Regional Veterinary Laboratory then fertility tests of the Hydatid cysts were carried out and the result were registered.

Laboratory examination

Laboratory examinations were carried out on all collected specimens to determine the fertility and sterility of the cysts. The contents of the cyst was aspirated with a syringe to decrease its pressure and collected in a graduated beaker and the rest of the fluid was then added to it and measure its volume and it was allowed to stay on incubator for 30 min at 36°C to settle the content and then about 10 ml of these sediment was poured to the test tube and centrifuged at 1000 rpm for 3 min to separate the contents clearly from the liquid part and the supernatant was discarded, but the sediment with some fluid was left in test tube examination was done under objectives of 40X magnification for the presence or absence of protoscolex (Gupta and Singla, 2012). The protoscolex which preset as white dots on the germinal epithelium or brood capsules for hydatid sands with in the suspension cysts was categorized as fertile and where its absence categorize the cysts as sterile or non fertile (McPherson, 1985).

Economic loss assessment

The total economic loss due to hydatidosis in cattle slaughtered at Adama municipality abattoir was estimated from the summation of annual organ condemnation cost (direct loss) and cost due to carcass weight reduction (indirect loss).

Direct loss

All organs namely liver, lung, heart, spleen and kidney which are positive for hydatidosis were totally condemned and conditions leading to partial condemnations were poorly recorded. The economic losses due to total/partial condemnation of organs due to bovine hydatidosis was then assessed using the following formula set by Ogunrinade and Ogunrinade (1980).

$ACL_1L_2HKC = P (CSR \times PL_1c \times L1c) + P (CSR \times PL_2C \times L_2C) + P (CSR \times PHC \times HC) + P (CSR \times PKC \times KC) P (CSR \times PSC \times SC)$.

Where ACL_1L_2HKSC = Annual cost of live, lung, heart, kidney and spleen condemned; CSR – average number of cattle slaughtered per year at a abattoir; P – prevalence of hydatidosis at Adama municipal abattoir; PL_1C – percentage of lungs condemned; L_1C – mean cost of one lung in Adama town; PL_2C – percentage of liver condemned; L_2C – mean cost of one lung in Adama town; PHC – percentage of heart condemned; HC – mean cost of one heart in Adama town; PKC – percentage of kidney condemned; KC – mean cost of one kidney in Adama town; PSC – percentage of spleen condemned; SC – mean cost of spleen in Adama town.

Indirect loss

A 5% carcass weight loss, due to hydatidosis in cattle, has been described by Polydrous (1992). So, the annual economic loss due to carcass weight reduction as a result of bovine hydatidosis was calculated as.

$ACW = CSR \times P \times BC \times CL \times 126 kg$

Where, ACW = annual loss from carcass weight loss due to hydatidosis; CSR = average number of cattle slaughtered per annum in Adama; CL = carcass weight loss in individual cattle due to hydatidosis; BC = average market price of 1 kg beef in Adama town; P = prevalence rate of hydatidosis at Adama abattoir.

Data analysis

Basic data entry and handling was done using MS-Excel. From row data collected, total number of cases showing hydatid cyst were determined.

Prevalence of hydatidosis was calculated as the number of cattle found to be infected with hydatid cysts expressed as the percentage of the total number slaughtered (Thrusfield, 2007), economic loss assessed by formula set by Ogunrinade and Ogunrinade (1980) and variation between origin were evaluated by Pearson's Chi-square (χ^2) and differences were regarded statistically significant if P <0.05 using STATA 7.0

RESULTS

Prevalence

Regular visit to Adama slaughter house during study period (November 2008 to May 2009) allowed examination of 500 cattle, of these 191 (38.9%) were found infected with hydatid cyst.

Observation during this period revealed that 166 (65.6%) lungs, 73 (28.9%) liver, 3 (1.16%) spleen, 9 (3.56%) kidney and 2 (0.79%) hearts were harbored with hydrated cyst representing a total 253 organs all together (Table 1).

Out of the total infected organs, the involvement of lung and liver accounted for 94.5%. In addition, pulmonary infection out weighted involvements of liver and other organs (Table 1). The frequency of distribution (infection rate) can also vary among different origin of animals in superiority of Arsi followed by Bale, Borena and Harar, respectively, even though the result was statistically insignificant (Table 2).

The total number of cysts found on each organ was in the order of 322 (72.9 %) in lungs, 105 (23.8%) in liver, 4 (0.9%) in heart in total cyst count being 442 (Table 1).

Table 1. Prevalence of bovine hydatidosis and organ involvement rate.

Organs involved	No. examined	No. Involved	Relative Prevalence (%)	Cyst count	
				Max. no of cyst/organ	Total
Lung	500	166	65.61	20	322
Liver	500	73	28.85	6	105
Spleen	500	3	1.16	2	4
Kidney	500	9	3.56	1	9
Heart	500	9	0.79	1	2
Total	500	253	100	20	442

Table 2. Prevalence of hydatidosis based on origin in the study area.

Results	Origin									
	Arsi		Bale		Borana		Harar		Total	
	No.	%	No.	%	No.	%	No.	%	No.	%
Positive animals	65	34.03	49	25.65	39	20.42	38	19.90	191	100.00
Negative animals	112	36.25	78	25.24	67	21.68	52	16.83	309	100.00
Total	117	35.40	127	25.40	106	21.20	90	18.00	500	100.00

Pearson chi^2 (χ^2) =0.8771, P=0.831.

Cyst characterization

Cyst size

An exceptionally large cyst was found measuring 15 cm in diameter and containing about 1.5 L of fluid. A considerable number of hydatid sands were recovered from it, which up on microscopic examination was classified as fertile and viable cyst. The remaining cysts were by far smaller than the above described one and were classified as: 153 (34.62%) small, 92 (20.81%) medium, 39 (8.82%) large and 158 (35.75%) calcified cyst (Table 3). The result revealed that small cysts represent the highest proportion, while large cysts are the least in terms of their prevalence (Table 3).

Fertility and sterility of cyst

Out of the total hydatid cysts recovered in this survey, 204 (46.15%) were found sterile, 80 (18.10%) fertile and 158 (35.74%) are calcified (Table 4).

Economic losses assessment

Assessment of the retail market prices of organs from averaged sized zebu in the study area revealed that the cost for lungs, liver, kidney, heart and spleen were indicated below (Table 5). The price of a kilo of beef is

about 55 Ethiopian Birr in average. Therefore, the calculated annual economic loss due to bovine hydatidosis at Adama slaughter house from organ condemnation are 3,069.71 Ethiopian Birr and from carcass weight loss is 168365.74 Birr mounting to a total loss of 171,436.36 Birr.

DISCUSSION

It was noted that *E. granulosus* recovered from geographic regions have shown considerable variation which may have important epidemiological implication. In addition, other factors such as difference in culture, social activities and attitudes to dogs in different regions may contribute to the variations in its prevalence (Arene, 1986).

In this study, a prevalence of 38.2% was seen which is very close (37.7%) to a finding by Yamane (1990) and slightly lower (48.7%) than that of Ahmed et al. (2016) in East Shoa. Barsisa (1994) in Nekemte reported a prevalence of 36.66%, Abduljewad (1988) reported 36.66% in Jima , Tamene (1986) 33.78% and Belina et al. (2012) in Bahir Dar. Still high prevalence values were also registered in other places: 63% of prevalence in Robe (Wubet, 1988), 54.8% in Arsi (Alemayehu, 1990), 55.71% in Debrezeit (Abera, 2007), 54.9% in BahirDar (Nebiyou, 1990) and 46.5% in Debrezeit (Yilma, 1984).

The high prevalence may be related to the presence of favorable factors for the propagation and maintenance of

Table 3. Cyst size and organ involvement frequency distribution.

Organs involved	Small		Medium		Large		Calcified		Total	
	No.	%	No.	%	No.	%	No.	%	No.	%
Lung	128	39.75	78	24.22	27	8.39	89	27.64	322	72.85
Liver	22	20.95	12	11.43	11	10.48	60	57.14	105	23.76
Spleen	0	-	2	50.00	1	25.00	1	25.00	4	0.9
Kidney	3	33.33	0	-	0	-	6	66.67	9	2.04
Heart	0	-	0	-	0	-	2	100.00	2	0.45
Total	153	34.62	92	20.81	39	8.82	158	35.75	442	100

Table 4. Distribution of cyst condition versus predilection site in affected animals.

Organs involved	Sterile		Fertile		Calcified		Total	
	No.	%	No.	%	No.	%	No.	%
Lung	163	50.62	70	21.74	89	27.64	322	72.85
Liver	35	33.33	10	9.52	60	57.14	105	23.76
Spleen	3	75.00	0	-	1	25.00	4	0.9
Kidney	3	33.3	0	-	6	66.7	9	2.04
Heart	0	-	0	-	2	100.00	2	0.45
Total	204	46.15	80	18.10	158	35.75	442	100

Table 5. Number of organs affected, % involvement and their current value in Adama market of cattle organs.

Type of organs	No. of condemned organs	Percentage	Price of each organ (Birr)	Total cost (Birr)
Lung	166	33.2	5.00	830
Liver	73	14.6	11.00	803
Spleen	3	0.6	1.00	3
Kidney	9	1.8	2.00	18
Heart	2	0.4	3.00	6

high level infection in the area. Moreover, the age of slaughtered animals is also anticipated as one of the reason contributing to the high prevalence of the disease in the area most of the slaughtered animals were old probably culled from productivity and, hence they were exposed over a longer period of time with an increased possibility of acquiring the infection. Studies conducted in New Zealand (1958) also strongly suggested that prevalence is heavily influenced by age. The result from this study later indicated that 9% of affected cattle were 1-2 years old. While 74% were 5yrs older. Another study reported a prevalence in calves as 7%, in cows 52.2%, in fattening bullocks 69.7%, in bulls and bullocks as 81.2% (Abebe and Yilma, 2011; Gracy, 1994).

A maximum of 20 cysts were recovered from a single lung in this study. This finding is nearly close to the findings of Fikre (1994) and Nebiyou (1990). A much higher and lower result was also found previously by

Tamene (1986), Wubet (1988), Feyissa (1987) and Barsisa (1994) who found 132, 5, 99 and 63 cysts per organ, respectively. Such variation in cyst abundances in an organ is explained as probably to the special distribution and infectivity of Echinococcus eggs (Gemmel, 1987).

In the present study, it was found that about 94% of the case hydatid disease involves the lungs and liver, although lung infection was relatively higher. This finding concord with the observations of other workers: Barsisa (1994), Nebiyou (1990), Abera (2007), Tamene (1986) Wubet (1988), Fufa and Debele (2013) and Lati et al (2015) for this reason, the explanation shows that these organs are the first capillary sites encountered by the migrating Echinococcus oncosphere.

In addition as to why lungs are organs much more affected than the liver is related to the slaughtered subject, as most animals were slaughtered with the age of above 5 years liver capillaries are dilated at older age that most oncospheres are easily pass directly to the lungs. This also facilitate the condition, then to the thoracic ducts and heart and finally to be trapped in the lungs.

In the present trial, higher number of medium and large sized cyst was found in lungs than in liver and most calcified cyst in liver. Similar observations were also described by other workers: Fikre (1994), Tamene (1986), Alemayehu (1990), Abera (2007) and Hagos (2007). The reason given for the occurrence of higher percentage of calcified cysts in the liver is associated with the relatively higher reticulo-endothelial cells and abundant connective tissue reaction of the organ (Gemmel, 1987); hence larger numbers of oncosphere are killed in this organs.

The study carried out to evaluate the condition of hydatid cyst revealed that rates of sterility and fertility vary among different organs. The finding of 46.25% sterile, 18.09% fertile and 35.74 calcified cysts may generally imply that most of the cysts in cattle are infertile. This finding is consistent with the observation of Fikre (1994), Barsisa (1994), Nebiyou (1990) and Wubet (1988). Conversely in Britain, up to 90% of the total cysts from cattle are said to be sterile. On the other hand, in some countries like South Africa, Belgium and Rhodesia, 96.9, 94.2 and 86.5%, respectively, of the uncalcified cysts were fertile (Arene, 1986). The variation in fertility rates in different geographic zone of the globe could be allocated to strain differences of *E. granulosus* (Arene, 1986) also strain of parasites and host can modify infectivity of parasite (Gemmel, 1987).

The economic loss due to bovine hydatidosis at Adama slaughter house from offal condemnations and carcass weight loss was estimated to be about 171, 436.36 Ethiopian birr per annum. These figures correspond to loss of 134.77 birr per head of slaughtered cattle. Interpretation of this result must be made with a very serious precaution particularly in light of the fact that in the study area, only few animals were brought to slaughter house for prevailing tradition in back-yard slaughtered. The calculated loss present is generally considered as by far lower than the real losses brought about by bovine hydatidosis.

Conclusions

Cystic echinococcosis/ hydatidosis is a disease of considerable importance both from public health and economic point of view. The prevalence of the disease and estimated corresponding economic losses in Adama municipal abattoir from offal condemnation and carcass weight loss were 38.2% and 171,436.36 ETB, respectively. Therefore, it is concluded that owing to the presence of socio- economic conditions that favors the propagation and maintenances of high level infection, and considering the incalculable indirect loss, hydatidosis

is one of the most economically important disease in Adama and its surrounding, warranting serious attention for its control and prevention.

Based on the results obtained and socio-economic realities in Adama town and its surrounding, the authors forwarded the following recommendations; public education of zoonotic importance, life cycle and economic importance of the disease through teaching at school for students, extension workers for farmer and other possible mass media (Radio, TV, etc); construction of abattoirs and provision of facilities such as well educated meat inspectors, construction of dog proof fence and construction of ideal disposal pits; imposing legislative measures that will put an end to back yard and road side slaughter activities and create favorable conditions for people to bring their animals to slaughter houses; control of dog population through killing of stray dogs in collaboration with rabies control campaign and detailed investigations for basic epidemiological factors governing the dissemination of hydatidosis/echinococcosis must be carried out.

CONFLICT OF INTERESTS

The authors have not declared any conflict of interests.

ACKNOLEDGEMENTS

The authors are grateful to all Adama Municipal Abattoir staffs and administrations workers for their kind cooperation during this research work.

REFERENCES

Abduljewad A (1988). Hydatidosis: prevalence of hydatidosis at Jimma Abattoir. DVM Thesis, AAU, FVM, Debrezeit, Ethiopia.

Abebe F, Yilma J (2011). Infection prevalence of hydatidosis (*Echinococcus granulosus*, Batsch, 1786) in domestic animals in Ethiopia, A synthesis report of previous surveys, JUCAVM, Jimma, Ethiopia. Vet. J.15:11-33.

Abera G (2007). Prevalence and economic significance of bovine fasciolosis and hydatidosis at Elfora Abattoir, Debrezeit, Ethiopia. DVM thesis, AAU, FVM, Debrezeit, Ethiopia.

Adem A (2006). Metacestodes of small ruminants: Prevalence at three export abattoirs (Elfora, Hashim & Luna) MSc. Thesis AAU, FVM, Debrezeit, Ethiopia.

Ahmed N, Diriba L, Eyob E, Birhanu A, Guluma A, Lamessa K (2016). Prevalence, organ condemnation and financial losses due to fasciolosis and hydatidosis in cattle slaughtered at Adama Manucipal Abbatior. African J. Basic Appl. Sci. 8(5):276-282.

Alemayehu L (1990). The prevalence of hydatidosis in cattle sheep goats and *E. granulosus* in Dogs in Arsi Administrative region. DVM thesis, AAU, FVM, Debrezeit, Ethiopia.

Arene GOI (1986). Prevalence of hydatidosis in domestic livestock in the Niger Delta. Trop. Anim. Health prod. 17(1):3-4.

Barsisa K (1994). Hydatidosis in Nekmete: Prevalence in slaughtered cattle and sheep. DVM thesis, AAU, Faculty of Veterinary Medicine, Debrezeit, Ethiopia.

Belina T, Alemayehu A, Moje N, Yechale A, Girma S (2012). Prevelance and public health significance of ovine hydatidosis in Bahir Dar Town,Ethiopia. J. Vet. Med. Anim. Health 4(8):110-115.

Chhabra MB, Singla LD (2009) Food-borne parasitic zoonoses in India: Review of recent reports of human infections. J. Vet. Parasitol. 23(2):103-110.

Eckert J, Deplazes P (2004). Biological, epidemiological, and clinical aspects of echinococcosis, a zoonosis of increasing concern. Clin. Microbiol. Rev. 17(1):107-135.

Feyissa R (1987). prevalence of hydatidosis at Nekemete Municipality slaughter house. DVM thesis, AAU, FVM, Debrezeit, Ethiopia.

Fikre L (1994). Hydatidosis in Nekemete prevalence in slaughtered cattle sheep, estimate economic loss and incidence in stray dogs. DVM thesis, AAU, FVM, Debreze Ethiopia.

Fufa A, Debele W (2013). Major causes of organ condemnation for cattle and its financial impact at Wolaita Soddo Municipality Abattoir, Southern Ethiopia. Glob. Vet. 11(6):730-734.

Gemmel MA (1987). Hydatidosis control a global review, Aus. Vet. J. 55:118-125.

Gracy JF (1994).Textbook of meat hygien. 6th ed.,Beilleir Tindall, London. P 517.

Gupta SK, Singla LD (2012) Diagnostic trends in parasitic diseases of animals. In: Veterinary Diagnostics: Current Trends. Gupta RP, Garg SR, Nehra V and Lather D (Eds), Satish Serial Publishing House, Delhi. pp. 81-112.

Hagos A (2007). Study on the prevalence and economic impact of bovine hydatidosis and Fasciolosis at Mekelle municipal abattoir. DVM thesis, AAU, FVM, Debrezeit, Ethiopia.

Hubbert WT, Culloch WF, Schnurrenberger AA (1975). Disease transmitted from animals to man 6th ed., U.S.A Charles Thomas publisher.

Jobre Y, Lobago F, Tiruneh R, Abebe G, Dorchies P (1996). Hydatidosis in three selectedregions in Ethiopia, an assessment trial on its prevalence, economic and public health importance. Revue Méd. Vét. 147:797-804.

Kebede N, Gebre-Egziabher Z, Tilahun G, Wossen A (2011). Prevalence and financial effects of hydatidosis in cattle slaughtered in Birre-Sheleko and Dangila Abattoir, North western Ethiopia. Zoonoses Public Health 58:41-46.

Kebede N, Mitiku A, Tilahun G (2010). Retrospective survey of human hydatidosis in Bahir Dar, North-Western Ethiopia. East Mediterr. Health J. 16:937-941.

Lati E, Biresaw S, Berhanu S, Eyob H (2015). Causes of organ condemnation, its public health and financial significance in Nekemte municipal abattoir, Wollega, Western Ethiopia. J. Vet. Med. Anim. Health 7(6):205-214.

McManus DP, Zhang WJ, Bartley PB (2003). Echinococcosis. Lancet 362:1295-1304.

McPheson LNL (1985). Epidemiology of hydatid disease in Kenya. A Study of the domestic intermediate hosts on Masailand Trans. R. Soc. Trop. Med. Hyg. 79(2):209-217

Nebiyou G (1990). Hydatidosis/Echinococcosis in cattle slaughtered at Bahir-dar Municipality slaughter house. DVM Thesis, AAU, FVM, Debre Zeit, Ethiopia.

NMSA (2016). National Meteorology Service Agency, 2015/2016, Addis Ababa, Ethiopia.

Ogunrinade A, Ogunrinade BI (1980). Economic importance of fasiolosis in Nigeria. Trop. Anim. Prod. 12:155-160.

OIE (2004). Hydatidosis: in Manual of Diagnostic Tests and Vaccines for Terrestrial Animals, 5th ed. http:// WWW.OIE.Int

Polydorous K (1992). Animal health and economics to Cyprus. Bull. Int. Epz. 939(5):981-992.

Sewell M, Brocklesby D (2002). Hand book on Animal disease in the tropics 4th ed. Billiard Tindall Great Britain. pp.117-119.

Soulsby EJK (1986). Helminthes, Arthropods and Protozoa of Domesticated Animals London: Bailliere Tindall. , London, UK. pp. 809.

Soulsby EJL (1982). Helminthes, Arthropods and Protozoa of Domesticated Animals, 7th Ed. pp. 119-127.

Tamene M (1986). A preliminary study of Echinococcosis /Hydatidosis in livestock (Cattle, Sheep, and Goats) in Gonder Administrative region. DVM thesis, AAU, FVM, Debrezeit, Ethiopia.

Thompson CRA, McManus DP (2001). Aetiology: parasites and life cycles, In J. Eckert, M. A. pp. 1-19.

Thrusfield M (2007). Veterinary Epidemiology second edition University of Edinburgh Black well science. pp. 180-188.

Urquahart GM, Armour J, Duncan JL, Dunn AM, Jennings FW (1996). Veterinary Parasitology Scotland, Black well science ltd. pp. 181-186.

Wubet M (1988). Preliminary study of hydatidosis in Arsi Administrative Region.The efficacy of Clinus-lotoidus seeds against E. Granulosus in pups infected experimentally in Hydatid materials. DVM thesis, AAU, FVM, Debrezeit, Ethiopia.

Yemane G (1990). Preliminary study on Echinococcosis Ruminant slaughtered at Nathereth Abattoir. DVM thesis, AAU, FVM, Debrezeit, Ethiopia.

Yilma J (1984). Economic Importance of bovine hydatidosis an assessment trial at Debrezeit Abattoir 2nd Students scientific Journey (SSJ), FVM, AAU, Ethiopia.

26

Prevalence, financial impact and public health significance of *Cysticercus bovis* at Bahir Dar Municipal Abattoir, Ethiopia

Birhanu Tamirat[1]*, Habtamu Tamirat[1] and Mu-uz Gebru[2]

[1]College of Veterinary Medicine, Mekelle University, Mekelle, Ethiopia. P. O. Box 2084, Ethiopia.
[2]College of Agriculture and Environmental Science, Bahir Dar University, Bahir Dar, Ethiopia.

A cross-sectional study was conducted from November 2016 to April 2017 to determine the prevalence of cysticercosis, asses the associated risk factors and public health importance of human taniasis at Bahir Dar municipal abattoir, Bahir Dar town. Active abattoir survey from local zebu cattle presented to Bahir Dar abattoir and questionnaire surveys data collected were analyzed using SPSS version 20. Out of 480 inspected animals, 20 animals had varying number of Cysticercus bovis with prevalence of 4.2% (20/480). Cyst distribution per organs were; tongue 12/20 (2.5%), shoulder 10/20 (2.08%), masseter muscle 7/20 (1.46%), heart 4/20 (0.8%) and liver 1/20(0.21%). From the total number of 119 *C. bovis* collected from the infected 20 cattle during the study period, 73 (61.3%) were found to be alive while the rest 46 (38.7%) were degenerative cysts. Cysticercosis prevalence showed that there was no statistically difference among age groups and body condition score with the occurrence of *C. bovis* ($p > 0.05$). Of the total 69 interviewed respondents, 30.4% (21/69) had contracted Taenia saginata infection. The prevalence of taeniosis showed significant difference ($p < 0.05$) with age groups, habit of raw meat consumption, toilet availability, sex and religion. However, there was no significance difference between marital status, educational level, knowledge of taeniasis and occupational risks ($p > 0.05$). The findings of this study indicated the importance of bovine cysticercosis and taeniosis in the study area. Therefore, attention should be given to the public awareness and routine meat inspection to be safe to public health and promote meat industry in the country

Key words: Abattoir, Bahir dar, *Cysticercus bovis*, prevalence, public health.

INTRODUCTION

Taenia saginata is a worldwide zoonotic cestode whose epidemiology is ethnically and culturally determined with estimation of 50-77 million cases of infestation worldwide with 50, 000 people dying from this problem annually. Both the adult and larvae formed hazardously affect the health of their respective hosts, either directly or indirectly, accompanied with several secondary infections, particularly in human hosts. The occurrence of larvae of *Cysticercus bovis* in cattle musculature causes cysticercosis while the adult worms in human small

*Corresponding author. E-mail: birhanutamirat606@gmail.com.

intestine cause taeniasis (Minozzo et al., 2002).

There are a number of zoonotic diseases that can be transmitted from animal to humans in various ways. Wide varieties of animal species, both domestic and wild, act as reservoirs for these pathogens (viruses, bacteria or parasites) which may be transmitted to humans (Sumbria et al., 2016). Given the extend of distribution of the animal species involved and the ineffective surveillance, prevention and control of zoonotic diseases pose a significant challenge (Meslin et al., (2000).

In the past, zoonotic diseases were limited to populations living in low- and middle-income countries, but the geographical limits and populations at risk are expanding and changing because of increasing international markets, improved transportation systems, and demographic changes (Chhabra and Singla, 2009). Most parasitic zoonoses are neglected diseases despite causing a considerable global burden of ill health in humans and having a substantial financial burden on livestock industries. Although the global burden for most parasitic zoonoses is not yet known, the major contributors to the global burden of parasitic zoonoses are toxoplasmosis, food borne trematode infections, cysticercosis, echinococcosis, leishmaniasis and zoonotic schistosomosis (Torgerson and Macpherson, 2011; Singla, 2012; Chhabra and Singla, 2014). Parasitic diseases are highly prevalent in Sub–Saharan Africa and incur severe economic losses by reducing productivity. *Taenia saginata* taeniasis / bovine cysticercosis is one of the major parasitic diseases, which does not only lead to economic loses, but also adversely affect public health.

Meat-borne diseases are common in developing countries including Ethiopia because of the prevailing poor meat handling, sanitation practices, inadequate food safety laws and lack of education for food-handlers (WHO, 2004). National Hygiene and Sanitation Strategy Program (WHO/FAO, 2005) reported that about 60% of the disease burden was related to poor hygiene and sanitation in Ethiopia.

In East African countries, prevalence rates of 30-80% have been recorded (Tembo, 2001). In developing countries, the incidence of human infection with *T. saginata* is usually high, with the prevalence of over 20 %; whereas in developed countries, the prevalence of cysticercosis is low, usually less than 1% (Urquhart et al., 1996).

In Ethiopia several authors have reported the prevalence of *T. saginata* taeniasis and cysticercosis with in a wide range of 2.5 to 89.41% and 3.11 to 27.6% prevalence, respectively (Dawit, 2004; Hailu, 2005; Abunna et al., 2008).

The problem of food borne parasitic zoonosis could be further complicated in Ethiopia by lack of efficient inspection at critical control points in abattoirs, lack of awareness and knowledge on the mode of transmission and public health hazard of these diseases as well as due to presence of widespread habit of raw meat consumption both in rural and urban communities. A

number of reports in Ethiopia indicated that, certain groups who had easy access to raw meat and meat products and those people with low level of formal education were reported to be more infected with meat parasitic zoonosis than those who had low access to raw and those with better education (Tadesse et al., 2012). This study aimed at determining the prevalence of *C. bovis* in cattle slaughtered at Bahirdar municipal abattoir, identify risk factors associated with cysticercosis and taeniasis and to estimate the prevalence of human taeniasis /*T. saginata* in the area.

MATERIALS AND METHODS

Study area

The study was conducted at Bahir Dar, the capital city of Amhara Regional State, located at 11°29'N latitude, 37°29'E longitude at about 565 km North-West of Addis Ababa from November 2016 to April 2017.

The altitude of the area is 1830 meter above sea level and has average annual rainfall of 1500 mm.The mean annual temperature of the study area is 23°C. Lake Tana and River Abay influence the climatic condition of the study area. The area has a mixed farming practice with crop and livestock production (Bard, 2009). Based on the Census conducted by the Central Statistical Agency of Ethiopia (CSA), Bahir Dar Special Zone has a total population of 221,991, of whom 108,456 are men and 113,535 women; 180,174 or 81.16% are urban inhabitants, the rest of population are living at rural kebeles around Bahir Dar (CSA, 2007).

Study population and study design

The study was a cross-sectional type in which a structured questionnaire survey and active abattoir survey was conducted. Animal study populations were cattle presented to Bahir Dar municipal abattoir for slaughtering. All cattle were local oxen that originated from Bahir Dar, Adet, Debre tabor and Este areas brought by the merchants. For human study population, residents of Bahir Dar town, were subjected to questionnaire surveys. The recruitment of volunteer individuals in the study was not based by age, sex, marital status, habit of raw meat consumption, education level and religion.

Sample size determination

The sample size was determined following the formula published in using the expected prevalence of bovine cysticercosis in Bahir Dar (19.4%) reported with 95% confidence interval at a desired absolute precession of 5%. Therefore, the required sample size was calculated according to the formula (Thrusfield, 2007 and Mulugeta, 1997):

$$N = 1.96^2 P_{exp} (1 - P_{exp})/d^2$$

Where, N = required sample size, P exp= expected prevalence, d = desired absolute precision and N = 1.96^2 x 0.194(1-0.194)/ $(0.05)^2$= 240 animals.

However, to increase the level of accuracy of prevalence determination, 480 animals were sampled and inspected during the study period for the presence of *C. bovis* cyst in different organs.

Sampling procedures

Active abattoir survey

The cross sectional study was conducted during meat inspection on randomly selected 480 cattle slaughtered at Bahir Dar municipal abattoir. Before slaughter, ante-mortem inspection was carried out and the tag number of each animal was recorded. According to the guideline (Ministry of Agriculture, 1972) for masseter muscle, deep linear incisions were made parallel to the mandible; the heart were incised from base to apex to open the pericardium and incise also made in the cardiac muscle for detail examination. Deep, adjacent and parallel incisions were made above the point of elbow in the shoulder muscle.

Examination of the kidney, liver, and the lung was also conducted accordingly.

All positive samples were transported to the parasitology laboratory of Bahir Dar regional laboratory for confirmation of cyst viability. The cysts were incubated at 37°C for 1 to 2 h using 40% ox bile solution diluted in normal saline.

After this, the scolex was examined under microscope by pressing between two glass slides. The cysts were regarded as viable if the scolex envaginates during the incubation period at the same time the scolex was checked whether it is *T. saginata* metacestode or others based on the size of cysticercus and absence of hook on the rostellem of the envaginated cyst (Gracey et al., 1999).

Questionnaire survey

To determine associated risk factors of taeniosis, 69 volunteer respondents were selected using simple random sampling methods based on willingness to participate on Questionnaire survey. Questionnaire survey respondents identified for this study were questioned on their habit of raw meat consumption, frequency of consumption, experience of taeniosis infection and finding of proglottids in their faeces, underwear, Religion (Christian and Muslim), educational status, age (less than 15 years, 16-30 years old and greater than 30 years old), sex, marital status, knowledge of *T. saginata* and toilet availability of respondents were registered as possible risk factors.

Data management and analysis

The data collected from the abattoir and questionnaire survey were stored into Microsoft excel. Statistical analysis was done using SPSS version 20. Chi-square (X2) test was used to determine the variation in infection, prevalence between body conditions, ages and origin. Statistical significance was set at P<0.05 to determine whether there are significant differences between the parameters measured between the groups.

The questionnaire data were also summarized and analyzed to the risk factors for human taeniasis using Chi Square(X2) SPSS, Version 20.

RESULTS

Active abattoirs survey

From the total of 480 inspected animals in Bahir Dar

municipal abattoir, 20 animals had different number of *C. bovis* with prevalence of 4.2% (20/480). In routine meat inspection, *C. bovis* was found in different organs with higher number of cyst in the tongue (12, 2.5%), shoulder (10, 2.08%), masseter muscle (7, 1.46%), heart (4, 0.8%) and liver (1, 0.21%) (Table 1).

Out of 119, *C. bovis* (73, 61.3%) were found to be alive while the rest (46, 38.7%) were degenerative cysts. The viable cyst detected in shoulder muscle (31, 72.1%), masseter muscle (16, 59.26%), heart (5, 55.6%), tongue (20, 51.3%) and liver (1,100%) (Table 2).Out of 118 (<5 years old), 237(6-10 years old) and 125 (>10years old) cattle 4 (3.4%), 10 (4.2%) and 6(4.8%) were positive for *cysts* respectively. There was no statistical difference for the three age groups and body condition score with the occurrence of *C. bovis* (p>0.05). The distribution of infection in cattle according to location was highest in cattle from Debretabor (15, 7.2%), followed by Adet (3, 3.1%), Este (2,1.6%) and Bahir Dar 0%. There was statistically significant difference in infected animal from different locations with the occurrence with *C. bovis* (P<0.05) (Table 3).

Questionnaire survey

From the total of 69 respondents interviewed in this study, 30.4% (21/69) had contracted *T. saginata* infection. Associated risk factors, age groups, frequency of raw meat consumption, sex, presence or absence of the latrine and religion showed statistically difference (p<0.05) in the prevalence of human taeniasis in this study. However, marital status, educational status, occupation and knowledge about the disease was not statistically significance difference (p>0.05) (Table 4).

DISCUSSION

Abattoirs survey of bovine Cysticercosis

The prevalence of bovine cysticercosis obtained in this study was 4.2% which is comparable to the report of Dawit (2004) (4.9%) at Gondor, Megersa et al. (2009) (4.4%) in Jimma, Belay and Mekelle, (2014) who reported (5.2%) in shire and Ibrahim and Zerihun, (2011) (3.6%) in Addis Ababa. However, slightly higher than the finding of Meron (2012) (2.5%) in Jimma, Adem and Alemneh (2016) (2.0%) at Gondar, Addisu and Wondimu (2015) (2.6%) in Batu, Bedu et al. (2011) (3%) in Zeway and Teka (1997) (2.2%) in Central Ethiopia. The present study was by far less than the report of other authors such as Getachew (1990) (13.8%) at Debre-Zeit, Regassa et al., (2009)(13.3%) at Wolaita, Birhanu and Abda, (2014) (19.7%) at Adama. The lower prevalence of cysticercosis in the study area could be due to the differences in the agro-climatic conditions, variation in personal and environmental sanitation, proper usage of latrine, culture

Table 1. Organs based prevalence of *C. bovis.*

Organ inspected	Number of animals inspected	Number of positive animals	Prevalence (%)
Tongue	480	12	2.5
Shoulder	480	10	2.08
Masseter	480	7	1.46
Heart	480	4	0.8
Liver	480	1	0.21

Table 2. The proportion of viable cysts is calculated from the total number of viable cysts as denominator.

Organ inspected	Number of cysts per organ examined	Number of viable Cysts per organ	Proportion of viable Cysts in each organ (%)
Tongue	39	20	51.3
Masseter	27	16	59.26
Liver	1	1	100
Heart	9	5	55.6
Shoulder	43	31	72.1
Total	**119**	**73**	**61.3**

Table 3. The associated risk factors of bovine cysticercosis.

Risk factor		Number of tested animal	Number of positive animals	Prevalence (%)	X^2	P-value
Age	<5	118	4	3.4		
	6-10	237	10	4.2	0.306	0.858
	>10	125	6	4.8		
Body condition	2	55	1	1.8		
	3	246	11	4.5	0.858	0.651
	4	179	8	4.5		
Location	Debretabor	207	15	7.2		
	Adet	98	3	3.1	9.459	0.024
	Bahirdar	51	0	0		
	Este	124	2	1.6		

and feeding habit of raw meat. Regarding the anatomical prevalence of cysts, tongue 12 (2.5%), shoulder 10 (2.08%), masseter muscle 7 (1.46), heart 4 (0.8%) and liver 1 (0.21%) (Table 1). The tongue and shoulder muscle have high blood circulation and high oxygen circulation are available and due to this they are frequently affected by cysts. The tongue was the most frequently affected organ and this is in line with the finding of Bedu et al. (2011) at Zeway. Shoulder, masseter muscle and heart were also predilection sites Zerihun (2011) in Addis Ababa.

The viability test showed that 73 (61.3%) of the 119 cysts were alive (Table 2). Shoulder muscle had the highest proportion of viable cyst (31, 72.1%) followed by masseter (16, 59.26%), heart (5, 55.6%) and tongue (20, 51.3%). Only one viable cyst was detected in liver. The shoulder muscles affected 72.1%; greater than the reports of Bekele et al. (2009) (46.3%) and Regassa et al (2009) (32%). The proportion of viable cyst in tongue was 51.3% which was comparable to the work of Hussein et al. (2011) (53.1%).

Questionnaire survey

The prevalence of human taeniasis differs from country to

Table 4. Associated risk factors of human taeniasis.

Variable		Number interviewed	Number positive	Prevalence (%)	X^2	P-value
Age	< 15	7	0	0		
	16-30	30	5	16.7	11.534	0.003
	> 30	32	16	50		
Sex	Male	40	18	45		0.002
	Female	29	3	10.3	9.536	
Religion	Christian	51	19	37.25		0.038
	Muslim	18	2	11.1	4.295	
Occupation	Government-employed	21	5	23.8		
	Private worker	30	12	40		0.316
	unemployed	18	4	22.2	2.305	
Education	Elementary	13	2	15.4		
	High school	20	4	20		0.102
	College	36	15	41.7	4.564	
Marital status	Married	28	10	35.7		
	Single	37	11	29.7		0.345
	divorced	4	0	0	2.127	
Habit of raw Meat	High	22	14	63.6		
	Medium	28	6	21.4		0.000
	Less	8	1	12.5		
	Non user	11	0	0	18.555	
Latrine	Have	61	16	26.2		0.036
	Do not have	8	5	62.5	4.395	
Knowledge	Have	38	15	39.5		
	Do not have	31	6	19.4	3.264	0.071

country, and it can vary within the same country. This might be the habit of raw meat consumption, knowledge about the mode of transmission of the disease and variation in personal and environmental sanitation. In the present study, the questionnaire survey revealed that the respondents disclosed the finding of proglottids in the faeces, underwear, in laboratory diagnosis facilities at health institution which indicates the presence of taneniasis. Accordingly, 30.4% (21/69) of surveyed individuals were previously affected with the disease. This result was lower than the work of Taresa et al. (2011) (64.44%) in Jimma, Megersa et al. (2009) (56.6%) in Jimma, Dawit (2004) (69.2%) in Gondar. The lower prevalence of T. saginata in this study might be the fact that some people are not willing to tell that they had contracted taeniais, poor environmental hygiene and

knowledge of the societies about taeniasis, way of transmission and variation in composition of the respondents, and the habit or culture of raw meat consumption may be low.

There was statistical difference of age groups, sex, religion, habit of raw meat feeding and toilet availability with the occurrence of taeniasis (p < 0.05). Older age groups (>30) have higher prevalence associated with long-term exposure and the habit of preferring raw meat consumption and also, older individuals can financially afford consuming raw meat mainly at butcher houses. The present study showed that taeniasis occurrence was higher in male. This might be due to the cultural and social factors in which the males are usually involved in slaughter houses and butchery as well has having access to the hotels meal. This result is in agreement with different reports in various parts of our country (Hailu, 2005) in eastern Shoa. The present study showed that there was higher prevalence of human taeniasis among individuals who often consume raw meat than those with occasional consumption. This was comparable with the report of Abunna et al. (2008). However, there was no statistical difference among marital status, education level, occupation and knowledge of taeniasis with occurrence of taeniasis (p>0.05).

During the studying period, there was total and partial condemned masseter muscle, shoulder muscle, tongue, heart and liver. Repetition of this reflected high economic loss annually. Besides the health or pathological impact of the problem on the exposed population, the cost of treatment to expel the parasite from the body is also high.

CONCLUSION AND RECOMMENDATIONS

Taeniasis and bovine cysticercosis are important zoonotic parasitic diseases in the study areas with prevalence of 30.4 and 4.2% respectively. Poor meat inspection procedures were applicable in Bahir Dar municipal abattoir. Consumption of raw and undercooked meat is the most important source of infection. Backyard slaughtering were also practiced which could be considered as the contributing factor for taeniasis. Religion, raw meat consumption, presence or absence of the latrine, age and sex were found to influence taeniasis. *T. saginata* is a medically and economically important parasite in humans. Infection with the *Cysticercus* larval stage in cattle causes economic loss in the beef industry. Based on the above conclusion, recommendations include backyard cattle slaughter should be discouraged, routine meat inspection procedure should be applied, the public should be made aware to use latrines, not to contaminate the environment with proglottids or *Taenia* eggs by defecating on pastures where cattle graze and further studies on the prevalence of taeniasis and cysticercosis should be encouraged in other areas.

CONFLICTS OF INTERESTS

The authors have not declared any conflict of interests.

ACKNOWLEDGEMENT

The authors are greatly gratitude to the staff of Bahir Dar Municipal Abattoir, Bahir Dar regional parasitology laboratory and College of Veterinary Medicine, Mekelle University for their kind reception, preparation of equipment, materials, logistic and financial support for the thesis work and the use of their laboratory.

REFERENCES

Abunna F, Tilahun G, Megersa B, Regassa A, Kumsa B (2008). Bovine cysticercosis in cattle slaughtered at Hawassa Municipal Abattoir, Ethiopia. Prevalence, cyst viability, distribution and its public health implication. Zoonosis Public Health 55:82-88.

Addisu D, Wondimu D (2015). Prevalence of *Taenia saginata* / cysticercosis and community knowledge about zoonotic cestodes in and Around Batu, Ethiop. Vet. Sci. Technol. 6:273.

Adem E, Alemneh T (2016). The occurrence of Cysticercus bovis at Gondar ELFORA Abattoir, Northwest of Ethiopia. J. Cell Anim. Biol. 10(3):16-21.

Bureau of Agriculture and Development (BARD) (2009). Bahir dar zuria woreda agricultural and rural development office, Bahir dar, Ethiopia. 106:97-103.

Bedu H, Tafess K, Shelima B, Weldeyohannes D, Amare B (2011). Bovine cysticercosis in cattle slaughtered at zeway municipal abattoir, prevalence and its public health importance. J. Vet. Sci. Technol. 2(108):2157-7579

Bedu H, Tafess K, Shelima B, Woldeyohannes D, Amare B, Kassu A (2011). Bovine cysticercosis in cattle slaughtered at Zeway municipal abattoir: Prevalence and its public health importance. J. Vet. Sci. Technol. 2(108):2157-7579.

Belay S, Mekelle BA (2014). Prevalence of Cysticercus bovis in Cattle at Municipal Abbatoir of Shire. Vet. Sci. Technol. 5(4):1.

Birhanu T, Abda S (2014). Prevalence, economic impact and public perception of hydatid cyst and *Cysticercus bovis* on cattle slaughtered at Adama Municipal Abattoir, South Eastern Ethiopia. American-Eurasian J. Sci. Res. 9(4):87-97.

Central Stastical Agency (CSA) (2007). Population and Housing Census Report, National. Available at: https://unstats.un.org/unsD/statcom/statcom_08_events/special%20events/population_census/docs/presentation%20at%20Stat%20Com-UN%20Samia1.pdf

Chhabra MB, Singla LD (2009) Food-borne parasitic zoonoses in India: Review of recent reports of human infections. J. Vet. Parasitol. 23(2):103-110.

Chhabra MB, Singla LD (2014) Leishmaniasis. In: Zoonosis: Parasitic and Mycotic Diseases, Garg SR (Ed), Daya Publishing House, New Delhi. pp. 134-147.

Dawit S (2004). Epidemiology of *T. saginata* and cysticercosis in North Gondar Zone, North west Ethiopia. DVM Thesis, Faculty of Veterinary Medicine, Addis Ababa University, DebreZeit, Ethiopia. 4(5):47-53.

Getachew B (1990). Prevalence and significance of Cysticercus bovis among cattle slaughtered at Debre zeit abattoir. Unpublished DVM thesis, Addis Ababa University, Faculty of Veterinary Medicine, Debre Zeit, Ethiopia.

Gracey F, Collin S, Hilly J (1999). Meat hygiene (10th ed.) W.B. Saunders Company. pp. 669-678. Available at: https://www.scribd.com/doc/48046190/meat-hygiene-gracey-10-edition

Hailu D (2005). Prevalence and risk factor for *T. saginata* cysticercosis in three selected areas of eastern Shoa. MSc Thesis, Faculty of Veterinary Medicine, Addis Ababa University, Debre-Zeit, Ethiopia.

Ibrahim N, Zerihun F (2011). Prevalence of *Tania saginata* cysticercosis in cattle slaughtered in Addis Ababa Municipal Abattoir, Ethiopia. Glob. Vet. 8(5):467-471.

Megersa B, Tesfaye E, Regassa A, Abebe R, Abunna F (2009). Bovine cysticercosis in cattle slaughtered at Jimma Municipal Abattoir, South western Ethiopia. Prevalence, cyst viability and its socio-economic importance. Vet. World 3(6):257-262.

Megersa B, Tesfaye E, Regassa A, Abebe R, Abunna F. (2009). Bovine cysticercosis in cattle slaughtered at Jimma Municipal Abattoir, South western Ethiopia: Prevalence, cyst viability and Its Socio-economic importance. Vet. World Res. 3(6):257-262.

Meron T (2012). Risk of human taeniasis and prevalence of bovine cysticercosis in Jimma town, Southwestern Oromia. MSc Thesis, Faculty of Veterinary Medicine, Addis Ababa University, DebreZeit, Ethiopia. Available at: http://etd.aau.edu.et/bitstream/123456789/5682/1/3.%20meron%20msc%20final%20thesis%202012.pdf

Meslin FX, Stohr K, Heymann D (2000). Public health implications of emerging zoonoses. Revue Scientifique et Technique-Office International des Epizooties 19(1):310-313

Ministry of Agriculture (1972). Meat Inspection Regulations. Legal notice No. 428 Negarite Gazexa. Addis Ababa, Ethiopia 14 (6):67-71.

Minozzo J, Gusso R, Castro D, Lago O, Soccol T (2002). Experimental bovine infection with *Taenia saginata* eggs: recovery rates and cysticerci location. Braz. Arch. Biol. Technol. 45(4):451-455.

Mulugeta A (1997). Bovine cysticercosis: prevalence, economic and public health importance at Bahir Dar Municipality Abattoir. DVM Thesis. Faculty of Veterinary Medicine, Addis Ababa University, Ethiopia.

OIE (World Organisation for Animal Health), WHO (World Health Organization) and FAO (Food and Agriculture Organization), (WHO/FAO, 2005). WHO/FAO/OIE Guidelines for the surveillance,prevention and control of taeniosis/cysticercosis. OIE, 12, rue de Prony, 75017 Paris, France.

Regassa A, Abunna F, Mulugeta A, Megersa B (2009). Major Metacestodes in cattle slaughtered at WolaitaSoddo Municipal abattoir, Southern Ethiopia. Prevalence, cyst viability, organ distribution and socioeconomic implications.TropicalAnimal Health Production.Pp.1495–1502. Available at: https://www.ncbi.nlm.nih.gov/pubmed/19353302

Singla LD (2012) Toxoplasmosis an opportunistic zoonosis: Disease manifestations and managemental issues. In: *Integrated Research Approaches in Veterinary Parasitology*, Shanker D, Tiwari J, Jaiswal AK and Sudan V (Eds), Bytes & Bytes Printers, Bareily. pp. 198-209.

Sumbria D Singla LD, Gupta SK (2016). Arthropod invaders pedestal threats to public vigor: An overview. Asian J. Anim. Vet. Adv. 11:213-225.

Tadesse A, Tolossa YH, Ayana D, Terefe G (2012). Bovine cysticercosis and human taeniosis in South-west Shoa zone of Oromia Region, Ethiopia. Ethiop. Vet. J. 17(2):121-133

Taresa G, Melaku A, Bogale B, Chanie M (2011). Cyst viability, body site distribution and bovine cysticercosis at Jimma, South West Ethiopia. Glob. Vet. 7(2):164-168.

Tembo A (2001). Epidemiology of Taenia saginata taeniasis and cysticercosis in three selected agro- climatic zones in central Ethiopia. M.Sc thesis, Faculty of Veterinary Medicine, Addis Ababa University.

Thrusfield M (2007). Veterinary Epidemiology. (3rded.). London, Blackwell Science. P 642. Avaliable at: http://eu.wiley.com/WileyCDA/WileyTitle/productCd-1405156279.html

Torgerson R, Macpherson N (2011). The socioeconomic burden of parasitic zoonoses, Glob. Trend Vet. Parasitol. 182(1):79-95.

Urquhart GM, Armour J, Duncan JL, Dunn AM, Jennings FW (1996). Veterinary Parasitology, 2nd ed., Black well science Ltd. London, UK.

World Health Organization (WHO) (2004). Developing and Maintaining Food Safety Control Systems for Africa Current Status and Prospects for Change, Second FAO/WHO *Global Forum of Food Safety Regulators*, Bangkok, Thailand. pp.12-14. Avaliable at: http://www.fao.org/docrep/meeting/008/ae144e/ae144e00.htm

27

Acetylcholinesterase, glucose and total protein concentration in the brain regions of West African dwarf goats fed dietary aflatoxin

Ewuola, E. O.* and Bolarinwa, O. A.

Animal Physiology and Bioclimatology Unit, Department of Animal Science, University of Ibadan, Ibadan, Oyo State, Nigeria.

A study was carried out on the effect of varied levels of dietary aflatoxin on acetylcholinesterase, glucose and total protein concentration in the brain regions of West African Dwarf goats. 20 West African Dwarf goats of about 5-6 months old were used for the trial and they were randomly allotted to four dietary treatments containing 0 (control), 50, 100 and 150 µg aflatoxin/kg diet. The animals were housed individually for the feeding trial in a completely randomised designed and the experiment lasted 12 weeks. At the end of the feeding trial, the animals were sacrificed and brain dissected into different regions. The different regions of the brain studied were medulla oblongata, amygdala, hippocampus, cerebral cortex, mid-brain, cerebellum, pons varoli and hypothalamus. Samples were collected from these regions and homogenised to determine acetylcholinesterase, glucose and total protein concentrations. Result showed that the acetylcholinesterase activity in the brain regions was not significantly influenced by the dietary aflatoxin among the treatments. Glucose concentration was significantly ($p < 0.05$) higher in the hypothalamus of animals fed 50 µg aflatoxin/kg and control diet than those fed 100 and 150 µg aflatoxin/kg. Total protein concentration in the medullar oblongata and the hypothalamic regions of the brain in animals fed 150 ppb was significantly ($p < 0.05$) higher than those on the control diet. The pH of the medulla oblongata, amygdala, hippocampus, cerebral cortex were significantly ($p < 0.05$) higher in goats fed 150 mg/kg than those fed the control diet. However, pH was not significant in the mid brain, cerebellum, pons varoli and hypothalamus among the treatments. This study suggests that dietary aflatoxin up to 100 ppb reduced glucose concentration in the hypothalamus and total protein in the medulla oblongata region of the brain with tendency to impair brain function.

Key words: Aflatoxin, West African Dwarf (WAD) goat brain, acetylcholinesterase, total protein.

INTRODUCTION

Aflatoxins are an important group of mycotoxin produced by the fungi *Aspergillus flavus, A. parasiticus* and *A. nomius* (Diaz et al., 2008). Other species of *Aspergillus* such as *A. bombycis, A. ochraceoroseus* and *A. pseudotamari* also produce aflatoxins (Bennett and Klich, 2003). On world-wide scale, the aflatoxins are found in

*Corresponding author. E-mail: eoewuola@gmail.com.

stored food commodities and oil seeds such as corn, peanuts, cottonseed, rice, wheat, oats, barley, sorghum, millet, sweet potatoes, potatoes, sesame, cacao beans, almonds, etc., which on consumption pose health hazards to animals, including aquaculture species of fish, and humans (Abdel-Wahab et al., 2008). The toxin is highly oxygenated, heterocyclic, difuranocoumarin compounds that could be present in human foods and animal feedstuffs. Health effects occur in fish, companion animals, livestock, poultry and humans because aflatoxins are potent hepatotoxins, immunosuppressant, mutagens, carcinogens and teratogens.

In the tropical regions, where the climatic conditions favour luxurious growth of Aspergillus spp, people rely on commodities such as cereals, oilseeds, spices, tree nuts, milk, meat and dried fruits that are potentially contaminated by aflatoxins (Strosnider et al., 2006). Animals are predominantly affected by the Aspergillus spp, metabolite through ingestion of contaminated diet. Aflatoxin is metabolized by cytochrome p450 group of enzymes in the liver, where it is converted to many metabolic products like aflatoxin 8, 9 epoxide, aflatoxicol, aflatoxin Q1, aflatoxin P1, and aflatoxin M1, depending on the genetic predisposition of the species. The amount of aflatoxin 8, 9 epoxide metabolite decides the species susceptibility as this can induce mutations by intercalating into DNA, by forming adduct with guanine moiety in the DNA (Smela et al., 2001).

There is currently lack of information on the aflatoxin effect on the brain of West African Dwarf (WAD) goats. The brain also operates as central control of movement, balance, memory, thought and emotion in the body of an animal (Taylor, 1998). Knowledge of the biochemical composition of the brain is therefore important. Some reports on the biochemical characteristics of the brains of farm animals have been documented, most especially for boars (Egbunike, 1981), pigs (Adejumo and Egbunike, 2001a) and rabbit (Bitto, 2008) but not in relation to aflatoxin effect.

METHODOLOGY

Experimental location and materials

This study was approved by our institutional committee on the care and use of animals for experiment. The experiment was carried out at the small ruminant unit of the Teaching and Research Farm, University of Ibadan, Ibadan, Nigeria. It is located at latitude 70° 20' N and longitude 40° 50' E. It is 200 m above sea level with average day time temperature of 23 to 27°C and relative humidity of 80 to 85%.

Clean maize grains were purchased from local market in Ibadan metropolis and sorted. Damaged, coloured and bad kernels were removed and disposed. Other ingredients used for the feeds were purchased from Kesmac Feed and Agric Consult feed mill, opposite University of Ibadan second gate, Ibadan.

Aflatoxin contaminated maize grains

Maize grain served as the aflatoxin carrier in the diets used for this

study. The maize grains used for the experiment was inoculated with toxigenic strain Aspergillus flavus predominant in Nigeria. This culturing and inoculation was done at the Plant Pathology Unit, International Institute of Tropical Agriculture, Ibadan, Nigeria. The concentration in the maize grains and the diet was determined as described by Suhagia et al. (2006).

Experimental animals

Total of 20 WAD bucks of 5 months old were purchased for the experiment. The weights of the animals ranged from 7-9 kg. The animals were acclimatized for 28 days at the experimental site for physiological adjustment to feed and environment. Concentrate diet and Gliricidia leaves were fed, and fresh water were provided for the animals throughout the experiment. The animals were vaccinated against peste des pesti ruminants and treated with ivomectin injection against endo and ecto-parasites. Other routine management practices were carried out during the experimental duration.

Experimental diets

Four diets were formulated to meet the nutrient requirement of the animals. Diet 1 which is the control in the experiment and contained cleaned maize without aflatoxin contamination. The contaminated maize grains were used in substitution for the uninfected maize grains to vary the concentration of aflatoxin among diets 2, 3 and 4. All diets were iso-nitrogenous (12.9% CP) and isocaloric (3.57kcal/g DE).

Treatment layout

Diet 1: Control diet without aflatoxin
Diet 2: Diet containing 50 ppb aflatoxin
Diet 3: Diet containing 100 ppb aflatoxin
Diet 4: Diet containing 150 ppb aflatoxin

Feeding trial

At the end of the acclimatisation period, 20 bucks were weighed and allotted randomly into four treatments such that each treatment has 5 animals housed individually in a completely randomised design. Dietary treatments 1, 2, 3 and 4 were represented with T1, T2, T3 and T4, respectively.

Dietary treatments were offered to the respective animals twice daily at 8.00 a.m. and 12.30 p.m. with their respective diets ad libitum. Feed supply was adequate and responsively supply as the bucks weight changes, since feed consumption would be expected to change with body weight. The experiment lasted for 12 wk, during which animals were fed concentrate as supplement to gliricidia sepium in ratio 2:3 of their body weight.

Brain regions assessment

At the end of the feeding trials the animals were sacrificed, head dissected to harvest the brain and the brain was separated into regions samples were taken from the following regions: amygdala, cerebellum, hypothalamus, hippocampus, pons varoli, mid-brain and medulla oblongata.

Total proteins concentration

The total protein concentrations in the regions were evaluated using

Table 1. Acetylcholinesterase (AchE, µmol/g/min) activity in the brain regions of West African dwarf bucks fed varied levels of dietary aflatoxins (Mean±SD).

Parameter	T1 (0 ppb)	T2 (50 ppb)	T3 (100 ppb)	T4 (150 ppb)
Medulla oblongata	0.85±0.85	0.29±0.04	0.51±0.16	0.42±0.34
Amygdala	0.57±0.83	0.25±0.17	0.51±0.16	0.22±0.10
Hippocampus	0.32±0.06	0.24±0.12	0.26±0.11	0.29±0.21
Cerebral cortex	0.65±0.53	0.34±0.23	0.32±0.26	0.16±0.14
Mid brain	0.38±0.32	0.22±0.11	0.69±0.64	0.81±0.72
Cerebellum	0.31±0.02	0.28±0.03	0.49±0.41	0.29±0.26
Pons varolii	0.28±0.12	0.42±0.25	0.66±0.95	0.25±0.16
Hypothalamus	0.19±0.09	0.29±0.02	1.08±0.90	0.48±0.39

the Biuret method as earlier reported by Adejumo and Egbunike (2001b). An automatic dispenser was used to measure 5 mL of Biuret reagent into a test tube and 10 µL of the homogenate will be added. The mixture was incubated at room temperature of about 25°C for 30 min. After incubation, the incubated mixture was poured into a clean cuvette. The side of the cuvette was thoroughly wiped with tissue paper before it was placed inside spectrophotometer at wavelength of 540 nm to determine the protein concentration. The blank was used to standardize the spectrophotometer. The standard was prepared using 0.1 mL of total protein standard and 5 mL of Biuret reagent.

$$\text{Total protein concentration} = \text{Absorbance of homogenate} \times 6 \text{ g/dL} / \text{Absorbance of standard}$$

Glucose concentration

The glucose concentrations in the regions of the brain were evaluated using the method as earlier reported by Bitto et al. (2009). 10 µL of the homogenate was introduced into a test tube and I mL of the glucose reagent was added. The mixture was incubated at 37°C for 10 min. Some of the incubated mixture was poured in a clean cuvette and read at wavelength of 500 nm.

$$\text{Glucose concentration (mg/dL)} = \text{Absorbance of homogenate} \times 100 / \text{Absorbance of standard}$$

***Acetylcholinesterase* concentration**

The regions were homogenized in 0.1 mL of phosphate buffer (pH 7.4) using Elvenjem glass homogeniser and latter assay for acetylcholinesterase (AChE) concentration was determined according to the calorimetric method as reported by Egbunike (1981) which measure the rate of hydrolysis and acetyl thiocholine iodine substrate to thiocholine and acetate using 5:5 dithiobis-2-nirobenzoate (DTNB) as the colour reagent. 2.6 mL of the buffer was pipette inside the cuvette. 100 µL of DTBN and 0.4 mL of the homogenate were added and the mixture was placed inside the spectrophotometer and this was standardized to zero after which 20 µL of substrate was added. The initial absorbance was read and after 4 mins the final reading was taken at a wavelength of 405 nm.

Data analysis

Data obtained were subjected to analysis of variance at p = 0.05 and means were separated using Duncan's multiple range tests of SAS (1999). SAS/STAT® (version 8.0) (SAS Institute, Cary, North Carolina, United States).

RESULTS

Acetylcholinesterase activity in brain regions of WAD goats

The effect of aflatoxin on the AChE activity in the brain regions of WAD bucks is as shown in Table 1. The result obtained showed that there was no significant difference the AChE concentration among the dietary treatments. The AChE in medulla oblongata, amygdala, hippocampus, cerebral cortex, mid-brain, cerebellum, pons varolis and hypothalamus was not significantly influenced by dietary aflatoxin among the treatments. The AChE observed in treated animals was not significantly different from the control.

Glucose concentration in the brain regions of WAD goats

The glucose concentration in the brain regions of WAD bucks fed varied levels of dietary aflatoxin is as shown in Table 2. The result obtained showed no significant difference in all the brain regions examined except hypothalamus among the treatments. It was observed that the glucose concentration in the hypothalamus of goats fed treatment 2 was not significantly different from those fed control diet. However, the value obtained for animals on T2 and T1 were significantly (p<0.05) higher than those fed treatments 3 and 4. The glucose concentration in hypothalamus of goats fed treatment 3 was not significantly different from those fed treatment 4.

The pH and total protein concentration in brain region of WAD goats

The pH of the brain regions of WAD bucks fed dietary

Table 2. Glucose concentration (mg/dL) in the brain regions of West African dwarf bucks fed varied levels of dietary aflatoxins (Mean±SD).

Parameter	T1 (0 ppb)	T2 (50 ppb)	T3 (100 ppb)	T4 (150 ppb)
Medulla oblongata	16.93±8.19	10.27±4.36	6.26±5.89	12.06±1.35
Amygdala	9.23±9.13	17.29±1.03	9.06±8.20	13.10±1.35
Hippocampus	2.39±2.79	6.52±3.54	16.57±4.40	21.31±18.38
Cerebral cortex	11.43±7.80	10.77±3.41	15.03±7.03	16.75±8.39
Mid brain	20.57±10.92	3.70±4.67	19.08±21.60	17.40±10.12
Cerebellum	17.71±5.01	15.54±11.03	13.07±4.41	16.61±2.57
Pons varolii	10.71±3.58	12.76±10.55	18.02±7.68	11.47±3.40
Hypothalamus	16.39±8.55[a]	12.33±8.32[a]	9.78±2.07[b]	8.55±4.30[b]

ab = means along the same row with different superscripts are significantly (p<0.05) different.

Table 3. The pH concentration of the brain regions of West African dwarf bucks fed varied levels of dietary aflatoxins (Mean ±SD).

Parameter	T1 (0 ppb)	T2 (50 ppb)	T3 (100 ppb)	T4 (150 ppb)
Medulla oblongata	7.30±0.17[b]	7.43±0.04[ab]	7.37±0.06[ab]	7.51±0.01[a]
Amygdala	7.33±0.06[b]	7.42±0.06[ab]	7.40±0.10[ab]	7.50±0.02[a]
Hippo-campus	7.37±0.56[b]	7.44±0.03[ab]	7.41±0.10[ab]	7.53±0.03[a]
Cerebral cortex	7.33±0.56[b]	7.43±0.10[ab]	7.39±0.12[ab]	7.50±0.02[a]
Mid brain	7.40±0.09	7.42±0.05	7.40±0.14	7.51±0.01
Cerebellum	7.33±0.06	7.43±0.15	7.41±0.11	7.50±0.03
Pons varolii	7.32±0.06	7.41±0.16	7.40±0.10	7.50±0.04
Hypothalamus	7.30±0.17	7.40±0.10	7.41±0.12	7.50±0.02

ab = means along the same row with different superscripts are significantly (p<0.05) different.

aflatoxin is as shown in Table 3. No significant difference was observed in the pH of mid-brain, cerebellum, pons varoli, hypothalamus of the animals among the treatments. However, there was significant (p<0.05) difference in the pH value of medulla oblongata, amygdala, hippocampus and cerebra among the treatments. The pH in these brain regions followed the same trend, and that of animal fed Treatment 4 were not significantly different from those fed treatments 2 and 3 but were significantly (p<0.05) higher than those bucks on the control diet.

The total protein concentration within the brain regions of the bucks fed varied level of dietary aflatoxin is as shown in Table 4. The amygdala, hippocampus, cerebral cortex, cerebellum and pons varoli of the animal fed dietary aflatoxin were not significantly different among the treatments.

However, total protein concentration in medullar oblongata of the animal on treatment 1 was significantly (p<0.05) lower than those on treatment 4 while those on treatments 2 and 3 were not significantly different from each other. Also, the hypothalamus of the animal fed treatment 4 which has the highest dose of aflatoxin recorded total protein concentration which was significantly (p<0.05) higher than goats fed treatments

1, 2 and 3. However, the total protein in hypothalamus of goats fed treatments 2 and 3 was not significantly different from the control.

DISCUSSION

The ability of aflatoxin producing fungi (*Aspergillus* flavus) to grow on wide range of food and feed stuffs under certain condition constitutes a threat to both animals and human (Sayed and Abeer, 2013). In developing countries where food availability often times are considered before food safety, there is a lack of legislation on acceptable limits for aflatoxin and population are undoubtedly exposed to high amount of aflatoxin (Williams et al., 2004). The AChE activity that was not significantly different among the brain regions for all the treatments indicated that the inclusion of aflatoxin level up to 150 ppb does not affect normal synthesis and catabolism of neurotransmitters (AChE) which could presumably be tolerated by the animal since it does not affect any brain region biochemicals. This could probably be that goat has higher resistance to aflatoxicosis than sheep and cattle. Adejumo et al. (2005) reported from the study on sex differences in acetylcholinesterase activity in Red sokoto

Table 4. Total protein concentration (g/dL) of the brain regions of West African Dwarf bucks fed varied levels of dietary aflatoxins (Mean ±SD).

Parameter	T1 (0 ppb)	T2 (50 ppb)	T3 (100 ppb)	T4 (150 ppb)
Medulla oblongata	1.24 ± 0.02^b	1.59 ± 0.89^{ab}	1.76 ± 0.17^{ab}	2.59 ± 0.60^a
Amygdala	0.66 ± 0.14	1.68 ± 0.78	1.11 ± 0.40	1.34 ± 0.56
Hippocampus	0.53 ± 0.62	1.30 ± 0.38	1.11 ± 0.40	1.34 ± 0.56
Cerebral cortex	1.48 ± 0.24	1.73 ± 0.25	1.27 ± 0.25	2.12 ± 0.28
Mid brain	1.05 ± 0.32	1.32 ± 0.35	1.02 ± 0.21	1.53 ± 0.86
Cerebellum	2.53 ± 0.00	1.68 ± 1.65	1.54 ± 0.30	1.53 ± 0.24
Pons varolii	1.27 ± 0.09	0.68 ± 0.05	1.28 ± 0.83	0.66 ± 0.47
Hypothalamus	1.35 ± 0.22^b	2.00 ± 0.50^b	1.54 ± 0.18^b	2.66 ± 0.10^a

ab = means along the same row with different superscripts are significantly ($p<0.05$) different.

bucks and does that the AChE maintains its characteristically low concentration in Red sokoto bucks brain. However, AChE concentration was highest in the mid brain, medulla oblongata, hippocampus of pig brain (Adejumo and Egbunike, 2002).

The lack of micro doses of dietary aflatoxin effect on the AChE activity in the cerebellum may be due to its involvement in locomotion and muscular activities which are maintained in the animal up till old age (Adejumo and Egbunike, 2004). In addition, the cerebellum itself is characterised by typically low AChE activities (Adejumo and Egbunike, 2002). The normal level of AChE reported for Red Sokoto goats was 4.32 ± 0.36 µmol/g/min (Adejumo and Egbunike, 2002).

The significant difference that was observed in the protein concentration in medulla oblongata and hypothalamus could be due to change in protein synthesis or metabolism and could be attributed to under nutrition or poor nutrient utilization as reported in these same animals (Ewuola et al., 2013). Aflatoxin has been reported to binds and interferes with enzymes and substrates that are needed in the initiation, transcription and translation process involved in protein synthesis. This may also be indicative of aflatoxin effect on the brain development as protein in the brain is important for it functions such as repair of worn-out tissues for growth, muscles development and it also binds to some minerals to ensure bioavailability of minerals for proper utilisation (Adejumo et al., 2005).

The total protein levels in the brain regions in the study were generally higher than the values reported for the brain regions of male porcine by Adejumo and Egbunike (2001, 2001a) and Bitto (2008) for rabbit bucks. This disparity may be due to species differences in biochemical characteristics of brain regions. Also, total proteins in the brain undergo major changes during development (Tucek et al., 1990) and such changes have been found to be unaffected by genetic or species effects amongst some ruminant (Adejumo et al., 2005).

There were no significant differences in glucose concentration of the different brain regions, except

hypothalamus. The significant difference in the hypothalamus may be due to its involvement in glucose transport, energy production and glycogenesis which was also observed by Sayed and Abeer (2013) male Sprague rat fed aflatoxin. It could also indicate that WAD bucks may have increased activities in their brain with respect to hormone secretion (Taylor et al., 1998) since hypothalamus is involved in the release of gonadotropin releasing hormones in the brain.

The glucose concentration in the hypothalamus region of animal fed 100 and 150 µg/kg aflatoxin significantly lower than those fed 50 µg/kg aflatoxin and the control diet could be an indication of hypothalamic hypoglycaemia probably induced by the toxin. This implies that glucose is low, psychological process requiring mental effort may be impaired. The result corroborates the finding of Ikegwuonu (1983) who reported that nerves tissue requirement for glucose molecules were reduced during aflatoxicosis. Glucose has earlier been reported to be the obligatory energy substrate for fuelling brain and it is entirely oxidised to carbon iv oxide and water for optimal use (Magistretti et al., 1999; Kong et al., 2002).

The alteration in the pH of medulla oblongata, amygdala, hippocampus and cerebral cortex among the treatments could be attributed to treatment effect induced by the toxin. However the observe values across the treatments were within the physiological range of 7.2-7.5 reported by Bermeryer (1974).

Aflatoxin does not have any significant effect on the brain pH, values obtained ranges from 7.3-7.5 in all the dietary treatments. The AChE is reported to be optimally active within a pH range of 7.2-8.5 (Bergmeryer, 1974). At a level beyond this range, AChE is inactivated (Bergmeryer, 1974), although WAD goats have been adjudged to be tolerable to aflatoxin.

Conclusion

Based on the results of this study, the acetylcholinesterase activity and total protein concentration for the treatments were not influence across the brain regions by the micro doses of aflatoxin up to 150 µg/kg. However, the animals on 100 and 150 µg/kg suffer hypothalamic hypoglycaemic condition in the brain which may impair psychological process and affect mental effort like coordination. This study suggests that dietary aflatoxin above 50 ppb reduced glucose concentration in the hypothalamus and total protein in the medulla oblongata region of the brain.

CONFLICT OF INTERESTS

The authors have not declared any conflict of interests.

FUNDING

This research did not receive any specific grant from any funding agency in the public, commercial or not-for profit sector.

REFERENCES

Abdel-Wahab M, Mostafa M, Sabry M., El-Farrash M, Yousef T (2008). Aflatoxins a risk factor for hepatocellular carcinoma in Egypt, Mansoura Gastroenterology Center study, (September-October 2008). Hepato-gastroenterology 55(86-87):1754-1759.

Adejumo DO, Egbunike GN (2001a). Age dependent change in the total protein concentrations in the brain regions and hypophyses of the pig, Int. J. Agric. Rural Dev. 5:19-26.

Adejumo DO, Egbunike GN (2001b). Effect of ovariectomy and testosterone and oestrogen administration on acetylcholinesterase activity and total protein in the brain regions and adenohypophyses of large white gilts. Trop. Anim. Prod. Invest. 4:77-81.

Adejumo DO, Egbunike GN (2002). Regional variation in acetylcholinesterase activity and total protein in the brain and hypophyses of large white boars managed under a hot humid environment. ASSET series A. 2(1):49-53.

Adejumo DO, Egbunike GN (2004). Changes in acetylcholinesterase activities in the developing and aging pig brain and hypophyses. Int. J. Agric. Rural Dev. 5:46-53.

Adejumo DO, Ladokun AO, Sokunbi OA (2005). Species differences in acetylcholesterase activity and total protein concentration in the brain and hypophyes of Red sokoto goats and Gudali Cattles, Asset Series A. 5(1):121-127.

Bennett JW, Klich M (2003). Mycotoxins. Clin. Microbiol. Rev. 16:497-516.

Bergmeryer HV (1974). Method of enzymatic analysis. 2nd Ed. vol. 2:831-853 Academic press inc. New York.

Bitto II (2008). Total protein and cholesterol concentration in brain regions of rabbits fed pawpaw peel meal. Afr. J. Biomed. Res. 11:73-78

Bitto II, Arubi JA, Gumel AA (2009). Reproductive Tract Morphometry and Some Haematological Characteristics of Female Rabbits Fed Pawpaw Peel Meal Based Diets. Afr. J. Biomed. Res. 9(3):199-204

Diaz DE Hopkins BA, Leonard LM, Hagler WM Jr, Whitlow LW (2008). Effect of fumonisin on lactating dairy cattle. J. Dairy Sci. 83(abstr.):1171.

Egbunike GN (1981). Regional distribution of acetylcholinesterase activity in the brain and hypophyses of crossbred European boars reared in the humid tropics. Acta Anat. 110:248-252.

Ewuola EO, Jimoh OA, Bello AD (2013). Growth response and nutrient digestibility of West African Dwarf goats fed micro doses of dietary aflatoxin. Sci. J. Anim. Sci. 2(11):316-322.

Ikegwuonu FI (1983). The neurotoxicity of aflatoxin B1 in the rat. Toxicology 28:247-257.

Kong J, Shepel PN, Holden CP, Mackiewicz M, Pack AI, Geiger JD (2002). Brain Glycogen Decreases with Increased Periods of Wakefulness: Implications for Homeostatic Drive to Sleep. J. Neurosci. 22(13):5581-5587.

Magistretti PJ, Pellerin L, Rothman DL, Shulman RG (1999). Energy on demand. Science 283:496-497

SAS (1999) Statistical Analysis Software. SAS/STAT user's guide. IAS Inst Inc. Cary, New York.

Sayed MR, Abeer MW (2013). Impact of 90 days oral dosing naturally occurring aflatoxin mixture on Sprague Rat neurochemistry and behavioural pattern middle east. J. Sci. Res. 14(2):228-232.

Smela ME, Sophie S, Curier E, Bailey A, John ME (2001). The chemistry and biology of aflatoxin B1. Carcinogenesis 22:535-545

Strosnider H, Azziz-Baumgartner E, Banziger M, Bhat RV, Breiman R, Brune M, DeCock K, Dilley A, Groopman J, Hell K, Henry SH, Jeffers D, Jolly C, Jolly P, Kibata GN, Lewis L, Liu X, Luber G, McCoy L, Mensah P, Miraglia M, Misore A, Njapau H, Ong C, Onsongo MTK, Page SW, Park D, Patel M, Phillips T, Pineiro M, Pronczuk J, Schurz RH, Rubin C, Sabino M, Schaafsma A, Shephard G, Stroka J, Wild C, Williams JT, Wilson D, (2006). Workgroup Report: Public Health Strategies for Reducing Aflatoxin Exposure in Developing Countries. Environ. Health Perspect. 114:1989-1903.

Suhagia BN, Shah SA, Rathod IS, Patel HM, Shah DR, Marolia BP (2006). Determination of gatifloxacin and ornidazole in tablet dosage forms by high-performance thin-layer chromatography. Anal. Sci. 22:743-745.

Taylor SJ, Green NPO, Stout GW (1998). Third Edition Biological Science Cambridge Low Price Editions. pp. 575-582.

Tucek S, Musílková J, Nedoma J, Proška J, Shelkovnikov S, Vorlícek J (1990). Positive cooperativity in the binding of alcuronium and N-methyl scopolamine to muscarinic acetylcholine receptors. Mol. Pharmacol. 38:674-680.

Williams JH, Phillips TD, Jolly PE, Stiles JK, Jolly CM, Aggarwal D (2004). Human aflatoxicosis in developing countries: a review of toxicology, exposure, potential health consequences, and interventions. Am. J. Clin. Nutr. 80:1106-1122.

28

Prevalence of bovine brucellosis, tuberculosis and dermatophilosis among cattle from Benin's main dairy basins

Nestor Dénakpo Noudèkè[1]*, Gérard Dossou-Gbété[2], Charles Pomalégni[2], Serge Mensah[2], Luc Gilbert Aplogan[3], Germain Atchadé[4], Jacques Dougnon[1], Issaka Youssao[1], Guy Apollinaire Mensah[2] and Souaïbou Farougou[1]

[1]Département de Production et Santé Animales, Ecole Polytechnique d'Abomey-Calavi, Université d'Abomey-Calavi, 01 BP 2009, Cotonou, République du Bénin.
[2]Laboratoire des Recherches Zootechnique, Vétérinaire et Halieutique (LRZVH), Centre de Recherches Agricoles d'Agonkanmey (CRA-Agonkanmey), Institut National des Recherches Agricoles du Bénin(INRAB), 01 BP 884 Recette Principale, Cotonou 01, Bénin.
[3]Laboratoire de Diagnostic Vétérinaire et Sérosurveillance des maladies animales de Parakou, Ministère de l'Agriculture, de l'Elevage et de la Pêche, Bénin.
[4]Laboratoire Vétérinaire de Bohicon, Ministère de l'Agriculture, de l'Elevage et de la Pêche, Bénin.

In order to determine the prevalence of bovine brucellosis, tuberculosis and dermatophilosis, a study was carried out in main dairy areas of Benin from April to September 2015. For brucellosis, 780 sera and 78 milk samples were analyzed by indirect enzyme-linked immunosorbent assay (iELISA). For tuberculosis, 780 cattle underwent a comparative intradermal tuberculin test and 78 milk samples were used for Ziehl-Neelsen's staining. About dermatophilosis, 78 samples of scabs were collected for Giemsa's staining. For brucellosis, the overall individual animal seroprevalence was 8.85%. The regions of Borgou with 19.33% and Atlantique with 0% prevalence showed significant differences (p <0.05) with the other regions. For tuberculosis, the overall individual animal prevalence was 2.18%. The regions of Borgou and Alibori, with 0% prevalence each, showed significant differences (p <0.05) with most other regions. Taking into account the individual animal prevalence, Zou (brucellosis 18.33%, tuberculosis 6.67%) and Plateau (brucellosis 10%, tuberculosis 6.67%) were the areas at risk for these two diseases. For dermatophilosis the overall herd prevalence was 23.08%. There was significant difference (p<0.05) between Alibori and Mono but also between Alibori and Zou. It is urgent, therefore, to put in place an adapted control strategy taking into account these geographical realities.

Key words: Brucellosis, tuberculosis, dermatophilosis, prevalence, cattle, Benin

INTRODUCTION

Brucellosis and tuberculosis are considered as the most important and prevalent zoonotic diseases (WHO, 2004). Both diseases are under control in developed countries, but remain prevalent in sub-Saharan Africa, affecting both livestock and human populations (Abbas and Agab, 2002; Schelling et al., 2003; Mostowy et al., 2005; Zinsstag et al., 2007). In addition to being a threat to public health, both diseases can have serious economic implications. Bovine tuberculosis has a negative impact on livestock production in developing countries by reducing production efficiency, seizure of carcasses or organs and restricting international trade. It has implications not only for the economies of livestock communities, but also for human health through the consumption of raw dairy products and / or close contact with infected animals or animal tissues (OIE, 2009). Brucellosis also causes significant reproductive losses in animals (Cutler et al., 2005). Bovine tuberculosis and brucellosis remain a major public and animal health problem in many developing countries, where cattle are a major source of food and income (Omer et al., 2000). Understanding the epidemiology of bovine tuberculosis and brucellosis is therefore essential to develop evidence-based disease control strategies. However, this information is insufficient in Africa's sub-Saharan. Therefore, appropriate preventive measures have not been taken (McDermott and Arimi, 2002). Bovine dermatophilosis is distributed worldwide, but mainly recorded in African countries (Kassaye et al., 2003; Kusina et al., 2004; Hamid and Musa, 2009). The disease leads to great economic losses in African countries due to inferior wool and leather quality, death and culling, decrease meat and milk production (Yeruham et al., 2000). Among the skin diseases, bovine dermatophilosis is one of the common economically important diseases of cattle with high economic significance in decreasing the productivity (Awad et al., 2008). As bovine tuberculosis and brucellosis, it is also a zoonotic disease.

Bovine tuberculosis, brucellosis and dermatophilosis are endemic in Benin. This is from the reports of the Direction of Animal Production (DAP) and authors mentioning cases from slaughter houses for tuberculosis and suspicions of clinical signs for brucellosis and dermatophilosis (Ali-Emmanuel et al., 2002; DAP, 2012, 2013, 2014, 2015, 2016). But there is no control program. However, in order to implement Milk and Meat Support Project (PAFILAV), it was imperative to investigate the current situation of the major pathologies affecting milk and meat production in the Project Intervention Zone (ZIP). The main objective of this project is to improve production systems and competitiveness of milk and meat sectors. Then, bovine brucellosis, bovine tuberculosis and bovine dermatophilosis have been retained to determine their prevalence throughout the national territory. These are diseases for which data on their prevalence in Benin are rare. Indeed, for bovine brucellosis, Akapko et al. (1984) found a seroprevalence of 10.4% in extensive herds. Koutinhouin et al. (2003) studies on herds supervised by Livestock Development Project gave a seroprevalence of 6.20 at 15.21%, while those of Adéhan et al. (2005) gave a seroprevalence of

2.06 to 3.4% on state farms. It should be noted that all these studies have focused on serum analysis only.

Concerning the prevalence of bovine tuberculosis, Farougou et al. (2006) conducted a study at the state farms of Samiondji and Bétécoucocu with single intradermal skin test. Prevalences obtained were 8.25 and 2.64% respectively for Samiondji and Bétécoucou. In addition, Dossou et al. (2016) conducted a study on milk through detection of *Brucella abortus* and *Mycobacterium tuberculosis* in the state farms of Kpinnou, Bétécoucou, Okpara and a private farm in Adjohoun, with no case of infection found. It is clear that all these previous studies, in geographical terms, took far more account state farms. No studies have considered both serum and milk for bovine brucellosis. Similarly, no studies have considered a comparative intradermal skin test and milk for bovine tuberculosis. Concerning bovine dermatophilosis there is no study about it prevalence in Benin. Thus, the aim of our study is to provide information on bovine dermatophilosis herd prevalence and to determine the bovine brucellosis and bovine tuberculosis in the Projet d'Appui aux Filières Lait et Viande (PAFILAV)'s ZIP with the identification of areas at risk through the analysis of serum and milk associated with comparative intradermal skin test.

MATERIALS AND METHODS

Study area

The PAFILAV's ZIP has 27 municipalities out of 77 of the country, and extends throughout the national territory. Benin is part of the intertropical zone. Depending on the latitude in which they occur, rainfall periods combine in different ways to define rainfall regimes. In the south of the 7° 45 'parallel is a bimodal regime with four (4) seasons, two dry and two rainy seasons. North of parallel 8° 30 ', there is a unimodal regime with two seasons, one dry season and one rainy season. Thus the South experiences a climate with four seasons: a great rainy season from April to July; a small dry season from August to September; a small rainy season from October to November and a great dry season from December to March. The North has two seasons: a dry season from November to early May and a rainy season from May to October. The administrative division of Benin comprises 4 hierarchical levels, which are in decreasing order: Regions, municipalities, districts, villages or wards. So we have 12 regions; 77 municipalities; 546 districts and 3557 villages/wards.

The intervention zones are targeted by region and municipality according to the potential in livestock and milk production. The study was conducted in 26 municipalities from eleven of the twelve regions of the country. These selected municipalities are 10 in the northern area and 16 in the southern and central areas of the country (Figure 1). These include:

1. Nikki, Kalalé, Parakou, Bembèrèkè, Gogounou, Tchaourou, Kandi, Banikoara, Bassila and Pehunco in the northern zone;

*Corresponding author. E-mail: noudnest@yahoo.fr.

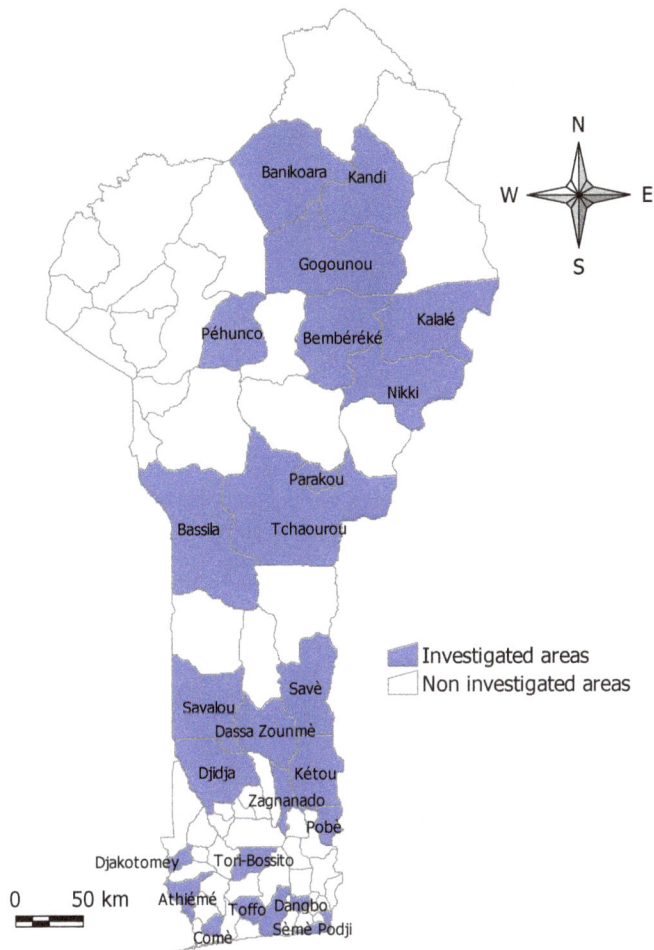

Figure 1. Map of Benin showing locations of the study area.

2. Djidja, Zagnanado,Djakotomey, Comé, Athiémé, Pobè, Kétou, Savalou, Dassa-Zoumè, Savè, Dangbo, Adjarra, Sèmè Podji, Abomey-Calavi, Tori Bossito and Toffo in the southern and central zones.

Sample collection

The sampling was carried out from April to September 2015. Respondents were selected based on their accessibility and availability to cooperate. Recruitment of animals for testing was based entirely on the owner's willingness. From the twenty-six (26) municipalities of the ZIP, three (3) herds were retained in each of them. Ten (10) identified animals were selected in each of those herds. In total, seventy-eight (78) herds and seven hundred and eighty (780) animals were included in the study (Table 1). On each of the 10 animals, blood is taken from the jugular vein and the two tuberculins are injected. In each herd, all animals with exudative dermatitis were examined. From these animals, three samples of scabs were collected in clean, sterile tubes for isolation of *Dermatophilus congolensis*.

For tuberculins' injection, animal is maintained in position of lateral decubitus. Two sites located to the right of the collar (the flat of the neck), at 20 cm intervals, were shaved and the thickness of skin is measured with caliper measurement. A first site is injected with 0.1 ml containing 2500 IU/ml bovine PPD. Similarly, 0.1 ml of avian PPD of 2500 IU/ml was injected into the second site. The

injection is done in the dermis using an insulin syringe. After 72 h, the skin thicknesses were measured at injection sites which are:

1. For bovine tuberculin (B): at the limit of the posterior and middle thirds of the neck and approximately equidistant from the upper and lower edges of the latter;
2. For avian tuberculin (A): in front of the preceding one, at the limit of the anterior and middle thirds of the neck, and approximately equidistant from the upper and lower edges of the latter.

In addition, once all herd cows are milked, 50 ml of the milk mixture is collected. During this study, 78 herds including 780 animals (595 females and 185 males) were investigated throughout the national territory (Table 1). For tuberculosis, 780 tuberculinations were performed with 78 samples of milk for Ziehl-Neelsen's staining. For brucellosis, 780 sera and 78 samples of milk were analyzed by indirect ELISA.

Analysis of samples

To analyze serum, milk and scab, the two veterinary laboratories of the country (Laboratory of Parakou and that of Bohicon) were involved.

For bovine tuberculosis

Reading was done 72 h later. We went back into the herd and we measured the skin thickness at the injection sites. The thickness differences between D_0 and D_3 were calculated:

$DB = B_3 - B_0$ for bovine tuberculin
$DA = A_3 - A_0$ for avian tuberculin

The interpretation of the measures is as follows:

If DB - DA is greater than 4 mm: Positive result
If DB - DA is less than 1 mm: Negative result
If DB - DA is between 1 mm and 4 mm inclusive: Doubtful result

The milk samples were subjected to Ziehl-Neelsen's staining.

For bovine brucellosis

Sera and milk were subjected to the indirect Enzyme Linked ImmunoSorbent Assay (iELISA) using *Brucella* smooth lipopolysaccharide (S-LPS) as an antigen. Indirect ELISA results were classified as positive or negative using the manufacturer's recommended values.

For dermatophilosis

Small pieces were taken from the underside of the scab and softened in a few drops of distilled water on a clean microscope slide; a smear was made and stained with Giemsa's staining as described by Scott (1988).

Statistical analysis

Data had been integrated into the Excel spreadsheet and then into the software R version 3.1.2. For brucellosis, individual and herd prevalences were calculated by dividing the number of positive iELISA cases by the number of animals or milk taken.

Table 1. Categories and number of animals sampled for tuberculosis, brucellosis and dermatophilosis according to locations in Benin.

Region	Municipalities	Sampled animal						
		Cow	Bull	Heifer	Bull-calf	Calf	Calve	Total
Alibori	Gogounou	18	1	3	1	4	3	30
	Kandi	18	6	0	0	4	2	30
	Banikoara	18	3	4	4	0	1	30
Atacora	Pèhunco	17	3	3	0	2	5	30
Atlantique	Abomey-Calavi	16	4	4	3	2	1	30
	Tori Bossito	18	2	5	4	0	1	30
	Toffo	18	3	6	3	0	0	30
Borgou	Nikki	12	0	5	10	2	1	30
	Kalalé	10	0	9	7	1	3	30
	Parakou	15	7	2	3	3	0	30
	Bembèrèkè	23	1	0	2	2	2	30
	Tchaourou	27	1	1	0	0	1	30
Collines	Savalou	19	2	2	2	1	4	30
	Dassa Zounmè	22	3	2	3	0	0	30
	Savè	20	4	4	2	0	0	30
Couffo	Djakotomey	16	2	6	3	2	1	30
Donga	Bassila	12	5	6	1	3	3	30
Mono	Comè	12	1	6	5	4	2	30
	Athiémé	10	4	8	4	1	3	30
Ouémé	Dangbo	13	0	5	4	3	5	30
	Adjarra	11	1	4	3	2	9	30
	Sèmè Podji	19	0	5	5	0	1	30
Plateau	Pobè	16	0	3	6	1	4	30
	Kétou	4	1	16	9	0	0	30
Zou	Djidja	15	3	5	1	4	2	30
	Zagnanado	22	0	6	2	0	0	30
Total		421	57	120	87	41	54	780

For dermatophilosis, herd prevalence was calculated by dividing the number of positive cases by the number of scabs taken.

For tuberculosis, differences in skin thickness were calculated. Results from the Ziehl-Neelsen's staining were recorded. Thus individual and herd prevalences were estimated by dividing number of positive cases by the number of tuberculinized animals or the number of milk taken.

In both cases, the individual prevalences obtained by region were compared two by two with Fisher's exact test. For each relative frequency, a 95% confidence interval (CI) was calculated using the formula:

$$CI = 1.96\sqrt{\frac{[P(1-P)]}{N}}$$

Where P is the relative frequency and N is the sample size.

RESULTS

Concerning brucellosis, the overall individual seroprevalence was 8.85%. There was significant difference by sex and also between cow and calve (p<0.05). Moreover, according to the regions, and overall, Borgou with 19.33% and Atlantique with 0% (Table 2) showed significant differences (p <0.05) with the other regions. Ouémé with 1.11% and Zou with 18.33% also showed some significant differences with the rest of the

Table 2. Prevalence of brucellosis infection among cattle from different regions of Benin.

Region	Individual seroprevalence (%)	Confidence interval	Milk prevalence (%)	Confidence interval
Alibori	10[a]	6.2	66.67[ac]	30.79
Atacora	6.67[a]	8.9	66.67[ac]	53.34
Atlantique	0[b]	0	22.22[cde]	27.16
Borgou	19.33[a]	6.26	66.67[acd]	23.85
Collines	3.33[bd]	3.66	33.33[ac]	30.79
Couffo	0[bd]	0	66.67[ac]	53.34
Donga	13.33[a]	12.16	66.67[ac]	53.34
Mono	6.66[cd]	6.33	16.67[ac]	29.82
Ouémé	1.11[bd]	2.18	11.11[be]	20.53
Plateau	10[a]	7.6	33.33[ac]	37.72
Zou	18.33[ac]	9.76	83.33[ac]	29.82
Total	8.85	2	46.15	11.06

Proportions in the same column followed by different letters differ significantly at 5%.

other regions. Furthermore there was no significant difference (p> 0.05) between the four northern regions (Alibori, Atacora, Borgou and Donga); whereas in the South, with Atlantique, Mono, Ouémé and Plateau, there were significant differences between them. The herd seroprevalence was 37.18% (95% CI 26.45 to 47.91%). The milk prevalence was 46.15% (95% CI 35.1 to 57.2%). It relates only to the cows of the herds investigated. Overall, the region of Ouémé had a significant difference with most other regions. No significant difference was observed between milk prevalence and herd seroprevalence.

Concerning tuberculosis, the overall individual prevalence was 2.18%. There is no significant difference between sex and categories (p> 0.05). But depending on regions, Borgou and Alibori, with 0% each (Table 3), showed significant differences (p <0.05) with most of the other regions. Plateau and Zou, with 6.67% each, also had some significant differences with the rest of the other regions. There was no significant difference (p> 0.05) between the four northern regions (Alibori, Atacora, Borgou and Donga). Moreover in South, with Atlantique, Mono, Ouémé and Plateau, there were no significant differences between them. The herd prevalence was 15.38% (95% CI 7.38 to 23.38%). The milk prevalence was 6.41% (95% CI 0.98 to 11.84%). It is also related to the cows of the herds investigated. There were no significant differences between regions. No significant difference was observed between milk prevalence and herd prevalence.

Concerning dermatophilosis, Table 4 presents the results of herd prevalence by regions. The overall herd prevalence was 23.08% (95% CI 13.73 to 32.43%). There was significant difference (p<0.05) between Alibori and Mono but also between Alibori and Zou. The four northern regions (Alibori, Atacora, Borgou and Donga) had the lowest rates. In addition, taking into account the individual prevalence, Zou (Brucellosis 18.33%,

Tuberculosis 6.67%) and Plateau (Brucellosis 10%, Tuberculosis 6.67%) constituted the zones at risk for these two diseases. In the same way, but to a lesser extent, there were also the regions of Mono and Ouémé. Two cows at Pobè and one at Comè were both positive for brucellosis and tuberculosis. Thus mixed prevalence rate was 0.38%. No herds were positive for these three diseases at the same time.

DISCUSSION

For bovine brucellosis, the overall seroprevalence was 8.85%. This result is similar to that obtained by Akakpo et al. (1984). Moreover, it is much lower than that obtained by Koutinhouin et al. (2003) and much higher than that obtained by Adéhan et al. (2005). The Borgou region had the highest rate (19.33%) and there were no significant differences between the four northern regions which showed significant differences with those of the South. It should be noted that the North is characterized by large herds, unlike the South. This would promote close contact between the animals. Furthermore, in this region of North, animals move a lot, especially transhumance in search of water and grazing, whereas in the South the herds are more sedentary. These two situations could favor transmission and maintenance of the disease at this level. This has been noted by some authors (Berhe et al., 2007; Ragassa et al., 2009; Matope et al., 2010; Makita et al., 2011; Megersa et al., 2011). Nevertheless, study of Cadmus et al. (2013) in Nigeria has shown a higher seroprevalence in sedentary herds compared to transhumants. Significant difference was found by sex. This is in agreement with studies of some authors (Traoré et al., 2004; Dinka and Chala, 2009; Adugna et al., 2013). between cow and calf/calve. Indeed, younger animals are more resistant to primary infection and eliminate Brucella sp. although sometimes latent infection occurs (Walker, 1999). According to Acha and Szyfres (1989), heifers

Table 3. Prevalence of tuberculosis infection among cattle from different regions of Benin.

Region	CIDT individual prevalence (%)	Confidence interval	Milk prevalence (%)	Confidence interval
Alibori	0[bc]	0	11.11	20.53
Atacora	0[ac]	0	33.33	53.34
Atlantique	3.33[ac]	3.71	0	0
Borgou	0[b]	0	13.33	17.20
Collines	0[bc]	0	0	0
Couffo	0[ac]	0	0	0
Donga	3.33[ac]	6.42	33.33	53.34
Mono	5[ac]	5.51	0	0
Ouémé	2.22[ac]	3.04	0	0
Plateau	6.67[ac]	6.31	0	0
Zou	6.67[ac]	6.31	0	0
Total	2.18	1.02	6.41	5.43

Proportions in the same column followed by different letters differ significantly at 5%.

Table 4. Prevalence of dermatophilosis infection among cattle from different regions of Benin.

Region	Herd prevalence (%)	Confidence interval
Alibori	0[b]	0
Atacora	0[a]	0
Atlantique	33,33[a]	30.79
Borgou	20[a]	20.24
Collines	33,33[a]	30.79
Couffo	0[a]	0
Donga	0[a]	0
Mono	50[a]	40.01
Ouémé	22,22[a]	27.16
Plateau	16,67[a]	29.82
Zou	50[a]	40.01
Total	23,08	9.35

Proportions in the same column followed by different letters differ significantly at 5%

andcows are classified as the most sensitive. In Africa, some authors have recorded rates ranging between 3 and 13% (Traoré et al., 2004; Boussini et al., 2012, Cadmus et al., 2013). These rates are relatively close to ours. In Ethiopia, Tschopp et al. (2013) found 1.7%. But in Zambia, Muma et al. (2013) found 20.7%. It should be noted that in this case, serum samples were taken only from cows. Our herd prevalence was 37.18%. This is close to the 45.9% found in Ethiopia by Asgedom et al. (2016). The prevalence after analysis of the milk was 46.15%. It is above the 16% found in Egypt by Wareth et al. (2014).

For bovine tuberculosis, although comparative intradermal tuberculin test gives more specific results than single intradermal tuberculin test (Monaghan et al., 1994), our study gave an overall prevalence of 2.18%. This rate is similar to that obtained by Farougou et al. (2006) in Bétécoucou farm which was 2.64%, but very far

from the rate they obtained in Samiondji's farm which was 8.25%. The highest rates were observed in the regions of the South. It was noted that in this region, there are sedentary herds. Indeed, prolonged contact could favor transmission by aerosols. Factors such as water sharing, grazing, or high promiscuity are potential risk factors for bovine tuberculosis transmission (Thoen and Bloom, 1995). This rate is close to that obtained by Asante-Poku et al. (2014) in Ghana which was 2.48%. However, in Burkina Faso, Traoré et al. (2004) found 27.7%. There is no significant difference about sex. This is in agreement with the study of Traoré et al. (2004) in Burkina Faso. The herd prevalence was 15.38% and the milk prevalence was 6.41%. This difference, although not significant, may be due to the fact that *M. bovis* is rarely isolated from milk, although it is known to be secreted in milk. However, it is not found in milk that has been stored for a few days probably because of competition with lactobacilli (Mariam, 2009). Moreover, the numerous doubtful cases can have several causes. Indeed, considering that the tuberculin test is not a perfect test, some animals would not have been detected, which can lead to an underestimation of the prevalence. In endemic areas, delayed hypersensitivity may not develop for 3 to 6 weeks after infection, and in chronically infected animals with severe disease, tuberculin testing may not respond (OIE, 2010). Thus, it is evident that the initial thickness of the skin fold could confuse the interpretation of reactivity to tuberculin. In Africa, some authors have found relatively low rates ranging from 2 to 6% (Boukary et al., 2011; Boussini et al., 2012; Katale et al., 2013; Muma et al., 2013). In contrast, in Nigeria, Okeke et al. (2014) found 16.17% with PCR on cattle lungs taken from slaughterhouses. In Ethiopia, Tschopp et al. (2013) found 0.3%. The mixed prevalence rate for brucellosis-tuberculosis was 0.38%. It is close to that observed in Burkina Faso by Boussini et al. (2012) which was 0.49%.

For bovine dermatophilosis, about herd prevalence, the four northern regions (Alibori, Atacora, Borgou and Donga) had the lowest rates. This could be in correlation with season. Indeed, it is warmer in the North (only one rainy season) than in the South (two rainy seasons). Dejene et al. (2012) have shown that there was a significant variation between seasons of the year and bovine dermatophilosis which is highly prevalent during the wet season than the dry season. The higher prevalence of the disease during the mentioned season is due to activation of the motile zoospores by rain and increased arthropods population (ticks) so that they may contribute to the occurrence of the disease. Ticks were present in most sampled herds. Furthermore tick *Amblyomma variegatum* had been associated with transmission of the disease (Morrow et al., 1993; Chatikobo et al., 2004) and there was also an association with tick *Boophilus annulatus* (Awad et al., 2008) for which macroclimatic factors play a great role in seasonal dynamics (Singh et al., 2000). In the same way the dry season in the north is usually a period of extensive bush burning. Wilson (1988) observed that the disappearance of vegetation in the dry season had a direct effect on the local abundance of questing adult ticks. He reported that tick abundance was reduced by as much as 88% following removal of vegetation by burning.

Conclusion

Knowledge of diseases is a crucial step in the development of prevention and control measures. This study suggests that the overall prevalence of bovine brucellosis, tuberculosis and dermatophilosis in Benin in general and in the PAFILAV's intervention area in particular is very high and requires urgent intervention. These three diseases are likely to pose a significant risk for the achievement of PAFILAV's objectives. Several recommendations can be made to minimize the risk of spread of these diseases between regions. The first and most important is to disseminate knowledge about brucellosis, tuberculosis and dermatophilosis. Then, educate herders and people involved in the cattle trade on risk factors. Finally train herders on how to deal with any signs of suspicion of disease in their flock. In addition, further studies are needed to determine the actual burden of these zoonoses on public health.

CONFLICT OF INTERESTS

The authors have not declared any conflict of interests.

ACKNOWLEDGEMENT

The authors are grateful to Projet d'Appui à la Filière Lait et Viande (PAFILAV) for financial support.

REFERENCES

Abbas B, Agab H (2002). A review of camel brucellosis. Prev. Vet. Med. 55(1):47-56.

Acha PN, Szyfres B (1989). Zoonoses and communicable diseases common to humans and animals. Paris: O.I.E. P 1063.

Adehan R, Koutinhouin B, Baba-Moussa LS, Aigbe L, Agbadje PM, Youssao AKI (2005). Prevalence of bovine brucellosis in Benin's State farms from 2000 to 2003. R.A.S.P.A. 3:3-4.

Adugna KE, Agga GE, Zewde G (2013).Sero epidemiological survey of bovine brucellosis in cattle under a traditional production system in western Ethiopia. Rev. Sci. Technol. 32(3):765-773.

Akakpo JA, Bonarel P, d'Almeida JF (1984). Epidemiology of bovine brucellosis in tropical Africa.Serological survey in Benin's Republic. Rev. Méd. Vét. 37 :133-137.

Ali-Emmanuel N, Moudachirou M, Akakpo AJ, Quetin-Leclercq J (2002). *In vitro* antibacterial activities of *Cassia alata, Lantana camara, Mitracarpus scaber, Dermatophilus congolensis* isolated in Benin. Rev. Elev. Méd. Vét. Pays Trop. 55(3):183-187.

Asante-Poku A, Aning KG, Boi-Kikimoto B, YeboahManu D (2014). Prevalence of bovine tuberculosis in a dairy cattle farm and a research farm in Ghana. Onderstepoort J. Vet. Res. 81(2):1-6.

Asgedom H, Damena D, Duguma R (2016). Seroprevalence of bovine brucellosis and associated risk factors in and around Alage district, Ethiopia. Springerplus. 5:851.

Awad WS, Nadra-Elwgoud, Abdou MI, El-Sayed AA (2008).Diagnosis and Treatment of Bovine, Ovine and Equine Dermatophilosis. J. Appl. Sci. Res. 4(4):367-374.

Berhe G, Belihu K, Asfaw Y (2007). Seroepidemiological investigation of bovine brucellosis in the extensive cattle production system of Tigray region of Ethiopia. Int. J. Appl. Res. Vet. Med. 5:65-71.

Boukary AR, Thys E, Abatih E, Gamatie D, Ango I (2011). Bovine Tuberculosis Prevalence Survey on Cattle in the Rural Livestock System of Torodi (Niger). PLoS One 6(9):e24629.

Boussini H, Traoré A, Tamboura HH, Bessin R, Boly H, Ouédraogo A (2012). Prevalence of tuberculosis and brucellosis in intra-urban and peri-urban dairy cattle in Ouagadougou's city in Burkina Faso. Rev. Sci. Tech. Off. int. Epizoot. 31(3):943-951.

Cadmus SIB, Alabi PI, Adesokan HK, Dale EJ, Stack JA, (2013). Serological investigation of bovine brucellosis in three cattle production systems in Yewa Division, south-western Nigeria. J. South African Vet. Assoc. 84(1):00-00.

Chatikobo P, Kusina NT, Hamudikuwanda H, Nyoni O (2004).A monitoring study on the prevalence of dermatophilosis and parafilariosis in cattle in a smallholder semi-arid farming area in Zimbabwe. Trop. Anim. Health. Prod. 36(3):207-215.

Cutler SJ, Whatmore AM, Commander NJ (2005). Brucellosis: new aspects of an old disease. J. Appl. Microbiol. 98:1270-1281.

Dejene B, Ayalew B, Tewodros F, Mersha C (2012). Occurance of Bovine Dermatophilosis in Ambo town West Shoa Administrative Zone, Ethiopia. American-Eurasian J. Sci. Res. 7(4):172-175.

Dinka H, Chala R (2009). Seroprevalence study of bovine brucellosis in pastoral and agro-pastoral areas of East Showa Zone, Oromia Regional State, Ethiopia. American-Eurasian J. Agric. Environ. Sci. 6(5):508-512

Direction of Animal Production (DAP) (2012). Statistical Yearbook of 2011. Benin. P 31.

Direction of Animal Production (DAP) (2013).Statistical Yearbook of 2012. Benin. P 31.

Direction of Animal Production (DAP) (2014).Statistical Yearbook of 2013. Benin. P 28.

Direction of Animal Production (DAP) (2015).Statistical Yearbook of 2014. Benin. P 25.

Direction of Animal Production (DAP) (2016).Statistical Yearbook of 2015. Benin. P 12.

Dossou J, Atchouké GD, Dabadé DS, Azokpota P, Montcho JK (2016). Nutritional and health quality comparative evaluation of milk from different breeds of cows in some Benin's breeding areas. Eur. Sci. J. 12(3).

Farougou S, Agbadjè P, Kpodékon M, Adoligbé C, Akakpo JA (2006). Prevalence of bovine tuberculosis in the state farms of Samiondji and Betecoucou of Benin. R.A.S.P.A. 4(1-2).

Hamid M, Musa MS (2009).The treatment of bovine dermatophilosis and its effects on some haematological and blood chemical parameters. Rev. Sci. Tech. Off. int. Epizoot. 28:1111-1118.

Kassaye E, Moser I, Woldemeskel M (2003). Epidemiological study on clinical bovine dermatophilosis in northern Ethiopia.Dtsch. Tierarztl.Wochenschr.110(10):422-425.

Katale BZ, Mbugi EV, Karimuribo ED, Keyyu JD, Kendall S, Kibiki GS, Faussett PG, Michel AL, Kazwala RR, Helden PV, Matee MI (2013). Prevalence and risk factors for infection of bovine tuberculosis in indigenous cattle in the Serengeti ecosystem, Tanzania. BMC Vet. Res. 9(1):267.

Koutinhouin B, Youssao AKI, Houéhou AE, Agbadjè PM (2003). Prevalence of bovine brucellosis in the traditional breeding farms supervised by the Project for Livestock Development (PDE) in Benin. Rev. Méd. Vét. 154(4):271-276.

Kusina NT, Chatikobo P, Hamudikuwanda H, Nyoni O (2004). A monitoring study on the prevalence of dermatophilosis and parafilariosis in cattle in a smallholder semi-arid farming area in Zimbabwe. Trop. Anim. Health. Prod. 36:207-215.

Makita K, Fèvre EM, Waiswa C, Eisler MC, Thrusfield M, Welburn SC (2011). Herd prevalence of bovine brucellosis and analysis of risk factors in cattle in urban and peri-urban areas of the Kampala economic zone, Uganda. BMC Vet. Res. 7:60.

Mariam SH (2009). Interaction between lactic acid bacteria and M. bovis in Ethiopian fermented milk. Appl. Environ .Microbiol. 75:1790-1792.

Matope G, Bhebhe E, Muma JB, Lund A, Skjerve E (2010). Herd-level factors for Brucella seropositivity in cattle reared in smallholder dairy farms of Zimbabwe. Prev. Vet. Med. 94(3-4):213-221.

McDermott JJ, Arimi SM (2002). Brucellosis in Sub-Saharan Africa: epidemiology, control and impact. Vet Microbiol. 20:111-134

Megersa B, Biff D, Niguse F, Rufael T, Asmare K, Skjerve E (2011b). Cattle brucellosis in traditional livestock husbandry practice in Southern and Eastern Ethiopia, and its zoonotic implication.Acta. Vet. Scand. 53:24.

Monaghan ML, Doherty ML, Collins JD, Kazda JF, Quinn PJ (1994). The tuberculin test. Vet. Microbiol. 40(1-2):111-124.

Morrow AN, Arnott JL, Heron ID, Koney EBM, Walker AR (1993).The effect of tick control on the prevalence of dermatophilosis on indigenous cattle in Ghana. Rev. Elev. Med. Vet. Pays Trop. 46:317-322.

Mostowy S, Inwald J, Gordon S, Martin C, Warren R, Kremer K, Cousins D, Behr MA (2005). Revisiting the evolution of Mycobacterium bovis. J. Bacteriol. 187:6386-6395.

Muma JB, Syakalima M, Munyeme M, Zulu VC, Simuunza M, Kurata M (2013). Bovine Tuberculosis and Brucellosis in Traditionally Managed Livestock in Selected Districts of Southern Province of Zambia. Vet. Med. Int. 2013:730367.

Okeke LA, Cadmus S, Okeke IO, Muhammad M, Awoloh O, Dairo D, Waziri EN, Olayinka A, Nguku PM, Fawole O (2014). Prevalence and risk factors of Mycobacterium tuberculosis complex infection in slaughtered cattle at Jos South Abattoir, Plateau State, Nigeria. Pan Afr. Med. J. 18(1):7.

Omer K, Holstand G, Skjerve E, Woldehiwet Z, MacMillan AP (2000).Prevalence of antiodies to Brucella spp in catte, sheep, goats, horses and camels in the State of Eritrea; influence of husbandry system. Epidemiol. Infect. 125:447-453.

Ragassa G, Mekonnen D, Yamuah L, Tilahun H, Guta T, Gebreyohannes A, Aseff A, Abdoel TH, Smits HL (2009). Human brucellosis in Traditional pastoral communities in Ethiopia. Int. J. Trop. Med. 4:59-64

Schelling E, Diguimbaye C, Daoud S, Nicolet J, Boerlin P, Tanner M, Zinsstag J (2003). Brucellosis and Q-fever sero prevalence of nomadic pastoralists and their livestock in Chad. Prev. Vet. Med. 61:279-293

Scott DW (1988). Large animal dermatology.Edition Sanders.Philapdelhia. pp.136-146.

Singh AP, Singla LD and Singh A (2000) A study on the effects of macroclimatic factors on the seasonal population dynamics of Boophilus micropus (Canes, 1888) infesting the cross-bred cattle of Ludhiana district. Int. J. Anim. Sci. 15(1):29-31.

Swai ES, Schoonman L (2010).The Use of Rose Bengal Plate Test to Asses Cattle Exposure to Brucella Infection in Traditional and Smallholder Dairy Production Systems of Tanga Region of Tanzania. Vet. Med. Int. 2010:837950

Thoen CO, Bloom BR (1995). Pathogenesis of Mycobacterium bovis In: Thoen CO, Steele JH, editors. Mycobacterium bovis Infection in Animals and Humans. First ed. Ames, Iowa: Iowa State University Press. pp: 3-14.

Traoré A, Tamboura HH, Bayala B, Rouamba DW, Yaméogo N, Sanou M (2004). Overall prevalence of major pathologies affecting cow milk's production in intra urban breeding system in Hamdallaye (Ouagadougou).Biotechnol. Agron. Soc. Environ. 8 (1):3-8.

Tschopp R, Abera B, Sourou SY, Guerne-Bleich E, Aseffa A, Wubete A, Zinsstag J, Young D (2013). Bovine tuberculosis and brucellosis prevalence in cattle from selected milk cooperatives in Arsi zone, Oromia region, Ethiopia. BMC Vet. Res. 9:163.

Walker RL (1999). "Brucella," in Veterinary Microbiology, C. H. Dwight and C. Z. Yuang, Eds. Blackwell Science, Cambridge, Mass, USA. pp. 196-203.

Wareth G, Melzer F, Elschner MC, Neubauer H, Roesler U (2014).Detection of Brucella melitensis in bovine milk and milk products from apparently healthy animals in Egypt by real-time PCR. J. Infect. Dev. Ctries. 8(10):1339-1343.

Wilson ML (1986). Reduced Abundance of adult Ixodesdammini (Acari: Ixodidae) following destruction of Vegetation. J. Econ. Entomol. 79(3):693-696.

Wold Health Organization (WHO) (2004).Report of the WHO/FAO/OIE Joint Consultation on Emerging Zoonotic Diseases, Geneva, Switzerland. P 72.

World Organization for Animal Health (OIE) (2009).Bovine brucellosis and bovine tuberculosis.In OIE Terrestrial Manual. Chapter 2.4.3.Paris: France.

World Organization for Animal Health (OIE) (2010).Manual of the Diagnostic Tests and Vaccines for Terrestrial Animals.vol. 1.Office International Des Epizooties.5th edition. Paris: France.

Yeruham I, Elad D, Perl S (2000). Economic aspects of outbreaks of dermatophilosis in first calving cows in nine herds of dairy cattle in Israel. Vet. Rec. 146(24):695-698.

Zinsstag J, Schelling E, Roth F, Bonfoh B, Savigny D, Tanner M (2007). Human benefits of animal interventions for zoonosis control. Emerg. Infect. Dis. 13:527-532.

29

Effect of *Securidaca longepedunculata* root-bark methanol extract on testicular morphometry of New Zealand rabbits

Chibuogwu Ijeoma Chika[1], Mathew Luka[1] and Ubah Simon Azubuike[2*]

[1]Animal Science Department, Faculty of Agriculture, University of Abuja, Federal Capital Territory, Nigeria.
[2]Department of Theriogenology, Faculty of Veterinary Medicine, University of Abuja, Federal Capital Territory, Nigeria.

The aim of this work was to determine the effect of the root-bark extract of *Securidaca longepedunculata* in the improvement of fertility in buck rabbits as envisioned by morphometric indices of the testes. Testicular morphometry of New Zealand rabbits was studied following treatment with different doses of the extract. The extract was administered *per os* in three doses of 0, 50 and 100 mg/kg body weight to three treatment groups of rabbits A, B, and C respectively for 29 days in a completely randomized designed (CRD). Eighteen mature buck rabbits between the ages of 18 and 24 months and with initial body weight (1.1 to 1.9 kg) were used. Each group comprised of three rabbits replicated twice. After the period of treatment, rabbits were weighed and sacrificed. Mean absolute paired testes weight, testes length and testes width were obtained and expressed relative to body weight at sacrifice. The results showed a significant difference in the mean relative paired testes weight, testes length and testes width between groups ($p<0.05$). The treated group given 50 mg/kg body weight of the extract had the highest mean absolute and relative paired testes weight of 3.325 ± 0.1349^a g and 0.2098 ± 0.0139^a % with mean absolute and relative testes length of 2.4522 ± 0.0250^a cm and 0.1538 ± 0.0040^a %. While the group given 100 mg/kg body weight of the extract had the lowest values of 2.634 ± 0.2762^b g and 0.1565 ± 0.0124^b % with mean absolute and relative paired testes length of 2.1600 ± 0.0807^b cm and 0.1299 ± 0.0039^b % respectively. It was concluded that administration of the extract at 50 mg/kg body weight yielded higher testicular parameters of buck rabbits. It was recommended that the use of the extract in bucks should be done with caution in relation to dose and length of treatment and that a detailed research should be carried out to evaluate the semen quality of bucks treated with 50 mg/kg the extract.

Key words: *Securidaca longepedunculata*, root bark, testes, morphometry, buck, rabbit.

INTRODUCTION

The increasing population in the developing countries has led to increase in demand for animal protein. Rabbit meat presents the most affordable source of animal protein to mitigate the problem of protein malnutrition in Nigeria.

*Corresponding author. E-mail: drubah2000@yahoo.com.

Rabbit production also provides high returns on investment, high quality meat products with high protein level of about 20.8%, low sodium, low fat and cholesterol levels which compares favorably with the local bush meat (Shinkut et al., 2016). The presence of caecal microbes enables the rabbit to digest large amounts of fibrous feed better than most non ruminant species (Taiwo et al., 1999). It is for this reason that the costs of beef, chevon, mutton, chicken and frozen fish are higher compared to rabbit meat (Shinkut et al., 2016). For efficient and maximum production of rabbits for meat, a thorough understanding of the reproductive potential of the rabbit is invaluable. The importance of the breeder male spermatozoa for fertilizing eggs is rivalled only by his genetic influence on the progeny performance. The basic knowledge of the morphometric characteristics of the reproductive organs is essential for reproductive assessment and prediction of sperm production, storage potential and fertilizing ability of the breeder male (Gage and Freckleton, 2003). Testicular morphometry and histological changes in rabbit bucks have been used to access the male reproductive status (Abadjieva, 2016).

The plant *Securidaca longepedunculata* is a plant commonly known as Violet tree in English and Krinkhout in Afrikaans. In Swahili it is known as Chipvufanaor mufufu. In Nigeria, the Hausas call it Uwarmaganigunar while the Ibos call it Ezeogwu, Fulani name is 'aalali' is a medium size tree measuring 8 to 9 m height with visible violet (or white) flowers, pale smooth bark, common in North-Central Nigeria, and is generally widespread in hot temperate part of Africa. When in flower the plant is distinctly ornamental. The fruits are round, with a characteristic membranous wing up to 45 mm, purplish green when young, becoming pale straw colored between April and August (Alqasim, 2013). The genus Securidaca comprises about 80 species, characterized by papillionaceous purplish flowers and mostly scandent shrubs and lianas, which produce compounds known as securixanthones with antimicrobial and antioxidant properties (Da Costa et al., 2013). *S. longepedunculata* stem bark and roots are still found amongst the most traded medicinal plants in Africa (Tabuti et al., 2012).

The root extracts are used for treating venereal diseases, skin cancer, skin infections, flu; they are also used for contraceptive purposes, abortion, constipation, coughs and fever. Other uses of the root extracts are sexual boost, toothache, tuberculosis, rheumatism, pneumonia, and as blood purifier and it is also used as an aphrodisiac for men (Mongalo et al., 2015). It is used in treating infections related to nervous and circulatory system, dysentery, malaria, typhoid and frequent stomach ache (Maroyi, 2013; Mustapha, 2013a, b).

Traditionally, the root and bark are taken orally either powdered or as infusion for abortion, infertility, venereal diseases, headache among other diseases (Nordeng et al., 2013). In Limpopo, the Venda people mix the powdered root with maize and sorghum beverages for sexually weak men (Togun and Egbunike, 2006). A root decoction may be drunk in beer as an aphrodisiac, for sexual impotence, toothache, fungal infections and malaria among other diseases (Maroyi, 2013; Ogunmefun and Gbile, 2012; Mongalo et al., 2015; Motlhanka and Nthoiwa, 2013). Moreover, the dried root is ground into powder, along with that of *Parkia biglobosa* and then taken with cow's milk as a sexual boost. The pounded root may be mixed with that of *Zanthoxylum humile* and taken with soft porridge to treat erectile dysfunction (Semenya and Potgieter, 2013). *S. longepedunculata* Fresen (Polygalaceae) is a multi-purpose plant with a long history of use in African traditional medicine to treat various sexually transmitted infections and other health conditions (Mongalo et al., 2015). Phytochemically, extracts from various parts of *S. longepedunculata*, especially the root bark, contain numerous valuable compounds including xanthones, some benzyl benzoates and triterpene saponins amongst others.

Toxicity studies, both *in vivo* and *in vitro*, revealed that extracts are only toxic at relatively high concentrations. Furthermore, extracts have antimicrobial, antioxidant, antiparasitic, anti-diabetic, anti-inflammatory, antimalarial, insecticidal, pesticidal, and anticonvulsant properties. Some African medicinal plants have been ethnobotanically and scientifically implicated in the treatment of a variety of human infections (Mongalo and Mafoko, 2013; Mongalo, 2013; Zongo et al., 2013). The pharmacology of these plants may be attributed to various classes of compounds occurring within these plants. In general, these medicinal plants may have relatively low toxicity (Belayachi et al., 2013). Fresh leaves are made into paste with little or no water along with the bark of *Gardenia erubescens* and *Jussiaea suffruticosa* with shea butter and applied externally to treat skin cancer and skin infections respectively (Mustapha, 2013a). Smoke from dry leaves is inhaled to treat headaches while the boiled leaves are taken orally for contraceptive purposes (Mustapha, 2013b). The leaves are either chewed fresh or both orally and nasally administered to treat infertility and to expel the placenta among other uses (Augustino et al., 2011). A decoction from the stem bark may be taken orally for abortion, infertility problems, venereal diseases and some other diseases (Kadiri et al., 2013). The powdered stem bark has antimicrobial activity against a variety of organisms including *Neisseria gonorrhea, Candida albicans, Trichomonas vaginalis* and the agent for syphilis (Hedimbi and Chinsembu, 2012). However there is a need to explore the biological activity of various extracts from the species against microorganisms such as, *Klebsiella granulomatis, Mycoplasma hominis,* Mobiluncus spp. and *Mycoplasma genitalium* as the most common causative agents of gonorrhea, bacterial vaginitis, donovanosis and other urogenital infections (Mongalo et al., 2015).

Plant part used for abortion is dried root boiled into

distilled water along with Lállè (Hausa name)/nalli (Fulani name) (leave of Lawsonia inermis) and a pap is made from the juice (Alqasim, 2013). Dried root, ground into powdered form along with Dóòráwà (Hausa name)/nareehi (Fulani name) (root of Parkia biglobosa) when mixed with cow's milk is also used as a sexual boost (Alqasim, 2013). The aqueous root and ethanol extracts yielded alkaloids, cardiac glycosides, flavonoids, saponins, tannins, volatile oils, terpenoids and some steroids (Haruna et al., 2013a; Auwal et al., 2012; Gbadamosi, 2012) while chloroform and ethanol extracts indicated flavonoids, saponins, coumarins, tannins and alkaloids (Adebayo and Osman, 2012). The aqueous root bark extract was slightly toxic to albino rats with an LD_{50} of 0.771 g/kg (Auwal et al., 2012), while Agbaje and Adekoya (2012) reported an LD_{50} of 3.16 g/kg when administered orally to rats. Moreover, acute toxicity studies of the aqueous whole root extract on mice revealed LD_{50} values of 1.740 and 0.020 g/kg for the oral and intraperitoneal application routes respectively (Adeyemi et al., 2010). Elsewhere, the 80% ethanol extract of the root bark exhibited an LD_{50} of 0.547 g/kg against albino mice (Keshebo et al., 2014). These findings may well suggest that the root bark extract has greater acute toxicity than the whole root extract following oral administration. Antifungal activity has been reported (Karou et al., 2012; Alitonou et al., 2012). Hyperglycemic activity has also been reported (Keshebo et al., 2014).

The inclusion effects of 0.5 ml/kg C. populnea extract and inclusion of S. longepedunculata showed that C. populnea plant extract enhanced the reproductive profiles of male and female C. gariepinus brood stocks and brought about a significant increase in egg weight but on the other hand the inclusion of S. longepedunculata caused a significant reduction in egg weight at the two different concentrations of the plant extract while fish on diet 4 (0.5ml/kg SL) showed the lowest fecundity count. The reduction could be attributed to the concentration of toxic substances in the leaves of the plant (Ademola et al., 2017). S. longepedunculata inclusion also improves spermatogenesis in low concentration but at high dose, there was low sperm count and low motility which could be as a result of toxicity of the extract (Akah and Nwambie, 1994). The testosterone, progesterone and estrogen values as well as the milt volume, sperm motility and milt count were significantly reduced (p<0.05) in fish fed with diet inclusion of 1.0 ml S. Longepedunculata (Ademola et al., 2017).

This also agreed with the finding of Dandekar et al. (2002) that S. longepedunculata contains some compounds that have negative effect on animal reproductive parameters. The possible mechanisms for the anti-gonad action of S. longepedunculata extract could be by exerting a direct inhibitory action on the testis which affects androgen biosynthesis pathways and the pituitary gland, thereby causing changes in Gonadotrophin concentrations and subsequent spermatogenic impairment or changing the concentration of neurotransmitters (Sarkar et al., 2000). A total of 61 plants species from 36 families were found to be used traditionally to treat male sexual disorders, of the 61 plant species, only S. longepedunculata is also traditionally used as a contraceptive. The common methods of application are decoctions and/or infusions in water, beer or milk taken orally (Abdillahi and Van Staden, 2012).

Erectile dysfunction (ED) is a neurovascular event and entails the inability to sustain an erection during coitus as well as a decreased libido. Findings indicated the use of 12 species, 10 of them with new documentations. Only Osyris lanceolata and S. longepedunculata were previously recorded in the treatment of ED (Lourens et al., 2015). S. longependunculata is believed to have an aphrodisiac property, may improve sperm quality and enhance fertility (Bahmanpour et al., 2006). Plants with aphrodisiac property may be useful in solving fertility problems (Bahmanpour et al., 2006).

The aim of this work was to determine the effect of the root-bark extract of S. longepedunculata in the improvement of fertility in buck rabbits as envisioned by morphometric indices of the testes.

MATERIALS AND METHODS

Study location

This study was conducted at the Rabbitry Unit of the University of Abuja Research farm, Abuja Nigeria. University of Abuja Nigeria is geographically located on latitude 8.941°N and longitude 7.092°E at an altitude of 300 m above sea level.

Experimental animals and management

The animal experiments followed the principles of the Laboratory animal care (Canadian Council on Animal Care Guide, 1993). Eighteen (18) mature buck rabbits between the ages of 18 to 24 months and with initial weight (1.1 to 1.9 kg) were obtained from a rabbit farmer in Jos, Plateau state, middle belt of Nigeria. Rabbits were housed in battery cages and acclimatized for one month. During the acclimatization period all the rabbits in this study were fed standard commercial feed containing 18% crude protein twice daily and clean tap water was provided ad-libitum.

Collection and identification of plant materials

S. longepedunculata was collected within the premises of the University of Abuja permanent site by the help of the local people. The plant was subsequently identified and confirmed by the Herbarium and Ethno-Botany Unit of National Institute for Pharmaceutical Research and Development Idu- Abuja (NIPRD), where a voucher specimen (NIPRD/H/6576) was deposited.

Processing of S. longepedunculata root-bark

Some roots from each S. longepedunculata plant were removed in such a way that the tree still remained alive. The roots were dusted and peeled to obtain the bark. The obtained root bark was cut into pieces, dried in the shade to minimize loss of volatile constituents and reduced to size with pestle in a mortar.

Extraction

The plant material (500 g) was extracted by cold maceration in methanol for 48 h and concentrated in a rotary evaporator at reduced pressure to obtain a dark brown mass of the crude methanol extract.

Experimental design

Eighteen (18) mature buck rabbits between the ages of 18 and 24 months and with initial weight (1.1 to 1.9 kg) were randomly allocated into three experimental groups (A, B and C) with three rabbits per group replicated twice.

Rabbits in group A (control), B and C were administered 0, 50, and 100 mg/kg body weight of *S. longepedunculata* root bark extract respectively *per os* with the aid of an improvised oral catheter for 29 days. At the end of the treatment, rabbits were weighed and sacrificed. Both testes in each buck were dissected out, freed of all connective tissues and blotted on paper to remove blood. Both testes from each buck were weighed to get the paired testes weight using a sensitive weighing balance (Ohaus SP-602 Scout Pro Digital Balance, USA) while testes length and width were measured using a vernier caliper (Series 530 - Standard Model, Mitutoyo, USA). Mean absolute paired testes weight, testes length and testes width were obtained and expressed relative to body weight at sacrifice.

Statistical analysis

Data collected was subjected to a one-way analysis of variance (ANOVA) using SPSS, Version 17.0. Mean differences with values of $P<0.05$ was considered statistically significant and was separated using Tukey's HSD test.

RESULTS

Extraction yield

The plant material (500 g) yielded 54.51 g (10.9%) of the crude methanol extract.

Effect of extract on testes morphometry

The absolute paired testes weight showed significant difference between treatments ($P<0.05$). The highest absolute paired testes weight occurred in the 50 mg/kg body weight group, while control group had the lowest (Table 1). Mean absolute paired testes weight in control group was statistically similar to that of rabbits in 100 mg/kg body weight group (p>0.05). The mean paired relative testes weight was significantly different between treatments ($P<0.05$). Rabbits in 50 mg/kg body weight group had the highest relative paired testes weight. The lowest relative paired testes weight was seen in 100

mg/kg body weight group. The absolute testes length was significantly different between treatments ($P<0.05$). Rabbits in group B had the highest paired absolute testes length while rabbits in the group C had the lowest absolute paired testes length. However, the absolute paired testes length of control rabbits was similar to those of rabbits in the group C.

The relative paired testes length was significantly different between treatments ($P<0.05$). Rabbits in the group B had the highest relative paired testes length but were statistically similar to the control group. The lowest relative paired testes length was seen in group C. There was no significant difference in the absolute paired testes width when rabbits in each group were compared ($P>0.05$). Significant differences were observed when the relative paired testes width between each group was compared ($P<0.05$). Relative paired testes width was highest in the control group followed by group B. Whereas the relative paired testes width of group C was the lowest.

DISCUSSION

The crude methanol extract yield obtained in this study agreed with the crude methanol extract value of (10.9%) reported by Okoli et al. (2006). The extract seems to have some anabolic effects considering the body weight of the control and the treated groups. The treated groups have significantly higher body weight than the control. This effect may be due to steroids present as part of the constituents of the extract. It has been reported that the aqueous root and ethanol extracts yielded alkaloids, cardiac glycosides, flavonoids, saponins, tannins, volatile oils, terpenoids and some steroids (Haruna et al., 2013a; Auwal et al., 2012; Gbadamosi, 2012). The knowledge of the ability of the testes to produce spermatozoa is of immense importance in rabbit breeding program. The higher values in relative paired testes weight, length and width observed in the present study with the introduction of *S. longepedunculata* extract at 50 mg/kg body weight is a pointer that *S. longepedunculata* root-back extract promotes testicular growth. This indicates that administration of *S. longepedunculata* root-back extract at 50 mg/kg body weight for 29 days may be good for the development of spermatogenic potentials of the buck as reflected on the paired testes weight observed in this study. This agrees with Akah and Nwambie (1994) who reported that *S. longepedunculata* inclusion also improves spermatogenesis in low concentration. Testes size is a good indicator of the present and future spermatozoa production of an animal (Morris et al., 1979; Perry and Petterson, 2001; Gupta and Mohanty, 2003; Togun and Egbunike, 2006). The knowledge of basic morphometric characteristics of the reproductive organs have been found to provide valuable information on the evaluation of breeding and fertility potential of animals.

Table 1. Mean±SEM testicular parameters of buck rabbits treated with *Securidaca longepedunculata* root bark methanol extract at sacrifice.

Testicular parameter	Doses of extract (mg/kg body weight of rabbit)		
	0	50	100
	Mean±SEM	Mean±SEM	Mean±SEM
Body weight (g)	1450 ± 50.00^b	1600 ± 44.72^{ab}	1666.7 ± 61.46^a
Absolute paired testes weight (g)	2.5855 ± 0.0981^b	3.325 ± 0.1349^a	2.634 ± 0.2762^b
Relative paired testes weight (%)	0.1783 ± 0.0026^{ab}	0.2098 ± 0.0139^a	0.1565 ± 0.0124^b
Absolute paired testes length (cm)	2.2108 ± 0.0468^b	2.4522 ± 0.0250^a	2.1600 ± 0.0807^b
Relative paired testes length (%)	0.1537 ± 0.0073^a	0.1538 ± 0.0040^a	0.1299 ± 0.0039^b
Absolute paired testes width (cm)	0.9472 ± 0.0073^a	1.0155 ± 0.0304^a	0.9347 ± 0.0368^a
Relative Paired testes width (%)	0.0657 ± 0.0020^a	0.0637 ± 0.0030^{ab}	0.0561 ± 0.0012^b

a-c = Means in the same row with different superscripts are significantly different (p<0.05).

The fact that the group that received 50 mg/kg body weight of the *S. longepedunculata* root-back extract resulted in absolute and relative paired testes weight which were greater than the control shows that the reproductive potential of these testes were higher compared to those that did not receive the *S. longepedunculata* root-back extract. Larger testes (without any abnormality) have been reported to produce more spermatozoa than smaller testes (Oyeyemi et al., 2002; Galmessa et al., 2003; Britto et al., 2004; de Soya, 2007). Testes weight had been reported to be positively correlated with sperm volume, mass motility, sperm concentration, and testosterone but negatively correlated with dead sperm cell and primary abnormality in male goat (Johnson et al., 1984; Rahja et al., 1995; Daramola et al., 2007).

The positive effect of 50 mg/kg *S. longepedunculata* on the testes morphometry may have been contributed by its antimicrobial, antioxidant and aphrodisiac properties. Rabbits are known to suffer venereal diseases which could influence the testes parameters. Sub clinical infections may not be noticed. It has been reported that the root extracts of *S. longepedunculata* are used for treating venereal diseases, syphilis, skin cancer, skin infections and serves as a blood purifier (Maroyi, 2013; Mustapha, 2013a; Mustapha, 2013b). A decoction from the stem bark may be taken orally to treat infertility problems, epilepsy and venereal diseases (Kadiri et al., 2013). The powdered stem bark is also mixed with hot water and taken orally to treat syphilis and gonorrhoea (Hedimbi and Chinsembu, 2012). In another perspective the aphrodisiac properties may be playing a role on the positive testicular parameters observed at 50 mg/kg. A root decoction may be drunk in beer as an aphrodisiac (Motlhanka and Nthoiwa, 2013).

The lower values in relative paired testes weight, length and width of the group given 100 mg/kg body weight could be due to testicular aplasia or atrophy. Morton (1988) reported that in sacrificed animals, a decreased weight of the testes indicates wide spread or diffuse loss

of seminiferous epithelial cells. 100 mg/kg body weight of the extract for 29 days yielded lower testicular parameters. The result of 100 mg/kg of the extract for 29 days having lower values of testicular parameters measured, may be due to some level of toxicity at that dose and this is in agreement with Mongalo and Mafoko (2013), Mongalo (2013) and Zongo et al. (2013). In these reports, toxicity studies, both *in vivo* and *in vitro*, revealed that extracts are only toxic at relatively high concentrations. The findings of the present studies also concur with the report that the pharmacology of these plants may be attributed to various classes of compounds occurring within these plants. In general, these medicinal plants may have relatively low toxicity (Belayachi et al., 2013). The findings in this study is supported by that of Auwal et al. (2012) who reported that the aqueous root bark extract was slightly toxic to albino rats with an LD_{50} of 0.771 g/kg, Agbaje and Adekoya (2012) reported an LD_{50} of 3.16 g/kg when administered orally to rats. Moreover, acute toxicity studies of the aqueous whole root extract on mice revealed LD_{50} values of 1.740 and 0.020 g/kg for the oral and intraperitoneal application routes respectively (Adeyemi et al., 2010). Elsewhere, the 80% ethanol extract of the root bark exhibited an LD_{50} of 0.547 g/kg against albino mice (Keshebo et al., 2014). These findings may well suggest that the root bark extract has greater acute toxicity than the whole root extract following oral Administration (Mongalo et al., 2015). Out of the 61 plant species, used traditionally to treat male sexual disorders, only *S. longepedunculata* is also traditionally used as a contraceptive (Abdillahi and Van Staden, 2012), they are also used for contraceptive purposes and abortion (Maroyi, 2013; Mustapha, 2013a; Mustapha, 2013b). These reports are pointers that this plant has toxic potentials. The inclusion of *S. longepedunculata* in a dietary supplement of *Clarias gariepinus* caused a significant reduction in egg weight and fecundity count at the two different concentrations of the plant extract. The testosterone, progesterone and estrogen values as well as the milt volume, sperm motility and milt count were significantly reduced (p<0.05) in fish fed with diet inclusion of 1.0 ml *S. longepedunculata* (Ademola et al., 2017; Ajiboye et al., 2012; Akah and Nwambie, 1994). This also agrees with the finding of Dandekar et al. (2002) that *S. longepedunculata* contains some compounds that have negative effect on animal reproductive parameters. The possible mechanisms for the anti-gonad action of *S. longepedunculata* extract could be by exerting a direct inhibitory action on the testis which affects androgen biosynthesis pathways and the pituitary gland, thereby causing changes in gonadotrophin concentrations and subsequent spermatogenic impairment or changing the concentration of neurotransmitters (Sarkar et al., 2000). 100 mg/kg body weight of the extract for 29 days of the experiment could be toxic enough to elicit the changes observed. The investigation of other parameters of fertilization is necessary for a complete understanding of the action of this extract in this dose and period of treatment.

Conclusion

The administration of 50 mg/kg body weight of methanol extract of *S. longepedunculata* root-bark extract for 29 days yielded higher values of some of the testicular parameters such as relative paired testis weight and relative paired testis length and may be applied to improve the reproductive capacity of rabbit bucks at that dose. It is recommended that the use of the extract in bucks should be done with caution in relation to dose and length of treatment and that a detailed research should be carried out to evaluate the semen quality of bucks treated with 50 mg/kg the extract to ascertain its effect on semen quality.

CONFLICT OF INTERESTS

The authors have not declared any conflict of interests.

REFERENCES

Abadjieva D, Grigorova SV and Petkova M (2016). Testicular morphometry and histology of rabbit bucks supplemented with iodine in drinking water. Asian J. Anim.Vet Adv. 11:491-497.

Abdillahi HS, Van Staden J (2012). South African plants and male reproductive healthcare: Conception and contraception. J. Ethnopharmacol.143:475-480

Adebayo OL, Osman K (2012). A comparative evaluation of in vitro growth inhibitory activities of different solvent extracts of some medicinal plants in Northern Ghana against selected human pathogens. IOSR J. Pharm. 2:199-206.

Ademola ZA, Muyideen OL, Luke IO, Funmileyi OA, Faith IJ (2017). Dietary effect of *Cissuspopulnea* and *Securidaca longepedunculata* aqueous leave extracts on reproductive, haematological and biochemical parameters of African catfish, *Clarias gariepinus* (Burchell, 1822) broodstocks. Aceh J. Anim. Sci. 2(1):1-11.

Adeyemi OO, Akindele AJ, Yemitan OK, Aigbe FR, Fagbo FI (2010). Anticonvulsant, anxiolytic and sedative activities of the aqueous root extract of *Securidaca longepedunculata* Fresen. J. Ethnopharmacol. 130:191-195.

Agbaje EO, Adekoya ME (2012). Toxicological profile of aqueous root extract of *Securidaca longepedunculata* Fresen (Polygalaceae) after 90-day treatment in rats. Int. J. Toxicol. Pharmacol. Res. 4:5-11.

Akah PA, Nwambie AI (1994). Evaluation of Nigerian traditional medicines: 1. Plants used for rheumatic (inflammatory) disorders. J. Ethnopharmacol. 42(3):179-182.

Alitonou G A, Koudoro A Y, Dangou J S, Yehouenou B, Avlessi F, Adeoti S, Menut C and Sohounhloue C K (2012). Volatile constituents and biological activities of essential oil from *Securidaca longepedunculata* Fresen, growing in Benin. St Cerc St CICBIA, 13:33-42.

Alqasim A M (2013). Ethno-medico-botanical Uses of *Securidaca Longepedunculata* Fresen (Family-Polygalaceae) from Keffi Local Government, Nasarawa State, Nigeria. J. Nat. Remedies 13(2):133-137.

Anticonvulsant, anxiolytic and sedative activities of the aqueous root extract of *Securidaca longepedunculata* Fresen. J. Ethnopharmacol. 130: 191-195.

Augustino S, Hall JB, Makonda FBS, Ishengoma RC (2011). Medicinal resources of the Miombo woodlands of Urumva, Tanzania: plants and its use. J. Med. Plants Res. 5:6352-6372.

Auwal SM, Atiku MK, Wudil AM, Sule MS (2012). Phytochemical composition and acute toxicity evaluation of aqueous root bark extract of *Securidaca longepedunculata* (Linn). Bayero J. Pure Appl. Sci. 5(2):67-72.

Bahmanpour S, Talae T, Vojdani Z, Panjehshashin M, Poostpasand A, Zareel S and Ghaemina M (2006). Effect of *Phoenix dactyliferera* pollen on sperm parameters and reproductive system of adult male rats. Iranian J. Med. Sci. 31(4):208-212.

Belayachi L, Aceves-Luquero C, Merghoub N, Bakri Y, de Mattos SF, Amzazi S, Villalonga P (2013). Screening of North African medicinal plant extracts for cytotoxicity activity against tumor cell lines. Europ. J. Med. Plants 3:310-332.

Britto IFC, Silva AEDF, Unainian MM, Dode MAN, Barbos RT, Kastelic JP (2004).Sexual development in early and late maturing *Bos indicus* and *Bos indicus× Bos Taurus* crossbred bulls in Brazil. Theriogenology 62:1177-2177.

Canadian Council on Animal Care Guide (1993). Available at: http://www.ccac.ca/Documents/Standards/Guidlines/Experimental_Animals_Voll.pdf .

Da Costa CS, De Aguiar-Dias ACA, Simões AO (2013). *Securidaca marajoara* (Polygalaceae), a new species from the Brazillian Amazon. *Phytotaxa*. 137:53-56.

Dandekar SP, Nadkarni GD, Kulkarni VS, Punekar S (2002). Lipid peroxidation and antioxidant enzymes in male infertility. J. Postgrad. Med. 48(3):186-189.

Daramola JO, Adeloye AA, Fatoba TA, Soladaye AO (2007). Effect of exogenous, melatonin on spermiograms of West African Dwarf Bucks. Process of 32nd Annual Conference NSAP-Calabar, March18-22 pp. 111-113.

de Soya P (2007). Testicular parameters and Sperm Morphology of Chinchilla Rabbit fed with different planes of soymeal. Int. J. Morphol. 25(1):139-144.

Gage MJG, Freckleton RP (2003). Relative testis size and sperm morphometry across mammals: no evidence for an association between sperm competition and sperm length. Proceedings of the Royal Society of London B: Biol. Sci. 270(1515):625-632.

Galmessa U, Raina VS, Mohanty TK, Gupta AK (2003). Seminal attributes related to age and scrotal circumference in diary bulls. Indian J. Dairy Sci. 56:376-379.

Gbadamosi IT (2012). Evaluation of antibacterial activity of six ethnobotanicals used in the treatment of infectious diseases in Nigeria. Bot Res. Int. 5(4):83-89.

Gupta AK, Mohanty TK (2003).Testicular biometry and semen quality in Karan Fries bulls. Indian J. Diary Sci. 56:317-319.

Haruna Y, Elinge CM, Peni IJ, Dauda D, Aiki F (2013a). In vivo trypanocidal effect of aqueous root extracts of *Securidaca longepedunculata* and its phytochemical analysis. Afr. J. Pharm. Pharmacol. 7:2838-2842.

Hedimbi M, Chinsembu KC (2012). An ethnomedicinal study of plants used to manage HIV/AIDS-related disease conditions in the Ohangwena region, Namibia. Int. J. Med. Plants Res. 1:004-011.

Johnson BH, Robinson OW, Dillard EU (1984). Body growth and testicular development in young yearling Hereford bulls. J. Anim. Sci. 39:213.

Kadiri AB, Agboola OM, Fashina FO (2013). Ethnobotanical survey and phyto-anatomical studies of some common plants used for the treatment of epilepsy in some rural areas of South West Nigeria. J. Pharm. Phytochemistr. 2:175-182.

Karou SD, Tchacondo T, Tchibozo MAD, Anani K, Ouattara L, Simpore J, de Sousa C (2012). Screening of Togolese medicinal plants for few pharmacological properties. Pharmacogn. Res. 4:116-122.

Keshebo D L, Choundhury M K and Dekebo A H (2014). Investigation on toxicity, hypoglycemic effect of the root bark of Securidaca longepedunculata Fresen (Polygalaceae) and determination of heavy metals. Ann. Biol. Res. 5:15-19.

Lourens JCE, Marthienus JP, Sebua SS (2015). Erectile dysfunction: Definition and materia medica of Bapedi traditional healers in Limpopo province, South Africa. J. Med. Plants Res. 9(3):71-77.

Maroyi A (2013). Traditional use of medicinal plants in South-central Zimbabwe: Review and perspectives. J. Ethnobiol. Ethnomed. 9:31

Mongalo NI (2013). *Peltophorum africanum Sond* [Mosetlha]: A review of its ethnomedicinal uses, toxicology, phytochemistry and pharmacological activities. J. Med. Plants Res.7: 3484-3491.

Mongalo NI, Mafoko BJ (2013). *Cassia abbreviate Oliv.* A review of its ethnomedicinal uses, toxicology, phytochemistry, possible propagation techniques and pharmacology. African J. Pharm. Pharmacol. 7:2901-2906.

Mongalo NI, McGawb LJ, Finnieb JF, Van Stadenb J (2015). *Securidaca longipedunculata*Fresen (Polygalaceae): A review of its ethnomedicinal uses, phytochemistry, pharmacological properties and toxicology . J. ethnopharmacol. 165:215-226.

Morris DL, Smith MF, Parrish WR, William JD, Wilbank JN (1979). The effect of scrotal circumference, libido and semen quality on fertility of American Brahaman and Santa Certudies Bull. *Process Animal management of the Society for Theriogenology*, Oklahoma City. 92:196-200

Morton D (1988). The use of rabbits in male reproductive toxicology. Environ. Health Perspect. 77:5-9.

Motlhanka DMT, Nthoiwa GP (2013). Ethnobotanical survey of medicinal plants Of Tswapong North, in Eastern Botswana: A case of plants from Mosweu and Seolwane villages. Europ. J. Med. Plants. 3:10-24.

Mustapha AA (2013a). Ethno-medico-botanical uses of *Securidaca longepedunculata* (Fresen) (Family Polygalaceae) from Keffi local government, Nasarawa State, Nigeria. J. Nat. Remed. 13:133-137.

Mustapha AA (2013b). Ethno-medicinal field study of anti-fertility medicinal plants used by the local people in Keffi local government, Nasarawa State, Nigeria. Int. J. Med. Plants Res. 2:215-218.

Nordeng H, Al-Zayadi W, Diallo D, Ballo N, Paulsen BS (2013). Traditional medicine practitioners knowledge and views on treatment of pregnant women in three regions of Mali. J. Ethnobiol. Ethnomed. 9(1):67

Ogunmefun OT, Gbile ZO (2012). An ethnobotanical study of anti-rheumatic plants in South Western States of Nigeria. Asian J. Sci. Technol. 4(11):63-66.

Okoli CO, Akah PA, Ezugworie U (2006). Antiinflamatory activity of extracts of root-bark of S. *longepeduculata fres.* (polygalaceae) Afr. J. Tradit. Compliment. Alternat. Med. 2(3):50-63.

Oyeyemi MO, Oke A, Olusola C, Ajala O, Oluwatoyin O, Idehen CO (2002). Differences in testicular parameters and morphological characteristics of spermatozoa as related to age of West African Dwarf bucks. Trop. J. Anim. Sci. 5(1):99-107.

Perry G, Peterson D (2001). Determining reproductive fertility in herd bulls. University of Missouri Agriculture publication. pp. 1-8.

Rahja TA, Johnson RK, Lunstra DO (1995). Sperm production in boar after nine generation of selection for increased weight of testis. J. Anim. Sci. 73:2177-2185.

Sarkar R, Mohanakumar KP, Chowdhury M (2000). Effects of an organophosphate pesticide, quinalphos, on the hypothalamo-pituitary-gonadal axis in adult male rats. J. Reprod. Fert. 118(1):29-38.

Semenya SS, Potgieter MJ (2013). Ethnobotanical survey of medicinal plants used by Bapedi traditional healers to treat erectile dysfunction in the Limpopo Province, South Africa. J. Med. Plants Res. 7:349-357.

Shinkut M, Rekwot PI, Nwannenna IA, Sambo SJ, Bugau JS, Haruna M J (2016). Serum enzymes and histopathology of rabbit bucks fed diets supplemented with *Allium sativum*. IOSR J. Agric. Vet. Sci. 9(6):91-95.

Tabuti JRS, Kukunda CB, Kaweesi D, Kasilo OMJ (2012). Herbal medicine use in the districts of Nakapiripirit, Pallisa, Kanungu and Mukono in Uganda. J. Ethnobiol. Ethnomed. 8(1):35.

Taiwo BBA, Ogundipe II, Ogunsiji O (1999). Reproductive and growth performance of rabbits raised on forage crops. In: The Nigeria Livestock Industry in the 21st Century. Proceedings of the 4th Annual Conference of the Animal Association of Nigeria (G. N. Egbunike and A. D. Ologhobo, editors). 14th-19thSeptember. IITA Ibadan, Nigeria. pp: 108-109.

Togun VA, Egbunike GN (2006). Seasonal variations in the sperm production characteristics of Zebu (white Fulani) cattle genitalia in the humid tropical environment. Middle-East J. Sci. Res.1:87-95.

Zongo F, Ribout C, Boumendjel A, Guissou I (2013). Botany, traditional uses, phytochemistry and pharmacology of *Waltheria indica* L. (syn. *Waltheria americana*): A review. J. Ethnopharmacol. 148:14-26.

30

Effect of topical application of mixture of cod liver oil and honey on old (chronic) wounds and granulation tissue in donkeys

Addisu Mohammed Seid

Department Of Veterinary Clinical Medicine, Faculty of Veterinary Medicine, University of Gondar, Ethiopia.

A comparative study was conducted from November 2015 to May 2016 with the objective of investigating the beneficial effects of the mixture of cod liver oil and honey (group 1) comparing with routine treatment (group 2), combination of chlorhexidine (0.3%) and cetrimide (3%) in healing of contaminated old wounds in donkeys at Bahir Dar, North western Ethiopia. Out of 18 donkeys, 12 (6 male and 6 female) were treated with mixture of cod liver oil and honey and 6 donkeys (3 male and 3 female) were routinely treated. At the 35th day of treatment in group 1, the areas of the wounds were markedly decreased from 4.2% to 66.7% and in group 2 from 66.7% to 85.7% out of 100% of the initial area. The treatment outcome between group 1 and group 2 were significantly different ($p<0.05$).In group 1, no swelling and hyperemia of perilesional skin appearance, no inflammatory exudate, reduced wound area and short time to clinical healing of wound were recorded after treatment. This study also demonstrated that difference in wound healing process between sex groups, in which wound healing in male was significantly ($p<0.05$) faster than female. Mixture of cod liver oil and honey is beneficial in treatment of old traumatized wounds in the donkeys. This effect was primarily mediated by formation of healthy mature scars, clinical healing in short period of time. The owners, institutions or organization working with donkeys and governments may use this mixture for treating old traumatized wounds.

Key words: Cod liver oil, donkey, healing, honey, wound.

INTRODUCTION

More than 72% of the world's equine population resides in developing countries kept for draft purpose (Swann, 2006). Ethiopia has more than 6 million donkeys, the second largest donkey population in the world next to China, 1.9 million horses and over 350,000 mules (FAOSTAT, 2012). Equines are important animals to the resource-poor communities in rural and urban areas of Ethiopia, providing traction power and transport services at low cost (Dinka et al., 2006).

In Ethiopia, the rugged terrain characteristics, absence of well-developed modern transport networks and the prevailing low economic status of the community necessitate the use of equines for transportation (Alemayehu, 2004). In rural and per-urban area, people

E-mail: addisvet838@gmail.com.

used equines to transport crops, fuel wood, water, building materials and people can be transported by carts or on their back from farms and market to the home (Mohammed, 1991).

Despite their uses, the husbandry practices of working equines are poor. Some methods of hobbling to restrain equines cause discomfort and inflict (Alujia and Lopez, 1991; Mohammed, 1991). As per Alujia and Lopez (1991) report, loading of donkeys without padding and over loading in long distance causes external injury on donkeys and mules. Poorly designed harnesses or yokes that may be healthy and ragged have an effect on the animal health and safety (Alujia and Lopez, 1991).

Wound is an open mechanical injury of the epidermis, underlying the tissues and organs. It is characterized by pain, and gaping bleeding functional disturbance. The most common cause of wounds in working equine are over loading, accidents, improper position of load predisposing to falling, hyena bites, donkey bites, injuries inflicted by horned Zebu (DACA, 2006). Some hobbling methods, inappropriate harnesses or yokes that may be heavy and ragged, long working hours may cause discomfort and inflict wounds (Mekuria et al., 2013).

Wounds are one of the primary welfare concerns of working equines (Sells et al., 2010). The type of wound in working donkeys includes tissue damage with or without blood or exudates or pus, abscess formation, or any secondary bacterial complication. Bites (lacerated wounds) will be identified by irregular edges with underlying tissues removed as well as hemorrhage (Sevendsen, 2008).

Wounds can be either traumatic or surgical in origin; both types can fail to heal and become chronic although traumatic wounds are more commonly affected by healing difficulties. The incidence and prevalence of traumatic wounds in equine is considered to be high (Singer et al., 2003) and a high percentage become chronic, adding more complexity to wound healing management strategies.

Skin lacerations and other traumatic injuries of the integument are frequently seen in equine practices and range from relatively minor cuts to severe, potentially debilitating injuries. The challenges facing the practitioner managing these injuries are numerous, and treatment is dictated by the nature and size of the wound, the area of the body on which the wound occurs, and several aspects of wound healing unique to horses. The age of the wound, integrity of the local blood supply, degree of contamination, location of the injury, skin loss, and local tissue damage must all be considered when deciding on the most appropriate method for managing a particular wound. In addition to biologic factors, the physical size of equine patients and the environment in which they are kept present unique management challenges not encountered in the treatment of soft tissue injuries in other species (Jeremy, 2006).Wounds are of great concern in donkeys as they affect animal productivity and

their treatment represents an economic burden to the owners particularly in developing countries (Magda and Khaled, 2011). Granulation tissue is the pebbly or granular appearing tissue which develops in healing wounds anywhere on the horse's body. It is composed of small blood vessels and fibroblasts, but has no nerve supply (Christina, 2002).

Treatment methods that are employed in the management of wounds focus on rapid and efficient evaluation, scrupulous, aseptic surgical techniques, and conscientious and prolonged aftercare (Griffiths et al., 2003).

Many therapeutic agents are used for topical treatment of wounds including yeast cell derivatives (Crowe et al., 1999), cod liver oil (Kietzmann and Braun, 2006), honey (Iftikar et al., 2009), sugar (Cavazana et al., 2009), corticosteroids (Jorissen and Bachert, 2009) and phenytoin (Qunaibi et al., 2009). Honey and cod liver oil are increasingly used as natural products and biological therapies in clinical practice. To accelerate wound healing, modern honey wound dressings have become more widely available and used in wound management (Zumla and Lulat, 1989). This is largely due to the growing clinical problems of antibiotic-resistant bacteria and the combined difficulties for the practitioners in managing chronic wounds such as burns and leg ulcers (Lay-flurrie, 2008). Besides antimicrobial effects of honey (Cooper and Molan, 1999), it has anti-inflammatory and antioxidant properties (Gheldof and Engeseth, 2002), promotes moist wound healing and facilitates debridement (Majtán, 2009; pieper, 2009). Cod liver oil is a nutritional supplement derived from liver of cod fish. It has high levels of omega 3 fatty acid, vitamin A and vitamin D. Terkelsen et al. (2000) reported that cod liver oil was beneficial in wound healing as it enhances epithelization and revascularization.

Management of wound in the study area was practice locally which leads to delay in clinical healing, development of old wounds with or without granulation tissue. Due to this poor practice, the owners lost their money, time, working efficiency, and the donkey itself.

Hence, considering the importance of donkey wound management, the topic was built up to investigate the beneficial effects of the mixture of cod liver oil and honey in the contaminated old wounds without any other topical disinfectants or antimicrobial devices. The general objectives of the study include, investigation of the clinical wound healing process with a mixture of cod liver oil and honey in treatment of old wounds and granulation tissue in donkeys and the specific objectives include evaluation of the time taken for clinical healing of old chronic wound.

MATERIALS AND METHODS

Study area

The study was conducted from November 2015 to May 2016 in and

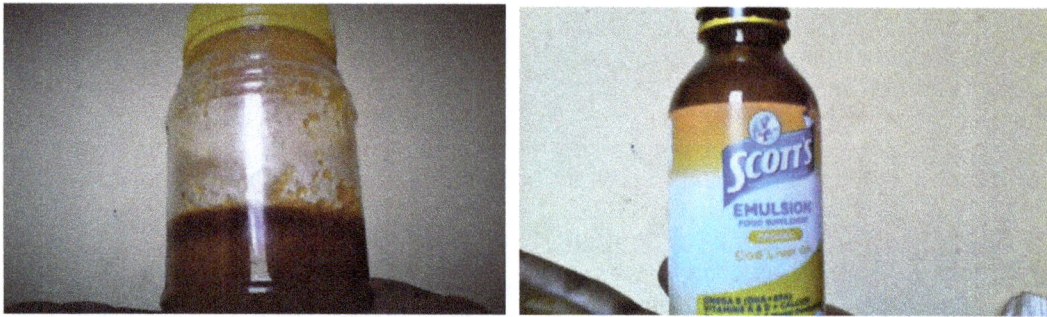

Figure 1. Natural bee honey (A) and cod liver oil (B).

around Bahir Dar (Amhara Region), North Western part of Ethiopia. It is located 564 km from Addis Ababa, capital of Ethiopia. The study area is covers a total of 197,199 hectares of land which has a summer rainy season with the highest rain fall between June and September (1200-1600 mm) and winter dry season (December to March) with mean annual temperature of 23°C. Located 11'29"N latitude, 37'29"E longitude and with altitude range of 1500-2300 meters above sea level (ANRSAB, 1999).

Topography of the area is characterized with slight slopping covering about 70% of a total land of area, and marked with Lake Tana and Abay River (ANRSAB, 1999). The land is covered by various, low woods, and mainly evergreen plants of various types of, with vegetation cover of land. The main agricultural product is teff, barley, sorghum, wheat, maize and all pulse crops (ANRSAB, 1999). The region has 1.4 million cattle, 1.3 million sheep and goats and 2.8 million equines of which the figure in Bahir Dar and its surroundings are estimated to have about 58 horses, 550 mule and 19517 donkeys (CSA, 2010).

Study population

The study was conducted on both sexes of the local breeds of donkeys affected with chronic and old wounds. Donkeys in the study area were mainly used for water, grain, stone, and fire wood transportation. Wounds are mainly due to car accident, heavy loading, loading without padding, improper tying of legs with rope and loading of hot flour. Those donkeys exposed to wound and/or granulation tissue were treated with cod liver oil and honey mixture (n=12) and with routine treatment (n=6) within a given time.

Selection of animals

A total of 18 adult donkeys of both sexes having wounds admitted in the Donkey Sanctuary Veterinary Service Centers for treatment of wounds were used.

Materials used during the study

Cod liver oil, tap water, natural honey, savlon (trade name), cotton gauze, ordinary ruler, shaving blades, 50 ml syringe, cotton and curved and straight scissors (Figure 1).

Treatment of old wounds in donkeys with mixture of cod liver oil and honey

12 donkeys (6 male and 6 female) were presented in the Donkey

Sanctuary Veterinary Service Center. After clinical examination, all donkeys were suffering with old and heavily traumatized wound along with the infection on the wound surface. Most wounds were located on the caudal back region of the donkeys. All of these wounds were caused due to heavy loading, loading without padding, improper loading of hot flour, and frequent loading with water for cultivation of chat in the area.

Treatment procedure

Before treatment history was recorded related to age, sex, breed and consent for treatment from the owner of the donkey was obtained. Treatment of wounds was carried out in the following steps: (1) the whole area around the wound up to about 5 cm length from the wound edges was clipped with curved scissor and shaved with shaving blade. (2) The Presence of Inflammatory Exudates (PIE) and Perilesional Skin Appearance (PSA) were assessed. (3) Its area was calculated by multiplying the two largest dimensions to assess the initial size and evaluate the progress in the healing process using ordinary ruler. (4) Grossly contaminated wounds were washed with slight warm water with body temperature water using syringe. (5) Then wound surface was covered with piece of gauze soaked in a mixture of an equal volume of cod liver oil and honey. The amount of the mixture varied according to the wound size. Generally, about 20 ml of the mixture will be used for 100 cm^2 dressing area on the body of the animal. (6) The frequency of changing dressing was decided with how rapidly the mixture is diluted with exudates. The bandage was changed daily up to seven days, every third day for two weeks and then once a week till clinical union of the wound took place. (7) At the end of treatment, the time required for clinical union of the wound, the remaining area, the perilesional skin appearance and the presence of inflammatory exudate were recorded.

Treatment of old wounds in donkeys with routine treatment savlon (chlorhexidine 0.3 + cetrimide 3%)

To investigate the whole effect of the mixture of cod liver oil and honey on the healing of wounds, its effects were compared with the routine treatment. Six donkeys (3 male and 3 female) with old wounds were prepared for this treatment. The wound area was aseptically prepared about a 5 cm from the edge of the wound. Hemorrhage was controlled by pressing of the wound surface for 10 minduring preparation. The wound surface was covered with piece of gauze soaked in savlon. The bandage was changed periodically daily for seven days, and every third day for two weeks and then once a week till the 35th day of treatment. In addition a combination of penicillin (8 mg) and dihydrostreptomycinsulphate (10 mg) per kg

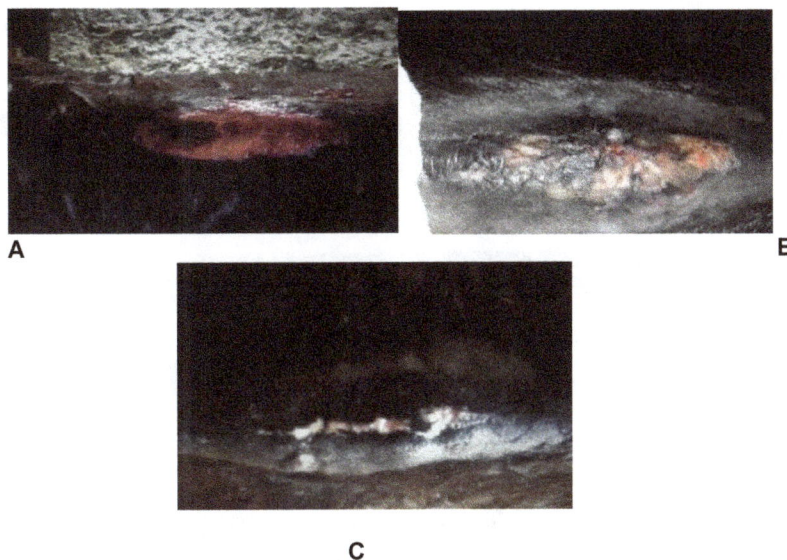

Figure 2. A. After cleaning with tap water. **B.** After one week of treatment with mixture of cod liver oil and honey. **C.** After three weeks of treatment with a mixture.

body weight or 1 ml penicillin and streptomycin per 25 kg bodyweight was given for three days to control the bacterial infection of the wound. The area of the wound, the time required for clinical union, PSA and PIE of the wound were recorded.

Statistical analysis

The data was entered into Mc-soft excel spread sheet and analyzed by STATA version 12.0. Independent t-test for the two groups of treatment and dependent t-test for sex difference within one group of treatment were utilized.

RESULTS

Treatment of old wounds in donkeys with mixture of cod liver oil and honey

The clinical healing of wounds in treated cases with the mixture of cod liver oil and honey took place in a period of time ranged from two to five weeks. It was found that surgical debridement at the beginning of treatment was important in most cases due to presence of granulation tissue. Washing of the wound with tap water was seen to be very successful in removal of debris, necrotic tissue and pus as well as helpful in refreshment of the wounds surface (Figures 2 and 3).

After one week of treatment, the wounds surface appeared bright red in color, moist and not elevated above wound edges. After two to three weeks of treatment, wounds in all cases showed cleanness and healthy surface and observable decrease in the wound surface. Wounds areas were markedly decreased after five weeks of treatment. After four weeks of treatment in

eight cases, the remaining wound areas out of 100% of the initial area were from 4.2 to 37.5% and there was no swelling and hyperemia at the perilesional skin appearance (PSA) and no inflammatory exudate (PIE) over the surface of the wound. The rest four cases showed that for 50 to 66.6% area from the initial area, there was mild swelling and hypereamia and thick crust over the wound surface (Table 1).

Wound healing difference between Sex group

Area, perilesional skin appearance (PSA), presence of inflammatory exudate (PIE) and time required to clinical union of wound were significantly different (p< 0.05) between both sex groups. In two cases, male donkeys showed remaining wound areas of 30 and 37.5% and in five cases, it was between 4.2 to 17% out of 100% of the initial area. The perilesional skin appearances and presence of inflammatory exudate in male were none except one which showed mild swelling and hyperemia and thick crust over the wound surface while in the female donkey, there was mild swelling and hypereamia and thick crust over the surface of the wound except one case which showed no exudate. The time required for clinical union in male cases took place between a time range of two to five weeks whereas in females four to five weeks.

Treatment of old wounds in donkeys with routine treatment savlon (Chlorhexidine0.3%+cetrimide 3%)

All treated cases with routine treatment, not showing

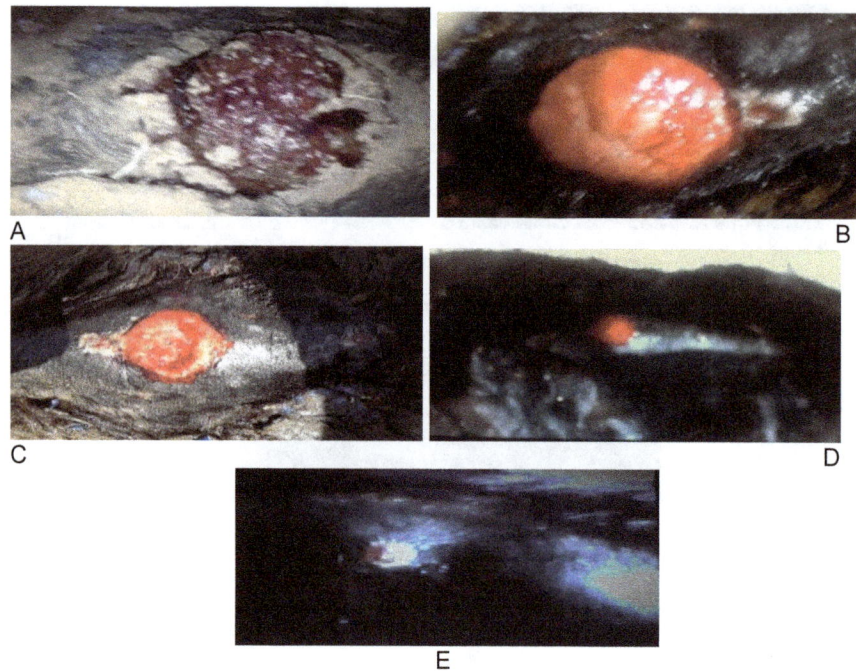

Figure 3. A. Before cleaning. **B.** After cleaning. **C.** After surgical removal of granulation tissue. **D.** After two weeks of treatment with mixture of cod liver oil and honey. **E.** After four weeks of treatment with mixture.

clinical union of wounds within a given period of time (35 days) and the area of wounds were not decreased(Figure 4). After six weeks of treatment only thick exudate was observed (Table 2).

Wound healing difference between two treatment groups

The times taken to clinical union of wound, area, perilesional skin appearance (PSA), and presence of inflammatory exudate (PIE) were significantly different (p< 0.05) between the two treatment different groups (Tables 3, 4, 5, 6, 7, 8, 9 and 10).

DISCUSSION

When treating equine wounds, the primary goal is to obtain rapid wound healing with a functional and aesthetically satisfactory outcome. Dressing are used to enhance and support the healing process by decreasing contamination, oedema or exudate, protesting against movement and further trauma and optimizing moisture, temperature, pH and gaseous exchanges at the wound site (Knottenbelt, 2003). Equines are known for their tendency to wound probably due to their inquisitive nature, large size and confinement in areas with potential obstacles such as metal or wire leads in their known

difficulties with healing. This study shows the beneficial effect of mixture of cod liver oil and honey in treatment of old traumatized chronic wounds in donkeys. In clinically treated wounds, it was found that surgical debridement washing with slight warm water were valuable steps in removing granulation tissue and debris and in minimizing infection. Formation of granulation tissue in wounds usually occurs as the result of weakness of the initial inflammatory response of wound which leads to chronic inflammation which further inhibits wound contraction and promotes exuberant granulation tissue formation (Wilmink and Weeren, 2005).

Application of mixture of cod liver oil and honey, after debridement, on and around the wounds, brought significance in the requirement of the infection, and observable decrease of wound surface after two weeks to five weeks of treatment. These effects of the mixture appeared to be mediated by the effects of honey, and vitamin A and omega-3 fatty acids in cod liver oil. Gethin et al. (2008) reported that honey dressings were associated with significant reduction in non-healed chronic superficial ulcers. Terkelsen et al. (2000) reported that vitamin A had an important role in accelerating wound healing process. McDaniel et al. (2008) reported that omega-3 fatty acids in cod liver oil can increase in the wound healing through increasing pro-inflammatory cytokines production at wound sites. After application of the mixture, all wounds were covered with protective bandages which were advantageous in controlling

Table 1. Area, PSA, PIE, time taken to clinical union of the wound in group 1.

Number	Sex	Area(size)of wound before treated with oil-honey mixture (cm²)	PSA before treatment	PIE before treatment	Area of after treatment (cm²)	PSA after treatment	PIE after treatment	Time taken to clinical union of wound (in weeks)
W1	M	4*3=12	Swollen and hypermia	Thin	2*1=2(17%)	No swelling and hypereamia	None	2
W2	F	7*4=28	Swollen and hypermia	Thin	5*3=15(53.6%)	Mild swelling and hypermia	Thick crust over the wound surface	4
W3	M	6*3=18	Swollen and hypermia	Thin	1*1=1(5.6%)	No swelling and hypereamia	None	3
W4	M	8*5=40	Swollen and hypermia	Thin	4*3=12(30%)	No swelling and hypereamia	None	3
W5	F	6*4=24	Swollen and hypermia	Thin	4*3=12(50%)	Mild swelling and hypermia	Thick crust over wound surface	5
W6	M	5*3=15	Swollen and hypermia	Thin	1*1=1(6.6%)	No swelling and hypereamia	None	3
W7	M	7*5=35	Swollen and hypermia	Thin	2*2=4(11.4%)	No swelling and hypereamia	None	3
W8	F	6*5=30	Swollen and hypermia	Thin	5*4=20(66.7%)	Mild swelling and hypermia	Thick crust over wound surface	5
W9	F	5*4=20	Swollen and hypermia	Thin	3*3=9(45%)	No swelling and hypereamia	Thick crust over wound surface	4
W10	M	4*3=12	Swollen and hypermia	Thin	1*0.5=0.5(4.2%)	No swelling hypereamia	None	5
W11	F	6*3=18	Swollen and hypermia	Thin	3*2=6(33.3%)	No swelling and hypereamia	None	4
W12	F	8*4=32	Swollen and hypermia	Thin	6*2=12(37.5%)	Mild swelling and hypermia	Thick crust over wound surface	5

bleeding, reducing the tendency for granulation tissue formation, absorbing exudates, keeping the wounds moist which helps epithelization, protecting the wound from contamination, dust and flies and keeping the topical mixture used better in contact with the wound surface. In wounds treated with routine treatment (group 2) there was very slow clinical healing process and not significant decrease in wound size when compared to those treated with the mixture (group 1). Similar observations reported by Iftikhar et al. (2010) found that honey increased epithelization in wound models in rats. Majtán et al. (2010) observed that honey increased metalloproteinase-9 in cultured human keratinocytes. Metalloproteinase-9 was observed to degrade type IV collagen in the basement membrane and further facilitate migration of keratinocytes (Kyriakides et al., 2009). Regarding cod liver oil, it was reported that topical application of cod liver oil ointment to surgically-induced full thickness

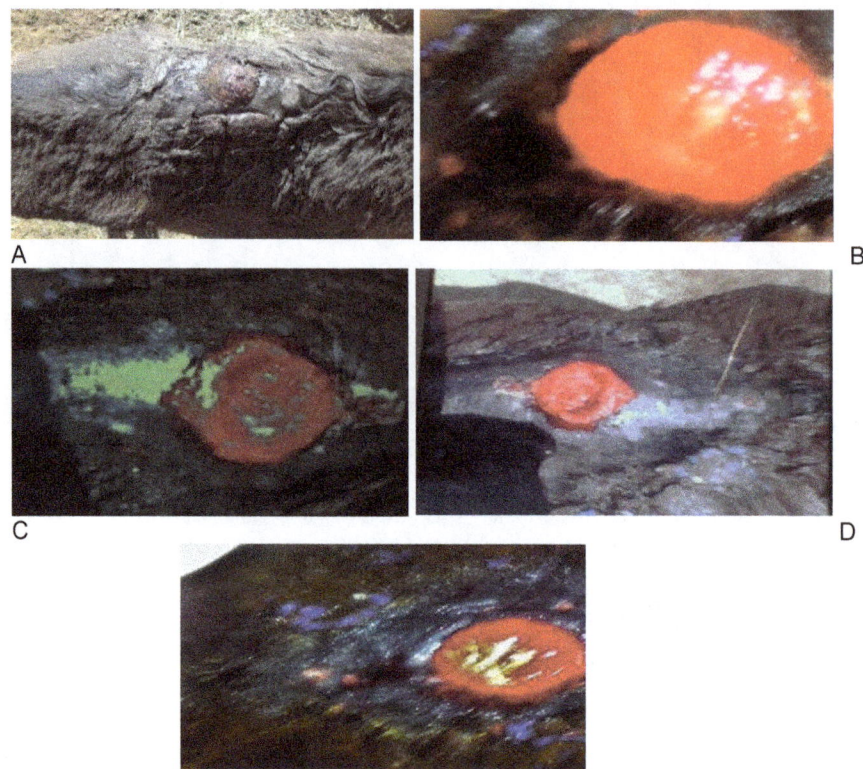

Figure 4. **A.** Before cleaning the wound. **B.** After cleaning. **C.** After surgically removing the granulation tissue. **D.** After three weeks of treatment. **E.** After five weeks of treatment.

Table 2. Area, PSA, PIE and time taken to clinical union of the wound.

Number	Sex	Area (size) of wound before treatment (cm²)	PSA before treatment	PIE before treatment	Area (size) of wound after treatment(cm²)	PSA after treatment	PIE after treatment	Time to clinical union of the wound (in weeks)
W1	F	7*2=14	Swollen and hyperemia	Thin	6*2=12(85.7%)	Swollen and mild hypereamia	Thick	No clinical union took pace
W2	F	6*2=12	Swollen and hyperemia	Thin	4*2=8(66.7%)	Mild swelling and hypereamia	Thick	No clinical union took pace
W3	M	5*3=15	Swollen and hyperemia	Thin	5*2-10(66.7%)	Mild swelling and hypereamia	Thick	No clinical union took pace
W4	M	6*4=24	Swollen and hyperemia	Thin	5*4=20(83.3%)	Swollen and hypereamia	Thin	No clinical union took pace
W5	M	4*3=12	Swollen and hyperemia	Thin	3*2=6(50%)	Mild swlling and hypereamia	Thick	No clinical union took pace
W6	F	3*2=6	Swollen and hyperemia	Thin	2*2=4(66.7%)	Swollen and hypereamia	Thin	No clinical union took pace

dermal wounds on the ears of mice resulted in faster epithelization than those coated with vaseline vehicle (Terkelsen et al., 2000). Vitamin A and D in cod liver oil are responsible for such effects. The mixture produced good results in clinically admitted wounds at the end of fourth week. This appeared due to formation of healthy scar that showed higher degree of maturity with an increasing number of fibrocytes and parallel collagen fibers.

This study also demonstrated some sex differences in

Table 3. Area of wound between group 1and 2 after treatment.

S/N	Group 1	Group 2
W1	2*1=2(17%)	6*2=12(85.7%)
W2	5*3=15(53.6%)	4*2=8(66.7%)
W3	1*1=1(5.6%)	5*2-10(66.7%)
W4	4*3=12(30%)	5*4=20(83.3%)
W5	4*3=12(50%)	3*2=6(50%)
W6	1*1=1(6.6%)	2*2=4(66.7%)
W7	2*2=4(11.4%)	
W8	5*4=20(66.7%)	
W9	3*3=9(45%)	
W10	1*0.5=0.5(4.2%)	
W11	3*2=6(33.3%)	
W12	6*2=12(37.5%)	

Table 4. Statistical analysis of area between group 1 and 2, ($p < 0.05$).

Variable	Obs	Mean	Std. Err.	Std. Dev.	[95% Conf.	Interval]
var1	6	1.5	0.34	0.84	0.62	2.38
var2	6	2.83	0.17	0.41	2.40	3.26
Diff	6	-1.33	0.49	1.21	-2.60	-0.06

Table 5. PIE between group 1 and 2 after treatment.

S/N	Group 1	Group 2
W1	None	Thick
W2	thick crust over the wound surface	Thick
W3	None	Thick
W4	None	Thin
W5	thick crust over the wound surface	Thick
W6	None	Thin
W7	None	
W8	thick crust over the wound surface	
W9	thick crust over the wound surface	
W10	None	
W11	None	
W12	thick crust over the wound surface	

Table 6. Statistical analysis of PIE between group 1 and 2, ($p < 0.05$).

Variable	Obs	Mean	Std. Err.	Std. Dev.	[95% Conf.	Interval]
var1	6	0.33	0.21	0.52	-0.21	0.88
var2	6	2.33	0.21	0.52	1.79	2.88
Diff	6	-2	0.37	0.89	-2.94	-1.06

clinical healing of wound. Clinical requirement of wound in male donkeys were significantly ($p<0.05$) faster than female donkeys. This may be due to the fact that in male there is larger dermal thickness compared to female, a parameter that has been reported to be under the influence of male hormones (Azzi et al., 2005). A direct

Table 7. PSA between group 1 and 2 of treatment.

S/N	Group 1	Group 2
W1	No swelling and hypereamia	Swollen and mild hypereamia
W2	Mild swelling and hyperemia	Mild swelling and hyperemia
W3	No swelling and hyperemia	Mild swelling and hyperemia
W4	No swelling and hyperemia	Swollen and hypereamia
W5	Mild swelling and hyperemia	Mild swelling and hyperemia
W6	No swelling and hyperemia	Swollen and hypereamia
W7	No swelling and hyperemia	
W8	Mild swelling and hyperemia	
W9	No swelling and hyperemia	
W10	No swelling and hyperemia	
W11	No swelling and hyperemia	
W12	Mild swelling and hyperemia	

Table 8. Statistical analysis PSA between group 1 and 2, ($p < 0.05$).

Variable	Obs	Mean	Std. Err.	Std. Dev.	[95% Conf.	Interval]
var1	6	0.33	0.21	0.52	-0.21	0.88
var2	6	1.5	0.22	0.55	0.93	2.10
Diff	6	-1.17	0.40	0.98	-2.20	-0.13

Table 9. Time taken to clinical union of the wound between group 1 and 2 of treatment.

S/N	Group 1	Group 2
W1	2 weeks	no clinical union took pace
W2	4 weeks	no clinical union took pace
W3	3 weeks	no clinical union took pace
W4	3 weeks	no clinical union took pace
W5	5 weeks	no clinical union took pace
W6	3 weeks	no clinical union took pace
W7	3 weeks	
W8	5 weeks	
W9	4 weeks	
W10	5 weeks	
W11	4 weeks	
W12	5 weeks	

Table 10. Statistical analysis of time taken to clinical union of the wound between group 1 and 2, ($p < 0.05$).

Variable	Obs	Mean	Std. Err.	Std. Dev.	[95% Conf.	Interval]
var1	6	1.33	0.21	.52	0.79	1.88
var2	6	3	0	0	3	3
Diff	6	-1.67	0.21	0.52	-2.21	-1.12

relationship between dermal thickness and collagen content, and thereby skin strength or mechanical resistance, has been suggested (Shuster et al., 1975). In relation to skin injury, the expression of collagen is markedly increased in fibroblasts in the dermis. This is followed by an extensive remodeling phase, in which the collagen content is degraded by the coordinated action of several collagenolytic proteases, whose expression and activation have been reported to depend on plasmin (Pins et al., 2000).

CONCLUSION AND RECOMMENDATIONS

This study demonstrated that cod liver oil and honey mixture was beneficial in healing of old traumatized wounds in donkeys before and after treatment, the time required to clinical healing of the wound, perilesional skin appearance and presence of inflammatory exudate. In conclusion, usage of mixture of cod liver oil and honey for old wound help in donkeys early clinical healing, reduce extra expenditure of money and time. Study also demonstrated that there was a significant difference in wound healing between sex groups.

Based on the important major findings and conclusion drawn, the following recommendations are forwarded: The owners, institutions or organization working with donkeys can use this mixture for treating old traumatized wounds as it enhances early wound healing, formation of healthy scar and can reduce risk of antibiotic resistance and also the knowledge of importance and usage of the mixture of cod liver oil and honey in wound healing may be transferred to the community for adoption.

CONFLICT OF INTERESTS

The author has not declared any conflict of interests.

ACKNOWLEDGEMENTS

My gratitude thank goes to Professor Rajendran Natarajan who seriously supported me throughout my thesis research. I would like to thank Assistant Professor Ashenafi Assefa. I would like to also thank Professor Ramaswamy, my friend Dr. Abebe Abuhay, Dr. Fentie Getnet and all the staff members of Faculty of Veterinary Medicine specially Department of Veterinary Clinical Medicine in University of Gondar.

Abbreviations: FAOSTAT, Food and Agricultural Organization Statistical; **DACA,** Drug Administration and Control Authority; **PSA,** perilesional skin appearance; **PIE,** presence of inflammatory exudate; **SIS,** small intestine submucosa; **LYCD,** live yeast cell derivatives; **BCE,** before christian era; **PI,** povidone iodine; **VEGF,** vascular endothelial growth factor; **ATP,** adenosine triphosphate; **DNA,** deoxyribonuclic acid; **MRSA,** methicillin resistant *Staphylococcus aureus*; **HP,** hydrogen peroxide; **ANRSAB,** Amhara National Regional State Agriculture Bureau; **CSA,** Central Statistical Agency; **CM,** centimeter; **ML,** milliliter; **MG,** milligram;

KG, kilogram.

REFERENCES

Alemayehu M (2004). The genetic resources perspective of equines in Ethiopia and their contribution to the rural livelihoods. ESAP Proceedings. P 81.

Alujia AS, Lopez F (1991). Donkeys in Mexico. *In*: Fielding D and Pearson, R.A (eds.). Donkeys, Mules and Horses in Topical Agricultural Development.*CTVM*, Edinburgh. pp.1-7.

ANRSAB (1999). Amhara National Regional State Agriculture Bureau. The Climatic and Geographical Description of Amhara Region.

Azzi L, El-Alfy M, Martel C, Labrie F (2005). Gender Differences in Mouse Skin Morphology and Specific Effects of Sex Steroids and Dehydroepiandrosterone. J. Invest Dermatol.124:22-27.

Cavazana WC, SimõesMde L, Amado CA, Cuman RK (2009). Sugar (Sucrose) and Fatty acid Compounds with Triglycerides on the Treatment of Wounds. Experimental Study in Rats, Anais brasileiros de dermatologia 84(3):229-236.

Christina C (2002). American Association of Equine Practitioners. AAEP's Horse Health Articles Search Engine.

Cooper R, Molan P (1999). The Use of Honey as an Antiseptic in Managing Pseudomonas Infection. J. Wound Care 8:161-164.

Crowe MJ, McNeill RB, Schlemm DJ, Greenhalgh DG, Keller SJ (1999). Topical Application of Yeast Extract Accelerates the Wound Healing of Diabetic Mice. J. Burn Care Res. 20(2):155-162.

Central Statistics Agency (CSA) (2010). Livestock population of Amhara Regional State.

Drug Administration and control Authority (DACA) (2006). Standard Treatment Guideline for Veterinary Practice of Ethiopia. pp. 209-211.

Dinka H, Shelima B, Abalti A, Geleta T, Mume T (2006). Socio-Economic Importance and Management of Carthorses in the Mid Rift Valley of Ethiopia. Proceedings of the 5th International Colloquium on Working Equines.

Food and Agricultural Organization Statistical Database (FAOSTAT) (2012). Food and Agricultural Organization Statistical Database. http://www.fao.org/corp/statistics/ access online/.

Gethin GT, Cowman S, Conroy RM (2008).The Impact of ManukaHoney Dressings on the Surface pH of Chronic Wounds. Int. Wound J. 5:185-194.

Gheldof N, Engeseth NJ (2002). Antioxidant Capacity of Honeys from Various Floral Sources Based on the Determination of Oxygen Radical Absorbance Capacity and Inhibition of in Vitro Lipoprotein Oxidation in Human Serum Samples. J. Agric. Food Chem. 50:3050-3055.

Griffiths DA, Simpson RA, Shorey BA, Speller DC, Williams NB (2003). Single-Dose Peroperative Antibiotic Prophylaxis in Gastrointestinal Surgery. Lancet 2(7981):325-328.

Iftikhar F, Arshad M, Rasheed F, Amraiz D, Anwar P, Gulfraz M (2010). Effects of Acacia Honey on Wound Healing in Various Rat Models. Phytother. Res. 24:583-586.

Jeremy V (2006). Principles of Reconstructive and Plastic Surgery. Equine Surgery (3rd eds.) P 254.

Jorissen M, Bachert C (2009). Effect of Corticosteroids on Wound Healing After Endoscopic Sinus Surgery. Rhinology 47:280-286.

Kyriakides TR, Wulsin D, Skokos EA, Fleckman P, Pirrone A, Shipley JM, Senior RM, Bornstein P (2009). Mice that lack matrix metalloproteinase-9 display delayed wound healing associated with delayed reepithelization and disordered collagen fibrillogenesis. Matrix Biol. 28(2):65-73.

Lay-flurrie K (2008). Honey in wound care: effects, clinical application and patient benefit. British J. Nurs. 17(11).

Magda MA, Khaled R (2011). Cod liver oil/honey mixture: An effective treatment of equine complicated lower leg wounds. Vet. World 4(7):304-310.

Majtán J (2009). Apitherapy-the role of honey in the chronic wound healing process. Epidemiologie, mikrobiologie, imunologie: casopis Spolecnosti pro epidemiologii a mikrobiologii Ceske lekarske spolecnosti JE Purkyne 58(3):137-140.

Majtán J, Kumar P, Majtán T, Walls AF, Klaudiny J (2010). Effect of honey and its major royal jelly protein 1 on cytokine and MMP-9 mRNA transcripts in human keratinocytes. Exp. Dermatol. 19(8).

McDaniel JC, Belury M, Ahijevych K, Blakely W (2008). Omega-3 Fatty Acids Effect on Wound Healing. Wound Repair Regen. 16:337-345.

Mekuria S, Matusala M, Rahameto A (2013). Management practices and welfare problems encountered on working equids in Hawassa town, Southern Ethiopia. J. Vet. Med. Anim Health 5(9):243-250.

Mohammed A (1991). Management and breeding aspects of donkeys around Awassa, Ethiopia. In Donkeys, mules & horses in tropical agricultural development: proc of a Colloquium organ by the Edinburgh School of Agric & the Cent for Trop Vet Med of the Univ of Edinburgh & held in Edinburgh, Scotland, 3rd-6th Sept 1990. [Edinburgh]: Centre for Tropical Veterinary Medicine c1991.

Pins GD, Collins-Pavao ME, Van De Water L, Yarmush ML, Morgan JR (2000). Plasmin Triggers Rapid Contraction and Degradation of Fibroblast-Populated Collagen Lattices. J. Invest. Dermatol. 114(4):647-653.

Qunaibi EA, Disi AM, Taha MO (2009). Phenytoin enhances collagenization in excision wounds and tensile strength in incision wounds. Die Pharmazie-An Int. J. Pharm. Sci. 64(9):584-586.

Sells P, Pinchbeck G, Mezzane H, Ibourki J, Crane M (2010). Pack Wounds of Donkeys and Mules in the Northern High Atlas And Lowlands of Morocco. Equine Vet. J. 42(3):219-226.

Sevendsen E (2008). The Professional Handbook of the Donkey. (4th eds). *London,* Whittet Books Limited.

Shuster S, Black MM, McVitie E (1975). The influence of age and sex on skin thickness, skin collagen and density. Brit. J. Dermatol. 93:639-643.

Singer ER, Saxby F, French NP (2003). A Retrospective Case-Control Study of Horse Falls in the Sport of Horse Trials and Three-Day Eventing. Equine Vet. J. 35(2):139-145.

Swann WJ (2006). Improving the welfare of working equine animals in developing countries. Appl. Anim. Behav. Sci. 100(1):148-151

Terkelsen LH, Eskild-Jensen A, Kjeldsen H, Barker JH, Hjortdal VE, (2000). Topical application of cod liver oil ointment accelerates wound healing: an experimental study in wounds in the ears of hairless mice. Scandinavian J. Plastic Reconstructive Surg. Hand Surg. 34(1):15-20.

Wilmink JM, van Weeren PR (2005). Second Intention Repair in the Horse and Pony and Management of Exuberant Granulation Tissue. Vet. Clin. North Am. Equine Pract. 21:5-32.

Zumla A, Lulat A (1989). Honey - A remedy rediscovered. J. Royal Soc. Med. 82:384-385.

Permissions

List of Contributors

J. K. Serem and R. G. Wahome
Department of Animal Production, University of Nairobi, Kangemi, Nairobi, Kenya

D. W. Gakuya
Department of Clinical studies, University of Nairobi, Kangemi, Nairobi, Kenya

S. G. Kiama and D. W. Onyango
Department of Veterinary Anatomy and Physiology, University of Nairobi, Kangemi, Nairobi, Kenya

G. C. Gitao
Department of Veterinary Pathology, Microbiology and Parasitology, University of Nairobi, Kangemi, Nairobi, Kenya

Haftay Abraha, Geberemedhin Hadish, Belay Aligaz, Goytom Eyas and Kidane Workelule
College of Veterinary Medicine, Mekelle University, Mekelle, Ethiopia

Mandefrot Meaza, Abayneh Keda, Biresaw Serda and Mishamo Sulayman
School of Veterinary Medicine, Wolaita Sodo University, Ethiopia

Tesfaye Wolde and Tigist Tamiru
Department of Biology, College of Natural and Computational Science, Wolkite University, Ethiopia

Jesca Nakayima, Daniel Aleper and Duke Okidi
National Livestock Resources Research Institute (NaLIRRI), Tororo, Uganda

Mary L. Nanfuka
National Animal Disease Diagnostics and Epidemiology Centre (NADDEC), Entebbe, Uganda

Alemayehu Lemma
Department of Clinical Studies, College of Veterinary Medicine and Agriculture, Addis Ababa University, Debre Zeit, Ethiopia

Sara González-Ruiz
Doctorado en Ciencias Biológicas, Facultad de Ciencias Naturales, UAQ, Mexico

Susana L. Sosa-Gallegos, Isabel Bárcenas-Reyes, Germinal J. Cantó-Alarcón and Feliciano Milián-Suazo
Facultad de Ciencias Naturales, UAQ, Mexico

Elba Rodríguez-Hernández, SusanaFlores-Villalva and Sergio I. Román-Ponce
Centro Nacional de Investigación Disciplinaria en Fisiología Animal-INIFAP. km 1 Carretera a Colón. Ajuchitlán, Querétaro, Mexico. Bovine tuberculosis (bTB) is a disease of cattle that presents

Temesgen Kassa Getahun, Tamirat Siyoum, Aster Yohannes and Melese Eshete
Ethiopian institute of Agricultural research, Holeta Agricultural Research Center, Holeta, Ethiopia

Adane Agegnehu, Basaznew Bogale, Shimelis Tesfaye and Shimelis Dagnachew
College of Veterinary Medicine and Animal Sciences, University of Gondar, Gondar, Ethiopia

M. A. Mousa
Nutrition and Clinical Nutrition Department, Faculty of Veterinary Medicine, Sohag University, Sohag, Egypt

A. S. Osman
Department of Biochemistry, Faculty of Veterinary Medicine, Sohag University, Sohag, Egypt

H. A. M. Abdel Hady
Bacteriology Department, Animal Health Research Institute, Egypt

Addis Kassahun Gebremeskel
School of veterinary Medicine, Hawassa University, Hawassa, Ethiopia

Abebaw Getachew and Daniel Adamu
College of veterinary medicine and animal sciences, University of Gondar, Gondar, Ethiopia

Anteneh Wondimu and Sagni Gutu
Haramaya University College of Veterinary Medicine, Dire Dawa, Ethiopia

Gianluca Pio Zaffarano, Benedetto Morandi, Fabio Ostanello and Giovanni Poglayen
Department of Veterinary Medical Sciences, University of Bologna, Ozzano dell'Emilia (BO), Italy

Alessia Menegotto
Conservation Global Agency for Environmental Gain npc, Company # 2010/018132/08, Knysna 6570, Garden Route, South Africa

Geoffrey Munkombwe Muuka, Ana Songolo, Swithine Kabilika, Harvey Sikwese, Benson Bowa and Obrien Kabunda
Ministry of Fisheries and Livestock, Central Veterinary Research Institute, Lusaka, Zambia

Abayneh Edget, Daniel Shiferaw and Shimelis Mengistu
College of Veterinary Medicine, Haramaya University, Haramaya, Dire Dawa, Ethiopia

Dereje Tulu
Ethiopian Institute of Agricultural Research, Tepi Agricultural Research Center, Tepi, Ethiopia
School of Veterinary Medicine, College of Agriculture and Veterinary Medicine, Jimma University, Jimma, Ethiopia

Benti Deresa, Feyisa Begna and Abiy Gojam
School of Veterinary Medicine, College of Agriculture and Veterinary Medicine, Jimma University, Jimma, Ethiopia

Ait Oudia Khatima and Khelef Djamel
National Veterinary Higher School of Algiers, Rue Issad Abbes, Oued Smar- Alger, Algeria

Karim Abdelkadir
National Veterinary Higher School of Algiers, Rue Issad Abbes, Oued Smar- Alger, Algeria
Laboratory of Research, Food Hygiene and Quality Assurance System (HASAQ), High National Veterinary School of Algiers, Algeria

Ubah Simon Azubuike
Department of Theriogenology, Faculty of Veterinary Medicine, University of Abuja, Nigeria

Rekwot Peter Ibrahim and Adewuyi Abdulmujeeb Bode
Artificial Insemination Unit, National Animal Production Research Institute, Shika, Zaria, Kaduna State, Nigeria

Ababa James Andrew
Veterinary Teaching Hospital, Ahmadu Bello University Zaria, Kaduna State, Nigeria

Mustapha Rashidah Abimbola
Department of Theriogenology and Production, Ahmadu Bello University, Zaria, Kaduna State, Nigeria

Helen Owoya Abah
Department of Veterinary Medicine, College of Veterinary Medicine, University of Agriculture Makurdi, Benue State, Nigeria

Paul Ayuba Abdu
Department of Veterinary Medicine, Faculty of Veterinary Medicine, Ahmadu Bello University, Zaria, Nigeria

Jibril Adamu
Department of Veterinary Microbiology, Faculty of Veterinary Medicine, Ahmadu Bello University Zaria, Nigeria

Bereket Molla
The Donkey Sanctuary Working Worldwide, Ethiopia Program, Ethiopia

Sefinew Alemu
University of Gondar, Gondar, Ethiopia

Haba Haile
University of Gondar, Gondar, Ethiopia
Gofa Universal College, Department of Animal Health, Sawla, Ethiopia

Zerihun Adugna Regasa and Belay Mulatea
Faculty of Veterinary Medicine and Animal Health, Wollo University, Ethiopia

Temesgen Kassa Getahun
Animal Health Research, Holeta Agricultural Research Center, Ethiopian Institute of Agricultural Research, Holeta, Ethiopia

Kidane Workelul Yalew, Yishak Tsegay, Haftay Abraha and Hailesilassie W/mariam
Department of Veterinary Medicine, College of Veterinary, Mekelle University, Kelamino, Mekelle, Ethiopia

Nesibu Awol
Department of Veterinary Medicine, School of Veterinary, Wollo University, Dessie, Ethiopia

Mulalem Zenebe Kelkay
Tigray Agricultural Research Institute, Mekelle, Ethiopia

Getachew Gugsa
School of Veterinary Medicine, Wollo University, Dessie, Ethiopia

Yohannes Hagos and Habtamu Taddelle
College of Veterinary Medicine, Mekelle University, Mekelle, Ethiopia

Cecilia Omowumi Oguntoye and Oghenemega David Eyarefe
Department of Veterinary Surgery and Radiology, University of Ibadan, Ibadan, Oyo state, Nigeria

Muhammadhussien Aman
Gindhir District Livestock and Fishery Resource Development Office, Bale Zone, Gindhir, Ethiopia

Diriba Lemma, Birhanu Abera and Eyob Eticha
Asella Regional Veterinary Laboratory, Asella, Ethiopia

Birhanu Tamirat and Habtamu Tamirat
College of Veterinary Medicine, Mekelle University, Mekelle, Ethiopia. Ethiopia

Mu-uz Gebru
College of Agriculture and Environmental Science, Bahir Dar University, Bahir Dar, Ethiopia

Ewuola E. O. and Bolarinwa O. A.
Animal Physiology and Bioclimatology Unit, Department of Animal Science, University of Ibadan, Ibadan, Oyo State, Nigeria

Nestor Dénakpo Noudèkè, Jacques Dougnon, Issaka Youssao and Souaïbou Farougou
Département de Production et Santé Animales, Ecole Polytechnique d'Abomey-Calavi, Université d'Abomey-Calavi, 01 BP 2009, Cotonou, République du Bénin

Gérard Dossou-Gbété, Charles Pomalégni, Serge Mensah and Guy Apollinaire Mensah
Laboratoire des Recherches Zootechnique, Vétérinaire et Halieutique (LRZVH), Centre de Recherches Agricoles d'Agonkanmey (CRA-Agonkanmey), Institut National des Recherches Agricoles du Bénin(INRAB), 01 BP 884 Recette Principale, Cotonou 01, Bénin

Luc Gilbert Aplogan
Laboratoire de Diagnostic Vétérinaire et Sérosurveillance des maladies animales de Parakou, Ministère de l'Agriculture, de l'Elevage et de la Pêche, Bénin

Germain Atchadé
Laboratoire Vétérinaire de Bohicon, Ministère de l'Agriculture, de l'Elevage et de la Pêche, Bénin

Chibuogwu Ijeoma Chika and Mathew Luka
Animal Science Department, Faculty of Agriculture, University of Abuja, Federal Capital Territory, Nigeria

Ubah Simon Azubuike
Department of Theriogenology, Faculty of Veterinary Medicine, University of Abuja, Federal Capital Territory, Nigeria

Addisu Mohammed Seid
Department Of Veterinary Clinical Medicine, Faculty of Veterinary Medicine, University of Gondar, Ethiopia

Index